UPLIFT
Secrets from the Sisterhood

"The morning I awoke from surgery, I knew no one who had ever had breast cancer. But by mid-morning, friends who'd had it began coming out of the woodwork! I was amazed. And appalled that no one had told me that women could actually live!"

—Jane Vaughan; diagnosed in 1991 at age 53; writer; Texas

"Think positive. Chemo is something they do *for* you, not *to* you. You are the aggressor. When you really feel lousy, you know that the weapon is doing a good job of attacking the enemy."

—Patricia Baker; diagnosed in 1993 at age 49; Massachusetts

"When you go for radiation, take a zip-lock bag with a moist washcloth and a shaker of pure cornstarch. Use them on your underarms in the changing room after treatment."

—Rayna Ragonetti; diagnosed in 1993 at age 52; executive; New York

"One Friday, in the midst of radiation, my husband kidnapped me and took me to a hotel for a romantic weekend away. It helped me to remember that I am a woman who is loved."

—Nancie Watson; diagnosed in 1995 at age 50; social worker; Pennsylvania

"I would have loved to talk with someone before I had treatment. The worst part was my imagination. But it's a lot like pregnancy; it's livable."

—Joy West; diagnosed in 2000 at age 34; advertising; South Carolina

BARBARA DELINSKY

UPLIFT

SECRETS FROM THE SISTERHOOD
of BREAST CANCER SURVIVORS

ATRIA PAPERBACK

New York London Toronto Sydney New Delhi

The author of this book is not a physician, and the ideas, procedures, and suggestions in this book are not intended as a substitute for the medical advice of a trained
health professional. All matters regarding your health require medical supervision.
Consult your physician before adopting the suggestions in this book, as well as about
any condition that may require diagnosis or medical attention. The author and publisher disclaim any liability arising directly or indirectly from the use of the book.

ATRIA PAPERBACK
A Division of Simon & Schuster, Inc.
1230 Avenue of the Americas
New York, NY 10020

First Atria Paperback edition September 2011

ATRIA PAPERBACK and colophon are trademarks
of Simon & Schuster, Inc.

For information about special discounts for bulk purchases,
please contact Simon & Schuster Special Sales at 1-866-506-1949
or business@simonandschuster.com.

The Simon & Schuster Speakers Bureau can bring authors
to your live event. For more information or to book an event
contact the Simon & Schuster Speakers Bureau at 1-866-248-3049
or visit our website at www.simonspeakers.com.

Manufactured in the United States of America

10 9 8 7 6 5 4 3 2 1

Library of Congress Cataloging-in-Publication Data

Delinsky, Barbara.
 Uplift : secrets from the sisterhood of breast cancer survivors / Barbara
Delinsky.—3rd ed.
   p. cm.
 Originally published: New York : Washington Square Press, 2001.
 1. Breast—Cancer—Popular works. I. Title.
 RC280.B8D415 2011
 616.99'449—dc23   2011023697

ISBN 978-0-7434-3136-1
ISBN 978-1-4516-5467-7 (pbk)
ISBN 978-0-7434-4005-9 (ebook)

Contents

Foreword

I am no bra-burner. I'm far too private a person for that. I've always been content working behind the scenes for the causes in which I believe. As a writer I've had the luxury of letting my characters do my bidding, whether that meant advocating safe sex, or open-mindedness, or the beauty of small-town life. I've been known to switch hairdressers when one takes to gushing on ad nauseam about my books, and I refuse to shop in bookstores where the booksellers hover so that I can't browse like a normal, everyday person. Because I *am* a normal, everyday person. And I like my anonymity.

For that reason, *UPLIFT* is an aberration for me. But if ever a cause was near and dear to my heart—and therefore worth the risk of putting my private self out there—breast cancer is it.

Breast cancer has been a player in my life since 1950, give or take. I can't tell you for sure, because my mother's hospital records don't go back far enough. When my sisters and I petitioned for a copy of them several years ago, the earliest ones we received were from 1951. That year, we were ages 8, 6 (me), and 5. According to what we've since learned from the occasional relative or friend, our mother was diagnosed two or three years before that.

We were 10, 8, and 7 when she died, but it wasn't until we were in our late teens that we learned she'd had breast cancer. It took my dad that long to say the word *cancer*, let alone *breast*. Things were different back in the forties and fifties, and it wasn't just my father. One of the early submitters to *UPLIFT*, Elinor Farber, a New Yorker who experienced breast cancer through her mother, had a similar experience.

"My mother was diagnosed with breast cancer forty-five years ago. Since there were no mammograms at that time, she was diagnosed with the help of a 'fluoroscope' machine. She had a radical mastectomy, followed by a series of X-ray treatments. There was no radiation treatment available back then. I was in seventh grade at the time. My sister, three years older than me, and I were both told of my mother's condition in hushed tones, and we were sworn to secrecy. I remember the panic and confusion that I felt. My mother, God bless her, lived for more than thirty years after her surgery, but she never spoke of her condition. She endured everything without the support of friends and neighbors, who were not told. I am so happy that breast cancer is no longer kept a dark secret. There is so much support now for women like my mother."

Indeed, there is. *UPLIFT* is a prime example of that. How did the book come to be? It was a total no-brainer that, as a novelist firmly ensconced in fiction, I simply didn't think to write—until the day last summer when I received one more note about Katherine Evans. Katherine is a character in one of my novels, *Coast Road*. She is the best friend of Rachel, the heroine, who is hurt in an automobile accident and lies in a coma through much of the book. Katherine is the one who notifies Rachel's ex-husband about the accident, and who tells Jack what Rachel's life has been like in the years since they divorced. Katherine also happens to be a breast cancer survivor, though the reader doesn't learn this until midway through the book, well after Katherine has been established as a woman who is vibrant and active, smart, attractive, and successful. At that midway point, we realize that she is grappling with the sexual ramifications of having had a bilateral mastectomy.

Readers have been applauding Katherine in their letters to me since *Coast Road* was first published in the summer of 1998. When I received that one more note last summer, the idea hit, and, in an instant, *UPLIFT* was born. In that instant, I knew that I wanted to write a book about all the other Katherines out there, because my readers seem so hungry for it. They like that Katherine is upbeat. They like that she has a productive life and that she isn't solely defined by having had breast cancer. They like that she is thriving physically. They say that she is an inspiration to them.

We are surrounded by people with a similar potential to inspire us. The problem is that we don't know it. We don't see all the women who have experienced breast cancer and moved on, whose lives are filled to overflowing with good stuff that has nothing to do with disease. When it comes to breast cancer, we hear about two kinds of women—those who are activists, often celebrities, and those who die.

Katherine is alive. I'm alive. Millions of other women are alive. If nothing else, this is what *UPLIFT* is about. Studies have shown that women consistently overestimate their risk of dying of breast cancer. No doubt, one of the reasons for this is that they've heard only about the Linda McCartneys of the world. They haven't heard about the Diane Cottings, the Ellie Anbinders, the Helen Kellys, or the Asha Mevlanas. They haven't heard about the Billie Loops, the Carolyn Steins, or the Willie Mae Ashleys. They haven't heard about the Barbara Delinskys.

I was diagnosed with breast cancer in 1994. Like so many women with a family history of the disease, I'd been waiting for it. Since I had been watched closely over the years, my cancer was caught early, picked up by a mammogram well before it was palpable. I had radiation the first year, then, when microscopic spots were found on the other breast the following year, a bilateral mastectomy and reconstruction. I told no one other than my family and a handful of friends about any of this.

There were reasons why I was silent. None had to do with embarrassment. Anyone who has ever read my books knows that I have no trouble saying the word *breast*. I certainly don't feel less of a person, or less of a woman, for having had breast cancer. Nor do I feel in any way responsible for bringing it on—though, years ago, this was indeed what women felt. No, I followed the "rules" and nursed my newborns, kept my weight down, got regular exercise, and ate broccoli. I also knew that, in truth, nothing I did was going to change something that might well be embedded in my DNA.

I suppose I could say that I kept my secret out of fear that it would hurt my career, and there was a bit of truth in that. But it wasn't the main reason.

The main reason why I didn't tell anyone outside that close circle of family and friends was that I didn't want to be seen as ill. I'd had something bad removed from my body. It was gone. I was well. I was writing up a storm, as prolific as always, and this, more than anything, eased the emotional fall-out of knowing that I'd had **IT**. When I went out, when I was with friends or colleagues, I didn't want their questions, however caring or well-meaning. I didn't want expressions of sympathy—or worse, pity. They would have been inappropriate and would have only cast an unnecessary pall on my day. I was enjoying myself—enjoying life too much to be talking cancer all the time.

Then why am I going public now? Perhaps because I'm far enough away from my diagnosis to know that others will know, as I do, that the cancer is gone. Perhaps because I'm far enough along in my career to know that publishers will buy my books and readers will read them whether I have a cold, a canker, or a cancer. Perhaps simply because I've gotten bolder since turning 50, so much bolder that I don't *care* who thinks what.

Actually, it's something else. In that Eureka! moment last summer, when *The Vineyard* was making its hardcover run on the *New York Times* list and yet one more reader wrote me about Katherine and *Coast Road*, I realized that I had the ears of millions of women and because of that *I could make a difference*. My readers look at my picture on book jackets, or talk with me at signings, and, like Katherine, see a woman who is healthy, vibrant, and strong. Telling them that I've had breast cancer and not only have recovered but am stronger than ever—that could make a difference to *them*. Additionally, there were three technical facts. First, I had the know-how to write a book. Second, I had contacts enough in the publishing world to get it in print. Third, thanks to the success of my fiction, I could afford to donate all of my proceeds to breast cancer research.

In that pivotal moment, it struck me that helping women with breast cancer, and in doing so raising money for research, was what I wanted to do more than anything else.

From the start, I knew just what the book would be. It would be the support group that I had never joined but could have used, the one that offered all the practical little secrets to survival that have nothing to do with doctors, machines, or drugs and everything to do with women helping women. But as support groups went, it would be unique in that it could be joined in total privacy, at any time of day or night, and selectively. It could also be consulted by the other people in our lives who are so important to us—our family, our friends, our co-workers. If they wanted to know how to help us—or how to help themselves through a rough period—this support group in book form would tell them.

I knew that I wanted my book to be written by women of every age and walk of life, because breast cancer doesn't discriminate. I wanted to give those women a voice, and I wanted to hear what they had to say myself—but only if it was positive. Time and again, I'd read studies showing the correlation between a positive attitude and the success of treatment. As far as I'm concerned, there is a correlation between a positive attitude and success in *life*. But still, when it came to breast cancer and the headlines in newspapers, the word was negative far more often than not. I'd read those headlines. We all have. Now I wanted to hear uplifting stories. I felt it was time to make the statement that . . . actually, Jane

Vaughan, a Texan who was diagnosed in 1991 at the age of 53, said it best.

"The morning I awoke from surgery, I knew no one who had ever had breast cancer. I assumed that everyone who had it died. By mid-morning, friends who'd had breast cancer began coming out of the woodwork. I was amazed. And appalled that no one had told me that women actually could live."

So there it was. *UPLIFT* had a face. In hindsight, I had no idea how much work was involved in a project of this scope—not that it would have discouraged me if I'd known. From the minute I conceived of this book, it was a passion for me. So I set to it, writing a detailed description of the project and a wide-ranging list of questions to spark the imagination of contributors. My assistant, Wendy Page, gave crucial help with this, as did my webmaster, Claire Marino, who took the material we'd written and designed a website that displayed it clearly and appealingly, with a submission form right there at the end.

One doesn't get submissions, though, without letting people know that a project exists. I began with a direct solicitation to my mailing list, which consists of the names of readers who have contacted me since my first book was published more than twenty years ago. My letter reached them during Breast Cancer Awareness Month in October 2000. It described *UPLIFT* and gave contact information—and the network began to grow. These readers told friends and relatives about the project. Some told reporters from their local papers, who wrote stories, which spread the word further. Others told their oncology nurses, who passed the information to other survivors, who passed the information to others still. Friends and readers sent me the names of yet more contacts, which my assistant pursued. We mailed out information on a daily basis, using breast cancer stamps whenever possible. My local post office has been cited as the national leader in sales of these stamps; I suspect *UPLIFT* may have helped.

UPLIFT doesn't pretend to be a scientific study. Once my initial mailing was done, I could no more control who learned about the project than I could control who chose to respond. The guidelines made it clear that the book would contain positives, rather than negatives, so nay-sayers no doubt took a pass. Likewise, the heavy concentration of recently diagnosed women suggests that those still visiting cancer centers on a regular basis were more apt to see the UPLIFT material on display there than those whose cancer experience was far in the past.

Fellow writers were instrumental in spreading the word about UPLIFT—from Elaine Raco Chase, who sent e-mail to her extensive mailing list, to Sandra Brown, who posted a note on her website, to Dorothea Benton Frank, who took time from a speech she was giving to distribute UPLIFT material at a luncheon for breast cancer survivors. The latter was probably the closest brush that UPLIFT had with traditional breast cancer organizations. From the start, I wanted this to be a grassroots effort. I wanted women like me, who are not typical activists, to have their say.

Submissions arrived one of three ways: via the website, via e-mail, or via the postal service. Some respondents followed the guidelines to the letter; others went off in a different direction. I was startled by the sheer length of some of the submissions—as long as ten typed pages, and that's not counting those who sent entire chapters from their journals! Some of the material was funny, some practical, some simply and solely uplifting. Jeryl Abelmann, a Californian who was diagnosed in 1986 at the age of 46, put it well in the hand-written note that prefaced her very normal-length submission: "Longer than a word . . . shorter than a thesis . . . from the heart!"

Submissions began arriving in mid-October. By mid-December, patterns had emerged. Certain topics, like hair loss, were hot ones. But as a cancer survivor who had never had chemo, I wanted to know about other things, too. So I fine-tuned the guidelines to encourage broader response. At the same time, I added questions on exercise and questions on the role of men in survivors' lives.

These questions yielded enthusiastic responses, particularly on the matter of men, which led to another modification. In January, with barely six weeks left in the submission process, I e-mailed all of those who had already submitted and invited the men in their lives to send along their own thoughts. As a result of the response to this e-mail, there is a specific chapter in *UPLIFT* for, by, and about men.

January became February. Just when I would be thinking that I'd seen and read everything there was to be said on a topic, survivors proved me wrong. They kept sending fresh material. Closing the submission phase at the end of February was hard to do, but it was necessary if I hoped to get the finished book to New York by the middle of May.

All told, I had more submissions than I'd ever hoped to receive. Though some were from friends and relatives of survivors, the bulk were from survivors themselves. They ranged in age at the time of diagnosis from eighteen to eighty, and were diagnosed as long ago as 1954. They came from every state in America, save six. There was even a submission from Canada.

Reading the submissions took several weeks. I selected those that were consistent with the spirit of the book and typed them up—no mean feat, since some submissions contained upward of a dozen separate elements. After printing out these many pages, I stood with a paper cutter and literally cut the submissions apart, so that I was left with strips of paper, each bearing a single entry and the name of its author.

Then the fun began. I put chapter signs around my dining room table, like place settings for guests, and walked around and around, back and forth, putting those strips of paper into the appropriate piles. There was overlap; my chapters were far from mutually exclusive. A funny story about wigs, for instance (and there are *tons* of those), could easily work in a chapter on hair loss or one on humor. So I put some in the first and some in the second. Same with submissions on regaining control and on staying positive; some thoughts definitely bear repeating, albeit in different women's voices. As the sorting went on and certain piles grew too large for a single chapter, I divided those submissions up into smaller topics.

Initially, I had hoped to give clever little titles to each of the chapters. But working now with the actual submissions, I realized that it was more important that readers know exactly what a chapter was about. Not every women needs chemo, or radiation, or a mastectomy. If a woman is grappling with lumpectomy and radiation alone, she doesn't need to hear about something she won't experience, like losing her hair. Push her too far when she's already strung tight, and she could freak out.

I know this. I've been there. When I was first diagnosed, the treatment plan was for a re-excision and radiation. Yet, in the midst of those seemingly endless hours waiting in examining rooms for the various doctors to stop by, the nurse came in to explain the use of drains. I'd been pretty together up to that point, but I came close to losing it then. My husband, who was with me, will attest to the fact that I went deathly pale. *No one told me about drains,* I fairly yelled. The nurse kindly said, *But you will have to deal with them after you've had your surgery.* I cried, *I'm only having a re-excision!* She paused, then asked, *Only a re-excision?* When I nodded, she apologized, packed up her demo drains, and left. Mind you, I did deal with drains after my surgery the following year, and they weren't so bad. But I was ready for them then, as I hadn't been ready the year before.

I feel strongly that *UPLIFT* is presented in a way that allows the reader to be selective. If she doesn't need chemo help, she doesn't have to read that chapter. If she isn't into religion, she can skip that one as well. If she doesn't have the peace of mind (a.k.a. attention span) to read more than five minutes at a time, *UPLIFT* allows for that, too.

This book is definitely informative, but its larger purpose is comfort. In order to be that, it must be nonthreatening. Beyond the clear labeling of chapters, this dictates the complete absence of medical talk. When I was going through treatment, I didn't read a single book, newspaper, or magazine article on breast cancer. I was too busy *having* it. I was walking a fine line between panic and calm, and I simply couldn't risk reading something that would upset me.

Pat Baker, my friend and a breast cancer survivor since 1993, puts it well. "In almost every book on breast cancer, there are elements that frighten a patient. One becomes wary of picking up the material. But your effort can bring only comfort."

I'm trying, Pat, I'm trying. There are so many positive things to say, and so many women anxious to *say* them. Mind you, we aren't Pollyannas. We are definitely grounded in reality. Ask any one of us to discuss the pros and cons of various treatment options, and we'll give you an earful. But not here. No, definitely not here.

By way of being assured comfort, readers of *UPLIFT* can pick and choose—pick and choose what chapters they read, pick and choose what submissions within a chapter they read, even pick and choose what tips they want to follow. On certain topics, those tips run the gamut. For instance, some women swear that going to chemo on a full stomach works best, while others advise eating lightly beforehand. Some women vow that joining a support group was the best thing they ever did, while others say that they did just fine without.

If this is confusing to readers, I apologize. All bodies are different; some stomachs will settle with saltines, while others need a chocolate shake. Likewise, all *people* are different; some thrive on joining groups, while others have neither the time nor the desire to belong. The point is that there are choices. If one option doesn't work, another will. There are no rights and wrongs here. When they are feeling overwhelmed, readers need to know that *there is a solution*. The hundreds of women who've submitted to *UPLIFT* are proof of that.

Orchestrating *UPLIFT* has been an incredible experience for me. For starters, in picking a name for the project to coincide with a web address, I learned more about trademark law than I ever wanted to know. Then there were the submitters to *UPLIFT*, women and men whose names and experiences became as familiar to me as those of my neighbors and whose enthusiasm has been a highlight of this project for me. I would also be remiss if I didn't mention the days when I shamelessly touted the book to my publisher—shamelessly, because for the first time in my career, I could brazenly promote one of my books, since there was absolutely no money in it for me. I still get a rush from that.

In truth, though, putting *UPLIFT* together hasn't always been easy. I was never one to fill my day with cancer. During all those years waiting for it to hit, I did what I had to medically, then went on with the rest of my life. Suddenly, with *UPLIFT*, I was immersed in cancer as I never had been when I was being treated, and it was hard. I have to confess that there were days last fall when I wondered whether I could do this—whether I could live and breathe the disease for the months that it would take to secure submissions and put together the book.

That fear passed, largely because of the wonderful people whose words constitute the body of this book. These people are upbeat. They are resourceful. They are intelligent, friendly, and warm. They are generous. And they are funny. Mostly, though, I was time and again humbled by their eagerness to share their experiences and their hope of making things easier for others.

I close this foreword by quoting three such extraordinary women.

Corinne Wood, Lieutenant Governor of Illinois, who was diagnosed in 1997 at the age of 42, wrote, "Since I made my story public, not a week has passed without people coming to me seeking information or wanting to share their experience. The impassioned testimonials I hear from husbands, wives, sisters, daughters, and friends help me to know I made the right decision in sharing my story. A generation ago, most people didn't talk about breast cancer. Many women suffered in silence, frustrated and alone, without access to information, counsel, or community support. We need to tell our stories. We need to humanize this disease. There is no shame in breast cancer; I want women to be proud to say, 'I am a breast cancer survivor. I beat this disease, and so can you!' "

Sheri Goodman, a social worker from New York, who was diagnosed in 1999 at the age of 50, wrote, "Breast cancer is no longer a covert disease that is accompanied by embarrassment or shame. It is a disease that strikes regardless of age, race, and socioeconomic status, and we can no longer ignore its presence. It is through the stories of breast cancer survivors that we are so well informed on this issue. I am only one survivor, but I represent the many who have not yet spoken. I am sharing my story now to show that there is indeed life after breast cancer. I am a wife, a mother, a sister, an aunt, a friend, a social worker . . . and will someday be a grandmother. Yes, I am a survivor. We all are."

And finally, Sallie Burdine, a survivor from Florida and mother of three young children, wrote, "I've often played this little mental game with myself in a crowded place like a shopping mall or an airport. I imagine myself yelling out, 'Hey! Who all here has breast cancer? Put your hands up!' And then maybe four or five women will slowly stop talking, walking, or whatever and look at me and raise their hands. We will simply smile warmly at one another, as if to say, 'We're okay, we're not alone, we can do this.' And then everyone goes on about their business, and I imagine we're all just a little bit stronger."

Here, then, is *UPLIFT*.

Barbara Delinsky
June 2001

Foreword to the Third Edition

UPLIFT was first published in September 2001, mere days before the terrorist strike that changed so many of our lives. Surviving 9/11 has much in common with surviving breast cancer. For one thing, we all now know of the fragility of life. For another, we feel the need to prioritize, to put on the front burner the things that mean the most to us. For a third, we are learning—still—that we can't live each day fearing a repeat of the past.

For that very reason, I did not include anything about recurrence in the original edition of UPLIFT. But several women caught me on it and said that there definitely are uplifting things to hear about recurrence. And there were. I discovered this when I solicited new material specifically on the subject. The second edition of UPLIFT, containing a chapter on recurrence, was published in May 2003.

Come September 2005, I realized that it was the fifth anniversary of UPLIFT's conception—and that I really wanted to know what was going on with those original UPLIFTers, five years later. So I wrote to them again and asked. And did they ever tell! The personal growth in those five years has been amazing—and so uplifting that I knew we had to go for a third edition.

I've had a wonderful time putting this new chapter together. I mean, what could be more gratifying than hearing about people who are living longer and longer, better and better, different and even more exciting lives after being treated for breast cancer?

Interestingly enough, I received as much input from people who hadn't been in the original UPLIFT as I did from people who had. It seems that the UPLIFT family is growing. And this is good. More and more of us are thriving.

So mark your calendars, guys. If this is the fifth anniversary, let's shoot for the tenth, then the fifteenth—unless, of course, there is a cure by that time, in which case UPLIFT will be totally obsolete. Wouldn't that be nice?

Barbara Delinsky
October 2006

Foreword to the
Tenth Anniversary Edition

When I first conceived of *UPLIFT*, we more often heard about people who died of breast cancer than those who survived. Not so now. Breast cancer has come out of the closet. Every spring and fall, there are walks all over the country. Year-round, we see pink tee-shirts, bumper stickers, ribbons, and hats. We see bald heads in the mall and the gym. We watch public figures thrive after a breast cancer diagnosis. We meet people, get to know them, and almost incidentally learn that they are survivors.

In that respect, *UPLIFT* is obsolete. Yes, nearly one in eight women will still develop breast cancer in her lifetime, but the vast majority will survive and go on to live long and happy lives. We know these women. They are our sisters, our neighbors, our friends.

And still, there is nothing more frightening than hearing the words, "You have breast cancer." This book is for all those who have felt the fear. It doesn't matter how many survivors we hear about on TV or read about in *People* magazine. We want to hear more. We want to hear about people like Linda Almond, who was diagnosed thirty-seven years ago, or Dorothy Coon, who was diagnosed thirty-six years ago, or Taylor Montagna, who was diagnosed twenty-nine years ago. There's Rita Madison, twenty-eight years ago   Lorraine Colavito, twenty-two years ago—Billie Bules and Doris Cantrell, both twenty years ago. Mary Ann Budnick and Susan Sanford are nineteen years out, Alyce Feinstein eighteen years, Pamela Lord sixteen years—I could go on and on. All are alive and well today. Take Bea Flannagan. Diagnosed thirty-nine years ago, she is currently traveling around the country doing breast cancer walks, hoping to reach every state in America "before my normal demise or lack of ability." You gotta love Bea.

That said, if you are newly diagnosed, you're likely in shock. You won't identify with these women today. But next week you will. And next month, next year, ten years from now? You'll identify, though you'll be too busy living your life to dwell on it.

As I write this, a recent report from the Centers for Disease Control says that one in twenty American adults is now a cancer survivor. We are everywhere. We are strong. We are happy.

For those moments when you need that little bit of extra convincing, I offer this Tenth Anniversary Edition of *UPLIFT*. Enjoy!

Barbara Delinsky
September 2011

1 • On Diagnosis

First Things First

Where was I when I learned that I had breast cancer? You may as well ask where I was when I learned that JFK had been shot. I will never forget either answer.

In the case of JFK, I was in college, returning to my dormitory after class to find the television on in the dorm living room and my friends gathered around it. I remember feeling total disbelief—that what had happened couldn't be so. It had nothing to do with political affiliation and everything to do with youth, vigor, and Camelot.

In the case of breast cancer, I felt no disbelief. I was working out in the basement of our home when my surgeon called to say that the results of my biopsy were in and that the tiny little granules she had removed from my breast were malignant. *She told you that on the phone?* Indeed, she did. It was just the right thing for me, and she knew it. She and I had been through biopsies together before. She knew that my mother had had breast cancer and that I'd been expecting it. She knew that the best approach to take with me would be the understated one. What she actually said was, "You've spent a lifetime waiting for the other shoe to fall, and now

1

that it has, it's a very small shoe. The cure rate for this is ninety-nine-point-five percent. Here is what I recommend . . ."

I listened. Then I hung up the phone and called my husband. Then I finished working out. In doing that, I was showing myself that I was healthy and strong, cancer and all. I needed to minimize the impact of what I'd learned . . . because just as a certain idealism had been lost when JFK was shot, so I knew that with a diagnosis of breast cancer, a part of my life was forever changed.

I was shaky as I climbed back up the stairs—and what had me most frightened wasn't the prospect of having a re-excision and radiation. It was phoning our three sons, who were in three different states, in college and law school at the time. I went about making dinner, a crucial same-old same-old, as I put through those calls, and as I talked with each son I had the first of many cancer experiences that weren't nearly as bad as I'd imagined. "Curable" was the word I stressed. My confidence was contagious.

MAKING DECISIONS

"When I was first diagnosed, I knew pretty much nothing about breast cancer—except that I didn't want it! By learning everything I could, I started to calm down, sort things out, and actively make decisions. Knowledge is power. It definitely makes you feel a little bit more in control of your life."

Deborah Lambert; diagnosed in 2000 at age 47;
medical secretary; Massachusetts

"The first thing I did when the doctor told me I had breast cancer was to sit down, since I was weak in the knees, then to get a pen and paper. As an educator I needed to get it all in print, to get it right. That served to calm me immediately."

Christine Foutris; diagnosed in 1999 at age 49;
teacher; Illinois

"When I woke up after a lumpectomy and learned that I had breast cancer, I was in shock. To show how little I knew, when my husband was visiting and offered me a sip from his drink, I declined, saying that we didn't know if he could catch cancer from my germs. After he left, I picked up a book that a friend had left. Opening it at random, my eyes caught the words, 'A cancerous cell is, in fact, a weak and confused cell.' That made both of us, I thought, and laughed heartily."

Carol Pasternak; diagnosed in 1986 at age 47;
artist; Ontario, Canada

"I was devastated when I got the diagnosis of cancer. I'd had my mammogram faithfully every year. I went home to prepare dinner in a sort of shock. As I stood at the stove I worried about what was going to happen and how I could handle it. Then, suddenly, a feeling of calm and peace came over me, and an inner voice said, 'You will be all right.' From that moment on, I knew I would survive."

Wendy Golab; diagnosed in 2000 at age 63;
nurse; Connecticut

"Realize that a diagnosis of cancer does not mean instant doom. You have time to investigate, reflect, get several opinions, and make careful decisions. Tell yourself this every morning, and tell everyone around you to keep telling it back to you."

Susan Stamberg; diagnosed in 1986 at age 48;
broadcast journalist; Washington, D.C.

"I didn't make any decisions about treatment until my children and significant other had been told. We all went to the surgeon's office together the next day. My children were all in their twenties. The home care nurse and I gave one daughter a crash course in Nursing 101 so that she could change my dressings, and they all took turns driving me to my doctor appointments and treatment. This was a reassurance for them that nothing was being kept from them."

Becky Honeycutt; diagnosed in 1995 at age 53;
licensed practical nurse; Indiana

"One of the very first things I did, after the words 'cancer' and 'radiation' were mentioned, was to get down to the local library to see what radiation entailed."

Deb Haney; diagnosed in 1996 at age 48;
administrative assistant, artist; Massachusetts

"When I was first diagnosed, I wanted information immediately. I wanted to know which treatment plan was right for me. I rushed out and purchased the largest book on breast cancer I could find and read it twice. I sought the advice of trusted family, friends, doctors, and breast cancer survivors. I made sure I was equipped with the best possible information, so that I could be my own best advocate."

Corinne Wood; diagnosed in 1997 at age 42;
Lieutenant Governor; Illinois

"Treat your diagnosis as a business problem. Do research. Use the Internet, and go through literature at the hospital resource room. Feeling in control is pretty important, so begin with a notebook. The inside cover should have the name and telephone numbers of each of your caretakers (doctor, nurse, etc.) as they come on the scene. The notebook can be sectioned to keep track of doctors' appointments, definitions, outside advice, and so on."

Anne Jacobs; diagnosed in 1999 at age 62;
managing partner, real estate; Massachusetts

"Try to attend lectures on breast cancer. All major hospitals have these programs. Just call the community relations director. Attend lectures on the side effects of treatment and the importance of good nutrition."

Ellen Beth Simon; diagnosed in 1998 at age 41;
lawyer; New Jersey

"When I went to appointments after the diagnosis, I always had two or three of the children with me and sometimes all of them. They had so many questions to ask and also wanted to make sure I understood all the doctor was saying. After a while, I went alone with just my husband. When the doctor came in and saw only the two of us, he started hunting in all the closets and cupboards and finally said, 'Okay, where are they hiding?' We got a big chuckle out of that."

Sally Martel; diagnosed in 1996 at age 60;
wife, mother, retired accountant; New Hampshire, Florida

"The hardest part of the whole mess was deciding what I wanted to do. I struggled with the decision-making process. Finally a dear, sweet lady said, 'Do your homework, make a decision, and don't look back. You can deal with whatever is up ahead when you get to it.' She was right."

Mitzi Scarborough; diagnosed in 1999 at age 37;
childcare provider; Arkansas

"How much do you really want to know? Be honest with yourself. Once you have the answer and know what your learning style is, find a survivor who is a match with you."

Kathy Weaver-Stark; diagnosed in 1991 at age 46;
insurance adjuster, instructor; Oregon

"I would have loved to talk with someone about all of this before I had surgery and treatment. The worst part was my imagination. I worried myself to death with chemotherapy horror stories. But it's a lot like pregnancy; it's livable, doable."

Joy West; diagnosed in 2000 at 34;
advertising account coordinator; South Carolina

"In deciding which option was best for me, I felt like I was looking at a Chinese menu. But what I found most comforting was that no matter who I talked to or what her own decision was, each felt confident of her decision even years later. Women even offered to show me their breasts. The idea of going to work without a bra began to sound pretty good."

Kathi Ward; diagnosed in 1994 at age 47;
merchandiser; South Carolina

"During the diagnosis phase, go to a fertility clinic for advice if you desire to have children after treatment for breast cancer."

Alexandra Koffman; diagnosed in 1997 at age 40;
registered nurse; Massachusetts

"When you're first diagnosed, you may find yourself reading books, watching videos, getting more and more information on your options. The important thing to remember is that you need to make the decision that's best for you. No one else can tell you that what you have decided to do is wrong, because there is no wrong, if this is what you want."

Glenda Chance; diagnosed in 2000 at age 38;
homemaker, mother, and wife; Ohio

"Be your own advocate. Do what feels right for you. Don't let anyone talk you into anything."

Rhonda Sorrell; diagnosed in 1998 at age 43;
special education teacher; Michigan

"Knowledge is power. The more educated you become, the less frightening the unknown is. Read, read, and read more. It helps!"

Cathy Hanlon; diagnosed in 2000 at age 42;
school researcher; New York

"Twenty-one years ago, when I was diagnosed, many people recommended that I read a particular book on breast cancer. It happens that the author's husband had left her following her diagnosis. I remember thinking how depressing that was. My husband was there. He was worried about me, and I was worried about him, since he looked like he'd been kicked in the stomach. I never had to even think about his leaving. I knew I was more to him than a pair of breasts, and any woman with a strong relationship should know so, too. It helped him that a family friend whose wife had recently had a mastectomy made the effort to talk to him. Marty isn't one who easily verbalizes his feelings, but having a friend who'd been through it was good for him."

Lynne Rutenberg; diagnosed in 1980 at age 35;
retired teacher; New Jersey

"Research everything about your disease. Ask questions. The ultimate decisions are yours to make. If you do your homework, you will feel that you have done the best for yourself and, ultimately, for all those who love and depend on you."

Christine Webber; diagnosed in 1998 at age 55;
registered nurse; Illinois

"Everyone handles traumatic situations differently. What is right for one can be wrong for another. I did everything I could not to dwell on my situation. I chose my doctors, got a second opinion, contacted the National Cancer Institute for the latest information, then I left it at that. A friend mailed me a book she had painstakingly highlighted to make the information she thought I needed more accessible—I never read it. People sent me articles, which I never read. I dressed up for every appointment, so my doctors and nurses would see what I looked like well and consider me a person who *would* be well. I was not in denial about having had breast cancer. Whenever I had a chance, I mentioned it to people. That was the promise I had made, the 'bargain' for my life . . . that I would spread the word that women had breast cancer and lived."

Jane Vaughan; diagnosed in 1991 at age 53;
writer; Texas

"I strongly recommend to anyone newly diagnosed that they join a clinical trials study. It is like having the undivided attention of a complete support system at all times."

Jacki Anthony; diagnosed in 1998 at age 48;
nurse; Massachusetts

"The four words that I live by: This too shall pass."

Suzanne Almond; diagnosed in 1996 at age 60;
secretary to the Special Services Director; New Hampshire

"Remember to thank your healthcare team as you navigate through the system of treatment. You would be surprised how much they worry about you as they plan your course of treatment."

Kathy Weaver-Stark; diagnosed in 1991 at age 46;
insurance adjuster, instructor; Oregon

HELPFUL LITTLE TRICKS

"Take another person with you to your doctor appointments to act as your advocate. They can ask questions you forget to ask and can make sure things are well explained. Also, take a list of questions with you, so you don't forget to ask the doctor something important. I know a woman who used to fax her questions in advance to her oncologist. Tape recorders are good for remembering the answers."

Sharon Irons Strempski; diagnosed in 1997 at age 52;
registered nurse; Connecticut

"My mother and my husband were with me at every doctor's appointment after my diagnosis. My mom kept a spiral notebook with her at all times to take notes. When we went for the first consultation to discuss the results of the pathology report, my mother had written down all the words that could possibly describe a tumor. When the doctor began, Mom just started circling words. This helped all of us to concentrate on what the doctor was saying. It was also helpful when reviewing later and doing research."

Jennifer Wersal; diagnosed in 2000 at age 30; marketing; Texas

"After my diagnosis, my dear friend and neighbor, Diane, came to the rescue. Because my husband and I were numb and couldn't 'hear,' Diane went with us to see three surgeons, a radiation oncologist, and a reconstructive surgeon. She took notes, and we discussed my options later. One surgeon also taped our consultation. I suggest to others that they take a tape recorder to all appointments, plus a 'Diane'—someone who loves you but can distance themselves."

Marianne Rennie; diagnosed in 1988 at age 39; cancer information specialist; Ohio

"Take a little tape recorder with you when you have your initial consultations with the surgeon and oncologist. Even if you have a friend or family member with you, there is just too much information to remember. I was able to replay the tape for my mother and sister, and it helped to answer questions that I had later on. There is just too much emotion going on to have to rely on your memory for technical terms and procedures."

Deb Haney; diagnosed in 1996 at age 48; administrative assistant, artist; Massachusetts

"When I was first diagnosed, a friend suggested I keep a journal of everything that was happening to me—what the doctor said, when and what the treatments were, and so on. I began doing that but found it to be too consuming. I was a pretty well-informed patient, and I didn't think I needed to concentrate on my cancer this way. Instead, I decided to keep a 'grateful journal.' Every day I wrote down five things that I was grateful for. Granted, some days it was difficult to meet that goal, but every day for nine months I wrote something. It was such a positive exercise during a difficult time in my life. When I read those journals now, they lift my spirits."

Susan Kowalski; diagnosed in 1997 at age 50;
college executive staff assistant; New York

"Form a phone tree. Then you only have to give an update to one person. Otherwise, the phone rings off the hook!"

Stephanie King;
friend of two survivors; New York

FINDING EARLY SUPPORT

"My husband was at home when I got the news. Our children were racing in the door from school, and at the same time the radiologist on the phone was confirming to me that I had cancer. I hung up and felt swallowed in confusion. My kids were rifling through the cabinets looking for snacks, and my husband was looking at the terror on my face, knowing in his heart what had just been said on the phone without hearing a word. Our children were eight and ten, and we decided that they needed to know. I made appointments with their teachers and explained the circumstances. With four months left in the school year, I knew I would need their help and support. I felt like I was assembling a team to go to war; it was empowering to have people on my side. When it came to the kids, we took them through each step separately so as not to overwhelm them—first surgery, then chemo, then radiation. Having information gave them the power to talk about the experience as we all went through it."

Cindy Fiedler; diagnosed in 1998 at age 40;
registered nurse, mom; Massachusetts

"I never hid my diagnosis. I cannot stress enough the importance of being open. It is amazing how many people will be there for you. The support of others is one of the greatest healers around."

Dee Pobjoy; diagnosed in 1999 at age 41;
sales clerk; Wisconsin

"At the time of my diagnosis, there were several other women in town who'd had breast cancer. One of them was a good friend and tennis partner of mine. She called and gave me a lot of support and advice. This helped me tremendously."

Polly Briggs; diagnosed in 1987 at age 41;
secretary; Mississippi

"On the day of my diagnosis, I phoned a friend who had gone through breast cancer three years before. She was very busy with work, but she gave me the time I needed. She told me that until I determined what my treatment should be, I would feel that I was totally out of control, but that once the decision was made, it would feel like a ton of bricks had been lifted off my shoulders. She was correct. I will always remember her last words. I said that I appreciated her time and long pep talk, and she said, 'You know, this is therapy for me, too.' "

Caroline C. Hudnall; diagnosed in 1992 at age 55;
retired legal tech in the Supreme Court of Alaska; Montana

"My surgeon told me I had breast cancer at 5 P.M. on a Monday and gave me until noon the next day to decide between mastectomy and lumpectomy. I knew what a mastectomy was, but I knew nothing about a lumpectomy. Frantic, I called two of my girlfriends, each of whom had a friend who'd had breast cancer. Both of these women called me that night. They offered no opinions but did give me the knowledge I needed to make the right decision for me. They were absolutely wonderful with their support before, during, *and* after the surgery. They also helped me understand the process of radiation. This is a scary experience. Without their help, it would have been much more stressful."

Rose Marie Clark; diagnosed in 1996 at age 50;
retired; New York

"When I was first diagnosed, I e-mailed a few friends to let them know. One friend who was not on my initial list e-mailed me to say, 'We're your friends in the bad times as well as the good!' After that, I gave my two closest friends permission to pass on my e-mail to anyone they felt it would help. The list grew over the next six months from fourteen to over two hundred. Discovering that people truly care about me was wonderful."

Deb Haggerty; diagnosed in 1999 at age 51;
professional speaker; Florida

"My feeling when I learned my diagnosis was, 'Why me? I have been a good person and had such a nasty marriage, and things are finally good in my world. Why now?' I was scared and cried in the parking lot. My boyfriend, Jerry, held me tightly and kept reassuring me that my cancer was curable. After surgery, the cards and phone calls were not to be believed. My bosses sent flowers and two huge live lobsters, which I loved!"

Sharon Daniels; diagnosed in 2000 at age 49;
hairstylist, wig store owner; Massachusetts

"Sleep didn't come easy for me after my diagnosis. Instead of sleeping pills, my husband and I started having a glass of wine before bedtime to help me relax. Every night while we drank wine, we talked, we read to each other, and we played games. This became a special time together when we shared our feelings, fears, and hopes for the future."

Julie Crandall; diagnosed in 1998 at age 31;
stay-at-home mom; North Carolina

"We had gotten two kittens a few weeks before I learned I had cancer. They were confined to the guest bedroom. Whenever I was feeling down, I would go in and lie on the bed with them. They would climb all over me, cheering me into a better mood. My husband referred to my going in there as 'opening a can of kittens.' "

Jeanne Sturdevant; diagnosed in 1990 at age 45;
artist; Texas

"Being a mother, wife, and nurse, I'd always been in the position of caring for everyone but myself. So I made an appointment with the social worker who was affiliated with the breast center I went to. Now, I must confess, I'm not one to share my feelings with a perfect stranger, but somehow I felt this was the healthiest thing to do. Though it was awkward and uncomfortable at first, I visited this social worker regularly. This helped me keep things in perspective. As time passed, I looked forward to our visits as a place where I could speak of what I feared or sing of my accomplishments."

Cindy Fiedler; diagnosed in 1998 at age 40;
registered nurse, mom; Massachusetts

GROWING BOLD

"When I awoke in the hospital after my mastectomy, the operating room nurse sat by my bed. A breast cancer survivor herself, she had been sent by my surgeon. Her advice was, 'When you need something from someone, ask.' My generation of women was taught to 'suffer silently,' not to complain or impose. An hour or so later, my husband called from his office a few blocks away to see how I was doing. I told him that I needed him, and he came immediately. Before the nurse's advice, I would have told my husband that I was okay—and then been miserable. Her advice has improved everything in my life!"

Jane Vaughan; diagnosed in 1991 at age 53;
writer; Texas

"Write all your questions down before your doctor's appointment. Make sure your doctor listens to you and doesn't talk down to you. If necessary, change doctors until you get the right one."

Ellen Beth Simon; diagnosed in 1998 at age 41;
lawyer; New Jersey

"If you think that something isn't right or hasn't been answered or resolved to your satisfaction, hang in there until you *are* satisfied— at *every* step of the way! When I had doubts about the way a technician was setting me up for radiation, I asked that he not work with me in the future. My request was respected. That was important."

Anne Jacobs; diagnosed in 1999 at age 62;
managing partner, real estate; Massachusetts

"The mammography technician who helped prep me for biopsy surgery was so kind that I have requested she do my mammograms each time I have gone back for followups. As a result, she and I have become friends."

Jeanne Sturdevant; diganosed in 1990 at age 45;
artist; Texas

"If a needle wire localization is being done before biopsy or lumpectomy, ask if it can be done in the supine position. Most modern breast centers can do this. I had to sit up for the first round, only minutes before my lumpectomy. Between the discomfort of the procedure and anticipating surgery afterward, I passed out cold! My surgery was canceled, and I had to return for it a week later. The second time went much better. It was easier being able to lie down."

Donna Barnett; diagnosed in 1999 at age 40;
registered nurse; California

"I refused to go back to the first radiation oncologist I saw, because he made me feel like a piece of meat. The second one was very sensitive to my feelings. He made a note on my radiation card that no male techs were to take care of me, and the female techs made a point of being busy with other things while I was undressing, thus making me feel less exposed. You have to speak up for yourself and let people know what your comfort levels are."

Sharon Irons Strempski; diagnosed in 1997 at age 52;
registered nurse; Connecticut

"Get a second opinion if you are unhappy with the first one. Do some reading, and speak up for what you want."

Mary Raffol; diagnosed in 1998 at age 44;
teacher; Massachusetts

"At no other time in your life will you have so much power and control over your own destiny; choose your health team well."

Kathy Weaver-Stark; diagnosed in 1991 at age 46;
insurance adjuster, instructor; Oregon

"I became bold enough to leave my first surgeon and radiation oncologist, because I didn't feel comfortable putting my life in their hands. At least, I still had *some* power."

Kathi Ward; diagnosed in 1994 at age 47;
merchandiser; South Carolina

"My first oncologist asked whether I wanted to take treatment, since there was no guarantee that it would help. My husband and I left that doctor and found another who said, 'You have a one in

eleven chance, and you might as well be that one.' His positive attitude lifted our spirits. A year later, when my treatment was done
and he told us there was no sign of cancer, I thanked him for sav-
ing my life. His reply was that my positive attitude had made the
difference. 'You knew you were going to get better, and you did,'
he said. Attitude is so important on everyone's part."

Florence Chandler; diagnosed in 1995 at age 66;

retired motel owner; Florida

ATTITUDE INDEED . . .

"The most constructive thing I did when I learned my diagnosis
was to continue to write out the invitations to my daughter's wedding shower."

Frances Gallello; diagnosed in 2000 at age 51;

mental health assistant; New York

"The best thing I did after being diagnosed was *not* to cancel a
planned bicycle trip. It did more for my optimism than anything
else could have done. Same thing with attending a neighborhood
party on the day I came home from the hospital. I refused to hole
up in self-pity."

Judith Ormond; diagnosed in 1996 at age 49;

symphony musician—piccolo; Wisconsin

"My husband, who is my best friend, took me for a walk in the
woods the day I was told I had a malignancy in my breast. He
knew that was where my spirit is most at peace."

Robin Smith; diagnosed in 2000 at age 53;

microbiologist, homemaker; New York

"I cried a lot during the two weeks between when I learned I had
breast cancer and the day I had the surgery. Once all the decisions were made and the surgery done, though, I considered my-

self 'on the road to recovery,' and I was determined not to cry or feel sorry for myself. I've always been an optimistic person and was determined to continue being that way. I considered what was happening to my body to be a temporary condition."

Patti R. Martinez; diagnosed in 1999 at age 54;
realtor; California

"Seven years ago, when I got my cancer diagnosis, I fell apart. I had no one to tell, my children were away at college, and I was by myself in the hills of Kentucky. I remember driving into the driveway and going straight to the barn to see my animals. My main concern was who was going to take care of them if I could not? My animals were the reason I was living in the county. They were part of my family. I went to visit a neighbor who was ninety-three years old at the time, and I had all the intentions of telling her what was wrong. When I walked in her house, though, she spoke before me. 'You know,' she said, 'some days God gives us a heavy load to carry, and we must do the best we can to tote it.' My neighbor died the following Sunday, and I still remember what she said. This is my eighth year since the diagnosis. My life has changed, and I have met wonderful people whom I would not have otherwise known."

Antonia Rhodes; diagnosed in 1993 at age 50;
Breast Cancer Outreach person; New York

"When I was diagnosed, I had just retired, and we had many plans for things to do. I found that continuing to work on those plans helped me to realize that this was just a bump in the road."

Monetta Lockey; diagnosed in 1997 at age 59;
retired teacher; Texas

"Even after my diagnosis, I went on a Caribbean cruise as planned. I continued with my regular schedule as soon as possible, seeing as many friends and relatives as possible so that they would know I was alive and well."

Carol Hattler; diagnosed in 1999 at age 65;
retired nurse; Virginia

"When I was diagnosed with breast cancer, I took six months' leave of absence from my job. During this time, amid surgery, chemotherapy, and radiation treatments, I discovered my creative side. I began to write poetry."

Mary Platt; diagnosed in 1998 at age 47;
radiology supervisor; South Carolina

"One strange thing. I cried when I was first diagnosed and never cried after that. Now, I cry at so many touching things. I feel that it's okay and healthy to do this. But I don't cry for myself. Not ever."

Sheila Roper; diagnosed in 1995 at age 57;
homemaker; New Hampshire

"When my doctor told me that I had breast cancer, I had a good cry. Then I decided that I wanted to live and would do everything necessary to achieve that goal."

Sandy Mark; diagnosed in 1998 at age 55;
administrative assistant; Connecticut

"When I was diagnosed, I kept three bits of advice in mind. First, stay in control. Second, be informed. Third, keep a positive outlook. After my surgeries, chemotherapy, and radiation, I add a fourth to the list. Be proud to be a survivor."

Helen Ann Kelly; diagnosed in 1996 at age 43;
teacher; New Hampshire

"My husband says that he got most of his comfort from me, because he felt that I was in control both of my disease and of the day-to-day workings of our lives. That was my goal—to keep everything at home operating as usual. The most contructive thing I did after hearing my diagnosis was to personally tell every friend, relative, neighbor, and co-worker of my diagnosis. As time passed, I kept everyone up to date with all the details, so that there would be no mystery or misunderstanding."

Deborah J.P. Schur; diagnosed in 1994 at age 43;

sales rep; Massachusetts

"A breast cancer diagnosis can be terrifying, especially because there is a lot of waiting—waiting for the mammogram results, waiting for the biopsy results, waiting to talk to the surgeon and plastic surgeon, and then waiting for the surgery. All this waiting can lead to a lot of stress and anxiety! Slow, desperate, and out of control were the feelings I was experiencing. It didn't take me long to realize that I had to take control or I would lose control. I believe the single most powerful thing I did to get through my breast cancer diagnosis was to concentrate on truly living and enjoying every day. For me this meant simply keeping very busy, doing things I enjoyed doing. The last thing I needed was time on my own. I took every opportunity I could to simply be with people—anybody and everybody. By forcing myself to be out in the world, surrounded by others, I was forced to look beyond myself. And did I ever keep busy! My husband and I took long bike rides, we went to the mall, we went out to eat, we went away every weekend—to the beach, to the mountains, anywhere, while we waited. It sounds so simple, but by keeping busy and active, I was reminding myself that life does go on. I did not feel ill; I felt good and healthy and alive. It was liberating to feel in control of my actions and my mind."

Julie Crandall; diagnosed in 1998 at age 31;

stay-at-home mom; North Carolina

"Being diagnosed at twenty-four, married, and taking care of a two-year-old can be overwhelming for anyone. Not me! When I found out I had cancer, I did not think I was going to die. I was just going to face the facts and beat this to the end, and that I did."

Candice Jaeger; diagnosed in 2000 at age 24;
wife, mother; Illinois

"I have always tried to live and eat healthily. Still, I found a lump in my breast. I had a mastectomy and reconstructive surgery. Since I am the mother of two daughters and have two granddaughters, I participated in a clinical study. I thought that if my participation could help at least one other person, it would all be worth while."

Nancy Ellis; diagnosed in 2000 at age 53;
quality technician; New York

"One year ago I was diagnosed
My life turned upside down
How do I feel about that?
I don't know.
Happy to be alive
I would be dead
If not for the check-up
How do I feel about that?
Grateful."

Cheryl Wilkinson; diagnosed in 1999 at age 45;
fast food; Ohio

"From the beginning, set your mind on one thought: I will beat this. It will not beat me."

Susan Schultz; diagnosed in 1990 at age 41;
special education teacher's aide; New York

"What worked for me? Never ever, *ever* thinking I would not survive."

Eleanor Anbinder; diagnosed in 1991 at age 50;
sales manager; Massachusetts

2 • Losing a Breast

Practical and Emotional

W hat to do? Lumpectomy? Mastectomy? Single? Double? Reconstruction with implants? Tissue flap reconstruction? No reconstruction?

So many questions, so many decisions. *UPLIFT* won't give you the answers. Nor does it discuss the medical merits of one procedure or another. It simply tells you of the decisions that different women made and why they are pleased with those choices.

I'm pleased with the choices I made. They were the right ones for me. As crass as it may sound, losing a breast was never something I spent much time thinking about. Before I was diagnosed, it was too *painful* a thought to dwell on. I had my mammograms and my physical exams, did everything I could medically to ensure early detection. Then I blotted it out. I figured I'd deal with it when and if I had to.

When I was first diagnosed and my surgeon recommended a re-excision and radiation, I happily went along with it. For those of you unfamiliar with the term, re-excision is a lumpectomy involving cells too small to be called a lump. My doctor predicted a high cure rate with this plan, and I had total faith in her. The following year, when cancerous cells were found in the other breast, she recommended mastectomy. Given that both of my breasts had now proved to be cancer-prone, I was content to get them gone.

My husband was more torn. Not long ago, when I asked him about this, he confessed that the idea of mastectomy had initially frightened him. I'd sensed that at the time, based on his repeated urgings that I not rush to a decision. But he hadn't been living with the specter of cancer all the many years that I had. Once he realized how much it meant to me to deal with it once and for all, he never looked back. He has been totally supportive, has never shied away from looking at my new breasts. If he finds them any less attractive than the old ones, he's never let on. And let's be honest, girls. Some things men simply can't hide.

No, I don't regret my decision to have the mastectomy. My only regret is that I didn't have it done the first year. This would have saved me the six weeks of radiation then, not to mention the struggle with reconstruction that came from trying to stretch my radiated tissue a year later. But we're all brilliant in hindsight. The truth is that I wasn't ready for a mastectomy that first year. If I'd done it then, I would have always wondered if it had been necessary. The bottom line here? I did what was right for me at the time.

That is what you all have to do. What was right for me isn't necessarily right for you. If you've just had a single mastectomy, you may want to skip the section on doubles. You've already made your decision; the surgery is done; second-guessing it won't accomplish a thing except make you a nervous Nellie.

UPLIFT looks at the positive side of losing a breast—but make no mistake. Surgery isn't fun. No one wants to have a mastectomy. No matter how you look at it, the procedure is barbaric. And I do miss my breasts. I miss the look of them, particularly in summer when women wear tank tops that show the gentlest curve of a breast. I miss them at night. They were sexual beings.

That said, I wouldn't want them back. They were lumpy. They were sore. They caused me worry for a long, long time, not to mention an increased insurance premium when the term "fibro-cystic disease" popped up. Then came cancer. I'd say that losing my breasts is a small price to pay for another forty years of life. Of course, I may rethink that in thirty years when my joints are stiff, my back is bent, and my daily worries center on constipation . . .

THE DIRTY DEED

"Amazon women used to remove a breast in order to shoot their arrows with better accuracy. I nursed all three of my sons and at 47 didn't need to have breasts any more."

Jane Royal-Davidson; diagnosed in 1996 at age 47;
educator; North Carolina

"My surgery was to be on November 7th—my birthday and my son David's birthday. I was turning forty-six, and he was turning eighteen. I said to him, 'I am so sorry that my operation is on our birthday.' His response was, 'Mom, I'm glad your surgery is going to be on our birthday. This is not a leg, or an arm or an eye. It is a breast. And, Mom, think of this as a rebirth. Because it *is* our birthday.' "

Jeryl Abelmann; diagnosed in 1986 at age 46;
elementary school teacher; California

"When my husband hugged me, I told him I was frightened. I shed a few tears. The image of how my breast would look after the surgery hit me. Charles reassured me that he would love me regardless of how it looked. When I apologized for crying, he said he was glad to see me finally acting 'normal' about the situation."

Sandy Williams; diagnosed in 1999 at age 51;
children's public services librarian; Texas

"As I prepared for my surgery I drew images of one-breasted women. Now why do they all tend to be warriors? I am a Sagittarian, and a mythical figure that has always held high significance for me is Chiron the centaur, the wounded healer. The version I created was Christon, a one-breasted female centaur, drawing back her bow unimpeded across the flattened right side of her chest. Yes, I've probably finally lost it, but paradoxically, along with the fear and sheer disbelief that I am actually about to have a breast cut off, I am feeling more free, and more truly myself than I have for a long time!"

Christine McNamara; diagnosed in 2000 at age 54;
retired physician; Florida

"The morning after my surgery, I was determined to be normal even though I could barely lift my arm. I put makeup on—the doctors were not going to see a sick woman when they came into my room. I think the surgeon and oncologist were very surprised!"

Marianne Rennie; diagnosed in 1988 at age 39;
cancer information specialist; Ohio

"There was a cleaning strike at the hospital, and my bathroom was filthy. So right after my surgery I cleaned the bathroom with my right arm, holding the IV pole!"

Aileen Pandapas; diagnosed in 1989 at age 41;
mom, volunteer, former secretary; Virginia

"The day after my mastectomy, I was taken to the rehab room to begin reactivating the muscles affected by the surgery under my arm for lymph node tests. During the wheelchair ride down several floors, I drooped and felt sorry for myself—an amputee without the strength to walk down the hall by herself. Did I ever get yanked back to reality fast! An eighteen-year-old boy learning to walk with a wooden leg was supporting himself on the bars and falling again and again. An older man was learning to walk with two wooden legs while his anguished wife watched his stumbling attempts. A multiple sclerosis victim was trying to activate dying muscles. It hurt a little as I walked my fingers up the wall, but at least I didn't need to learn how to navigate without a vital appendage. After all, I had nursed my three children. These breasts had fulfilled their purpose."

Lorraine J. Pakkala-Lintala; diagnosed in 1992 at age 62;
editor, author; Florida, New York

CLOTHES, PILLOWS, AND BRAS . . .

"The daughter of a breast cancer survivor gave me a button-front nightshirt to wear in the hospital. The morning after my surgery, I washed up and put on this bright nightshirt. I felt feminine again. The button-front allowed me to deal with the drains."

Sheila Levine; diagnosed in 1992 at age 43;
teacher; Maryland

"My favorite piece of clothing right after surgery was my husband's tee-shirt. It was so comfortable."

Barbara C. Sumner; diagnosed in 1982 at age 59;
homemaker; New Hampshire

"I had a bilateral mastectomy and felt like I was a tangle of drains and tubing. I found that the easiest way to deal with the drains was to string all of them on a long shoelace and tie it around my waist."

Linda Dyer; diagnosed in 1993 at age 40;
magazine editor; New Jersey

"I bought some large button-front men's shirts to wear after my surgery. They were comfortable and easy to get in and out of."

Val Long; diagnosed in 1999 at age 47;
administrative assistant; Massachusetts

"Because I had mobility problems with my arm, I was overanxious to succeed in putting on a tee-shirt. Well, I did it . . . but then I couldn't get it off! I live alone. I ended up wearing the tee-shirt for a few days."

Judith Ormond; diagnosed in 1996 at age 49;
symphony musician—piccolo; Wisconsin

"What really helped after surgery was a foam wedge. I had a double mastectomy, reconstruction, and a hysterectomy all in one surgery. So it wasn't easy to lie flat in bed. The foam wedge can be turned several ways to allow for easier positioning and more comfortable sleeping. I had also purchased three house dresses that had snaps in the front, top to bottom. They were easy to get in and out of, and were washable."

Gwen Loverink; diagnosed in 1994 at age 34;
police dispatcher; California

"My mother made me a small pillow to put between my arm and rib cage for the days following my surgery. It made sleeping more comfortable. I was warmed by this loving gift, and have passed it, and other pillows, along to friends facing breast surgery."

Marcia Gibbons; diagnosed in 1991 at age 52;
artist; Maine

"I had massages before surgery and resumed as soon after as I could. There are massage therapists trained to work with cancer patients."

Anne Jacobs; diagnosed in 1999 at age 62;
managing partner, real estate; Massachusetts

"I applied a form of aloe vera gel (available at health food stores) to the incision every day. There were no puckers, red marks, or problems at all."

Lorraine J. Pakkala-Lintala; diagnosed in 1992 at age 62;
editor, author; Florida, New York

"I didn't undress in front of anyone, and even with my husband it took me six months. He was fine with it, but I wasn't. It's good for new patients to know that the scar fades and diminishes an awful lot from the original look."

Irene Louise; diagnosed in 1995 at age 41;
retired executive secretary; Pennsylvania

"My husband rigged up 'training equipment' for me. It was a clothesline and pulley over a clothes rod, so I could pull my arm up and exercise the arm muscles. It was in a walk-in closet. That closet became my sanctuary—a good place to hide, cry, and curse."

Earlene Smith; diagnosed in 1985 at age 52;
part-time postal worker; New Hampshire

"After eight weeks post-op of not being able to raise my arms much, I went to physical therapy. I have four children, and I needed to be able to do things. Over the next month, I regained ninety-eight percent of my presurgery movement. However, when I got the green flag to drive, I was intimidated. I found that using a flat, square pillow between my body and the seat belt gave me a real security boost. I got a lot of funny looks from other drivers, but it was worth the independence I gained."

Linda Caradec; diagnosed in 1999 at age 41;
microbiologist; Texas

"When my daughter arrived to take me home after my mastectomy, I made a bizarre joke about my double-breasted coat being useless now. She took in the situation in an instant. 'Welcome to reality,' she said. 'Shelly (her sister) and I have had to stuff our bras since we were twelve.' Whipping the curtain around us, she yanked tissues from the box and started stuffing my empty bra cup. In no time she had constructed a size 38B. I was in awe at her expertise. 'I've had lots of practice,' she said smugly, and we went home."

Lorraine J. Pakkala-Lintala; diagnosed in 1992 at age 62;
editor, author; Florida, New York

"When I had my surgery twenty years ago, I remember being afraid to look at my incision. Also, I wore a bra stuffed with Kleenex for *months* until the school nurse told me of a special store where I could be fitted for a prosthesis. If she hadn't suggested it, I'd probably still be using Kleenex!"

Hope Cruickshank; diagnosed in 1975 at age 54;
retired secretary; Massachusetts

"The best purchase I made after my mastectomy was a good breast prosthesis. When I received my new breast form and walked out of the shop, I felt complete. My daughter said that I'd been going around with my head down and would not look at people. Wearing the new breast form, I held my head high. I knew that I looked like everyone else, and I felt in balance again. No one had told me that I would feel *out* of balance after having one breast removed, but I did. I didn't realize how much until I got my prosthesis and the problem was solved."

A survivor; diagnosed in 2000 at age 50;
teacher's aide; Illinois

"Being fitted for a prosthesis was quite interesting. The fitter explained that there are over five shapes of breasts. She found my shape, size, and a corset-looking bra, and made me put it on then and there. The fit was perfect, a perfect three-pound balance. When I got dressed and left the fitting room, my daughters couldn't tell which was the new breast. We went out to a very fancy restaurant to celebrate. Later, I found the 18-Hour Bra much more comfortable than the more expensive medical one."

Lorraine J. Pakkala-Lintala; diagnosed in 1992 at age 62;
editor, author; Florida, New York

"I refused to let the surgery get in my way. So six days after I got home, my friend and I went to the mall to buy some pretty night-gowns. Though I couldn't stand up straight, the fresh air felt wonderful, and I proved to myself that I could do it. Seven weeks after the surgery, I played golf. Hey, I could do that, too, and my right arm worked!"

E. Mary Lou Clauss; diagnosed in 1991 at age 55; homemaker, retired registered nurse; Pennsylvania

"During my rehab, I thought I would never be able to use my left arm again. Well, let me tell you, that left arm is now used for car-rying around five grandchildren and for swinging a golf club."

Joanne Bellontine; diagnosed in 1982 at age 39; consultant, recruiter; New York

"For five years following my mastectomy (without reconstruction), I had some pain or discomfort with my bras. Several months ago, the pain specialist at my family doctor's office suggested I try a sports bra. I went to the dealer where I purchased my mastectomy bra and found that they did not have a sports bra to offer. So I went to Kmart and purchased one there. At first, I pinned the prosthe-sis to the bra, since there was no pocket for it. Then one day I for-got to pin it in, and I was surprised at the end of the day to find that it had stayed in place all day with no problem. I love the sports bras. I no longer have any pain or discomfort, the strap is out of the trench on my shoulder, and the sports bras are not expensive."

Margaret Leggett; diagnosed in 1995 at age 58; retired personnel technician; Florida

"In 1985, I had a mastectomy. As I began to heal I knew it was time to buy a prosthesis, but I kept procrastinating, pretending I was too busy with the approaching holiday season. I found a comfortable blouse with a right-hand pocket where I could stuff Kleenex, so I bought half a dozen in various colors. I wore them to work with loose jackets to camouflage my lopsided figure. My husband, Ted, had been especially supportive throughout the preceding months, combining loving tenderness with pragmatism, but I felt his attention was waning. One Saturday he said, 'Come on, we're going shopping. No questions or excuses!' He drove to the poshest section of Coral Gables, parked on Miracle Mile, and escorted me into an exclusive lingerie salon. Stylish suburban women were trying on sheer negligees and lacy underthings. I felt like a fish in a bicycle shop. Then Ted asked for someone by name, and I realized he had called ahead for an appointment. A lady showed me into a private dressing room and fitted me for my prosthesis and mastectomy bras. She couldn't have been kinder or more professional. I joined Ted at the cash register as she brought my purchases— in a plain white box—from the back room. 'Gift wrap them, please,' Ted said, getting out his credit card. In front of the store, he handed me the gaily wrapped package, gave me a deep kiss, and winked. 'Merry Christmas!' Now, even after years of enjoying my reconstructed bustline, I still remember one of my cherished gifts."

Nancy Sena; diagnosed in 1985 at age 46;
retired counselor; Florida

ALL IN THE FAMILY

"My fifteen-year-old daughter's response to my approaching mastectomy? 'So you'll be uni-boobed!' "

Mindy Greenside; diagnosed in 2000 at age 48;
midwife; Maryland

"My husband emptied and measured the drain tubes when I got home from the hospital. He was there for me all the time."

Rebecca Clarkson; diagnosed in 1997 at age 45;
trucking; Utah

"My grandmother was an amazing lady. At the age of 89, she had a double mastectomy. Less than two hours after the surgery, she was out of recovery and being wheeled into her room. She immediately began giving orders. 'My teeth are in that drawer—I need them,' 'Where is the telephone—I want to call my friend Jenny to tell her that the food at this hospital is better than the food at her hospital.' She recovered quickly and came home several days later. I went with her to be fitted for her prostheses. She had always been a very large breasted woman, and she now chose a smaller size. Once they arrived in the mail, she wore them all the time. She said that if she had known they would look so much better, she would have done this years ago!"

Marianne McCaskill;
granddaughter of Anita Lundberg; California

"I quickly lost my self-consciousness about undressing in front of others, because my husband and my neighbor changed my bandages. They stood there gazing and talking about how good it looked, and this was good for me, because I hadn't been afraid of the word 'cancer.' I had feared how my husband would accept my disfigurement. I should have known better, as he loved me, not only my breast. He was my rock. He never let me think about losing a breast, just about beating the odds."

Jacqueline Durant; diagnosed in 1994 at age 68;
retired; Massachusetts

"My husband was wonderful. His sense of humor helped me tremendously. He frequently hid my prosthesis or walked around with it on his prematurely balding head. He made it comfortable for all six of the children to look at the prosthesis, feel it, and look at me without it. He was so wonderful with my body that I never felt less of a woman. We were both so grateful that I was alive, that losing a breast was not devastating."

Cornelia Doherty; diagnosed in 1985 at age 45;
mother, widow, speaker; Massachusetts

"To all women who are single or divorced and have had breast cancer, do not be afraid. You are not just a breast. You are a beautiful woman and will find a loving man who will love you for you. Real men don't care about your scars. Everyone has baggage."

Miriam Cooper; diagnosed in 1982 at age 36;
housewife, mother, volunteer, real estate agent; New Jersey

"Day after day following my mastectomy, I looked in the mirror and saw this disfigured woman, and I became depressed. My husband, noting the change in me, asked what was wrong. When I told him how I felt about myself, he took me in his arms and said, 'I didn't marry you thirty years ago because you had two breasts. I married you because I loved you, and I will love you till the day I die, whether you have one breast or none.' This was what I needed to hear to become a whole person once again."

Frances Meadow; diagnosed in 1973 at age 50;
retired business owner; Florida

"Neither my husband nor I misses my breasts. We considered it a good trade for survival and peace of mind."

Wanda Null; diagnosed in 1986 at age 41;
librarian; Massachusetts

"My husband has been wonderful. He says he doesn't even see the scars that go across my breasts. They are there and probably always will be, but he is just grateful I am here to help raise our children."

Tresa Johnson; diagnosed in 1999 at age 23;
executive secretary; Oklahoma

"From the day of my diagnosis, I vowed that I would take each step to survival one step at a time. After each step comes a big reward. I try to think of fun things I can do with my husband that remind us we have so much more living to do. Just five days after my lumpectomy, we took a trip to London for a week. It was the best thing we could have done! Although I was recovering from surgery and was a little sore being bounced around in London cabs, I was living life! After chemo, there will be another trip before radiation. Having this to look forward to really helps."

Helen Lawlor; diagnosed in 2000 at age 43;
medical communications; New York

SWEET SINGLE

"After the operation, I was able to make fun of myself, such as telling my brother that I went in for a breast reduction, and they made a mistake and took it all!"

Jacqueline Durant; diagnosed in 1994 at age 68;
retired; Massachusetts

"I was determined that if I was going to give up a breast, I was going to get something out of it. So, not only did I ask my plastic surgeon to make my other breast match the new one, I asked her to fix my earlobes, so that I could wear pierced earrings again!"

Rosamary Amiet; diagnosed in 2000 at age 48;
program manager; Ohio

"My boyfriend was with me when the doctor told me I had breast cancer. He said that all he heard was, 'It's curable,' and that was enough for him. I sometimes talk about my different breast in front of others, and he says, 'Doesn't bother me. I always preferred the other one, anyway.' "

Sharon Daniels; diagnosed in 2000 at age 49;
hairstylist, wig store owner; Massachusetts

"I don't care if other women see me undressing at the Y with only one breast. I'm just thankful to be alive!"

Billie Loop; diagnosed in 1997 at age 63;
housewife; Missouri

"To destroy a bosom is a form of mental rape.
Were I younger and had life ahead
I would resent the need that made it necessary
To invade my person.
However, cancer forces reality.
Medical skill keeps me alive.
My gratitude bows to surgeons.
Forgiveness is my pride."

Barbara M. Wells; diagnosed in 1999 at age 78;
mother, writer; New Hampshire

"This is for anyone who is contemplating having reconstruction surgery after a mastectomy. As the Nike ad says, 'Just Do It!' Before my surgery, I didn't take the time to consider reconstruction. For two and one-half years, I wore a special bra with my prosthesis, and I knew that many women were doing the same thing. But eventually the idea of replacing my 'flat' side with a 'bump' began to appeal to me more and more. I was only in my early fifties, and had decided that there was no reason why I would not live a normal life span. So I had an implant inserted and later had a nipple areola reconstruction. After my experience, I would recommend reconstruction for anyone who may be wondering if it is worth the surgery. Vanity is not the issue here, but there is nothing like being able to dress without special 'equipment.' Life continues to be better and better each day!"

Gail Blackmer; diagnosed in 1997 at age 50;
paraprofessional, teacher's aide; Florida

"The upside to having reconstructive surgery is that your breast will never sag!"

Debby Whittet; diagnosed in 1996 at age 43;
household technician, part-time library worker; Michigan

"I waited eighteen months before I had the courage to go for reconstructive surgery, and then I had a tissue flap reconstruction. It was a rough operation, worse actually than the mastectomy, but well worth it. I feel much better than when I was wearing a prosthesis. And I got a tummy tuck in the process!"

Rebecca Clarkson; diagnosed in 1997 at age 45;
trucking; Utah

"I decided to have reconstruction for balance. I only had one breast removed and didn't want to be lopsided. I thought briefly about a prosthesis, but decided I wanted something more permanent. I had this vision of coming home from vacation having left it in the room. I imagined having to call the hotel and ask if anyone had found a breast in room 123."

Val Long; diagnosed in 1999 at age 47;
administrative assistant; Massachusetts

"It really helped for me to go into the hospital with two breasts and come home with two breasts. I had reconstruction that used my own muscle and tissue. I'm very happy with the results. My breast looks normal again, and this makes me feel complete."

Gwen Loverink; diagnosed in 1994 at age 34;
police dispatcher; California

"When I was diagnosed with breast cancer, I did not panic. I simply made up my mind to do everything I could to beat it. I had a mastectomy and reconstruction, and this made me feel whole again. It has been more than two years now, and I am healthy and happy."

Ann Gordon; diagnosed in 1998 at age 73;
retired business executive; Florida

TWO'S A COUPLE

"Both of my breasts had been cystic, and I'd had questionable lumps removed from both over many years. So it made sense to me to stop living with the emotional roller coaster and have both breasts removed in a single surgery. It is a wonderful feeling to be finished with that part of my life."

Carol Hattler; diagnosed in 1999 at age 65;
retired nurse; Virginia

"Waiting for breast cancer to arrive provided me with the opportunity over many years to decide what I would do about it. My sister Adelaide was diagnosed with breast cancer twenty years before I was, and my sister Elizabeth two years before I was. Although I only had cancer in one breast, I had both removed. Being pragmatic, I never liked wearing a bra, and I couldn't imagine always being unbalanced. Now I can run like I did when I was ten years old."

Cleves Daniels Weber; diagnosed in 1999 at age 60;
owner, metaphysical bookstore; Hawaii

"I was diagnosed at 35. I was fortunate enough to have doctors who caught the disease early, but when it came to treatment, I told them I wanted a double mastectomy. I had been packing a 44DD for most of my life, and being free of the cancer seemed to be a good trade-off. I walked around the month after my surgery wearing a tee-shirt, and I felt like a little kid. I wouldn't say that I have been worry free, especially being in my late 30s and dealing with my boyfriend, but guess what? We are both appreciative of the fact that I am here."

Marian Anne Miziorko; diagnosed in 1995 at age 35;
tax assessor; Pennsylvania

"When it came to reconstruction, I only went for a small bulge so that I wouldn't be so flat. Now, when I look at my chest, I think that I look like a female athlete. I do not miss my old lopsided breasts, and I love not having to wear bras. I feel alive and more feminine. I feel free!"

Carol Hattler; diagnosed in 1999 at age 65;
retired nurse; Virginia

"Twelve years ago, I had breast cancer in both breasts. I had reconstruction and loved it. I had always been a D-cup, so surgery was my salvation—getting rid of those *big* breasts!"

Mary Ann Lee; diagnosed in 1988 at age 46;
tax collector; North Carolina

"I have to say that with everything I went through, I did get beautiful breasts."

Tobi Stelzer; diagnosed in 1997 at age 40;
teacher; New Jersey

"The first time I saw my sister-in-law after her reconstructive surgery (after a double mastectomy at the age of 27), I found I was trying very hard not to glance down at her chest. But finally, I couldn't contain myself any longer and admitted this ... to which Barbra replied, 'Here,' as she proudly opened her jacket to reveal a tight sweater through which I could see the shape of her breasts. 'They're great, aren't they?' And I have to admit, they *were* great!"

Wendy Page;
sister-in-law of Barbra Marcus Kolton

"The thing that helped me get over being self-conscious was having reconstruction. It was a big boost to my morale. After it was completed, I went to Victoria's Secret and bought a sexy bra, garter belt, and hose. I wore them for my husband on our twenty-fifth wedding anniversary."

Polly Briggs; diagnosed in 1987 at age 41;
secretary; Mississippi

"The upside of my reconstruction was that after years of suffering gravity's pull, I could now go without a bra."

Barbara Moro; diagnosed in 1999 at age 57;
law secretary; New Jersey

WHO NEEDS BREASTS!

"For those who may wonder whether everyone has reconstruction, I did not, and I have never regretted it. I still feel feminine and sexy. Occasionally I may mention to my husband that perhaps I should have at least thought about reconstruction, and he responds, 'Why?' For several years I would look in the mirror after bathing and wonder when the scar and/or the absence of a breast would bother me. In nine years it never has. The only thing the scar does is remind me how lucky I am."

Jane Vaughan; diagnosed in 1991 at age 53;
writer; Texas

"I was diagnosed in 1993 and had a modified radical mastectomy. After two and a half years, I brought closure to my yearning for reconstruction by deciding against it and, instead, getting a tattoo etched on my mastectomy side. It is a very tasteful scene of a rufus-back hummingbird sipping nectar from a rose-vine type of plant, and a monarch butterfly is hovering close by. I've been able to display my tattoo to a diverse audience, and it has proven therapeutic for the viewer as well as for myself."

Kathy Kirkley; diagnosed in 1993 at age 40;

registered nurse, emergency nurse, mother, wife; Montana

"I don't have any breasts, and I don't care. I don't have to wear a bra, and I can jog without pain. I know that people love me for what's on the inside, not for my physical appearance."

Cindy Bird; diagnosed in 1998 at age 39;

human resources generalist; Colorado

"I have a very positive outlook in life. So when all the bandages were taken off, I said, 'Sue, be strong with the help of God. When you look into the mirror, you now have one smiley and one hung low, but you are alive.' "

Suzanne Almond; diagnosed in 1996 at age 60;

secretary to the Special Services Director; New Hampshire

"Not long after my surgery, my partner and I attended a women's retreat. During the course of the weekend, many women took their clothes off and jumped into the swimming pool. Of all the different body shapes, I noticed two women, one who had a single mastectomy and the other a bilateral. And there I stood trying to muster enough courage to do the same. I was waiting for the sun to disappear or some act of Mother Nature that would force all these women out of the pool. Heather was already in the pool waiting for me. Slowly, I undressed and entered the pool. Within minutes the tears started to roll down my cheeks. No one stared, no one turned away so as not to see my bare chest. It was okay even without a couple of body parts."

Carol Snyder; diagnosed in 1992 at age 47;

special education teacher; New York

"I had several male friends, co-workers, who were so supportive that it brought tears to my eyes. One even went to counseling so that he could help me. He was very comfortable discussing anything and everything, a true and rare friend. Thus far, the men I've told about my mastectomy have shrugged, telling me that I'm more than the sum of one body part. Frankly, I'm surprised, given how our society places an enormous value on breasts. But I'm not complaining. Perhaps our men are enlightened somewhat after all."

Marti Devich; diagnosed in 1980 at age 34;
sales, business owner, writer; Minnesota

". . . Mastectomy.
What a horrible word.
An ending—the removal of something so essential to
    womanhood.
But is it?
No, I think not.
Womanhood stems from our hearts and minds.
If necessary, I would sacrifice my breast to preserve my life."

Mary Platt; diagnosed in 1998 at age 47;
radiology supervisor; South Carolina

3 • Radiation

Soaking Up the Rays

W hen I learned that my treatment plan called for thirty sessions of radiation—five sessions a week for six weeks—I was dismayed. This would mean driving forty-five minutes each way, to the hospital and back, every day. Forget cancer; Boston traffic is stressful to me in and of itself. Besides, I was in the middle of writing a book, which typically requires my uninterrupted concentration from eight in the morning until six at night. Radiation would take a two-hour chunk out of that time, day after day.

How to turn that into a plus? I could request an early morning or late afternoon session, but those slots were in high demand by women who held jobs with less flexible hours than mine. I had the luxury of being my own boss. Taking that in its broadest sense, I simply shifted my thinking.

I planned my sessions for two in the afternoon. I worked at my computer until I had to leave for Boston, then used the driving time not to stress about traffic or cancer but to mull over what I'd written, speak changes into a mini-recorder, and plot out what I would write when I got home. Know what? There wasn't the slightest blip in my productivity during that entire six-week span.

With a few exceptions when my sons were home on vacation and drove me in, or when my husband met me at the hospital, or when a friend insisted on coming, I went to radiation alone. Just like finishing up on the weight machine after getting the phone call that said I had *it*, this meant a lot to me. I've always been independent—have always hated imposing on people. Driving myself to daily treatments was consistent with this, particularly since the radiation itself took no time at all. My being the driver was also another reminder to myself, and to my husband, my sons, and the few friends who knew, that I was healthy, strong, and as good as ever.

Having experienced radiation, I felt particularly strongly about the need for a chapter on it in *UPLIFT*. When I was told not to use deodorant, for example, I had no idea what to use in its place. The doctors shrugged, as did the radiation techs. They didn't know. But the sisterhood does. The little section on deodorant gives a handful of different options from women who have personally tried each one out.

Various submissions gave various reasons why traditional deodorants are banned during radiation. After reading one explanation too many, I sent a frantic e-mail to a friend whose husband is a radiation oncologist. As he explained it, the high density of trace metals in traditional deodorants can sensitize the skin, making it more likely to get irritated and even burned. Doctors believe that these metals seep into the skin so that they cannot be completely washed off before daily treatments. Hence, the ban.

A final word, while I have your attention. Tattoos. Typically, these are applied during the planning session before the start of radiation. They take seconds to apply and hurt only as much as an elastic band might if it were snapped against the skin. I won't explain their purpose, since Deb Haney has explained it so well in the section on tattoos. Suffice it to say that most women don't mind them at all, which I think is the best way to be. They aren't obtrusive. As many women point out, they are a badge of courage—a reminder that you've had something and been cured. In that, they serve a positive purpose.

I wish I could be as accepting as these women. But I'm not.

Oh, getting those tattoos was a piece of cake—though I have to say that I hadn't realized, until mere minutes before mine were applied, that they were part of the process. No one had told me that, and I was irked. But there were two other things that bothered me more.

First, I had always wanted a tattoo but hadn't had the courage to get one. Nice girls didn't do that, or so the story went; classy women didn't do it either. But suddenly it seemed unfair that I didn't have the tattoo I wanted, while I *did* have ones that I *didn't* want.

Second, one of the seven little blue dots that had been permanently inked into my skin was smack in the middle of my chest. I only had to wear a gently scooped-neck shirt, and there it was, like the mark of Cain. Please know that I wasn't embarrassed to have people see it—and even if I was, no one ever noticed mine, and I do wear my share of scooped-neck shirts. That dot might have easily passed as a birthmark. It was truly tiny.

The problem was me. I was dealing with breast cancer by doing everything medically that I could while keeping the rest of my life the same as ever—but there it was, that tattoo, staring back at me in the mirror every day, reminding me of what I'd had.

But I knew what I'd had—"had" being the operative word. The cancer was gone; I wanted the tattoo gone, too. It had served its purpose. I didn't see why I needed to keep it.

So I acted. First, I made an appointment at a laser center that advertised tattoo removal. It turned out that the removal of those tiny blue dots took mere seconds each. When I pulled out my wallet to pay, the doctor said, "No charge. You didn't ask for those tattoos. You shouldn't have to pay to have them removed."

Second, I got my own tattoo—one that I wanted—one that I see in the mirror every day and have never yet regretted. Nope. I'm not telling what it is or where, only that it brings great pleasure to my husband and me.

MAKING IT EASIER

"Different family members and friends went with me for my radiation treatments. We always went out for breakfast afterward."

Sharon Erbe; diagnosed in 1999 at age 54;
nurse educator; New York

"For my first radiation treatments, I had to travel two hundred miles each day. We lived in a rural area in southeast Missouri, and our friends and neighbors got together without my knowledge and scheduled one of them to drive me each day so that my husband could continue to work. I never knew who would drive up to take me until whoever it was arrived."

Kathleen Griffith; diagnosed in 1976 at age 42;
bookkeeper; Arizona

"I continued to work during my treatments, but I took off every Friday, when I had either treatment or blood testing. When it came time for radiation, I shortened my workday so that I could have treatment and be home before the kids got off the bus."

Deborah J.P. Schur; diagnosed in 1994 at age 43;
sales rep; Massachusetts

"Each day that I went for a treatment, there was a small anonymous gift waiting for me at my place at the kitchen table. The gifts were placed after I retired at night, and before I arose at 6 A.M. After about 3 weeks, I realized that there was a let-down feeling on Saturdays and Sundays because there was no gift. These were really little things like a fancy pencil or a small notebook, but they lifted my spirits. It was not until after all the treatments that I was told that one daughter had the idea and started the 'gift bag' to have something for another daughter to put out each night."

Lela Quimby; diagnosed in 1985 at age 56;
retired teacher; California

"I love lattes and looked forward to the treat every day after radiation."

Marge Fuller; diagnosed in 1994 at age 63;
Yakima school district, retired; Washington

"During radiation, I visualized myself on a beach under the healing light of the sun. I felt strength moving through me. My treatments were done in February. My family held an *indoor beach party* to celebrate."

Sharon Erbe; diagnosed in 1999 at age 54;
nurse educator; New York

"In the midst of radiation, my wonderful husband, who is my rock, kidnapped me one Friday and took me to a hotel for a romantic weekend away just for us. It helped me to remember that I am a woman who is loved."

Nancie Watson; diagnosed in 1995 at age 50;
social worker; Pennsylvania

TATTOOS

"The reason you get tattooed is that, with permanent marks to align the machines on, they can radiate the exact same area each day. But I had never heard about the tattoos before radiation, and my mind raced off in all directions. I pictured myself with a HUGE BLACK domino shape tattooed on one side of my chest— big round black dots that would be with me forever, like giant cards out of Alice in Wonderland or a funky biker tattoo. My fear stayed with me until the day I went in for orientation and tattooing at the radiation center. Much to my relief, the technician was a sensitive young girl, and the tattoos she made were no larger than tiny pinpricks."

Deb Haney; diagnosed in 1996 at age 48;
administrative assistant, artist; Massachusetts

"I had always said that when I turned forty, I would get a tattoo, but I chickened out. Well, hey, I did get my tattoos. I thought it was kind of neat."

Dee Pobjoy; diagnosed in 1999 at age 41;
sales clerk; Wisconsin

"I recently read of some women who want to get their radiation tattoos removed. I say, 'no way!' These are a symbol of all I've been through and have overcome."

Fran Hegarty; diagnosed in 2000 at age 47;
librarian; Massachusetts

"I hate my tattoos. I notice them every day, and they remind me that I have had breast cancer. But they also remind me that I am very lucky and I am a survivor."

Suzanne Pollock; diagnosed in 1995 at age 50;
stationer; North Carolina

"What to do with my tattoos? I have three down the center of my chest. My friend says I should make the top one into a dolphin diving down into my breast."

Pam Waddell; diagnosed in 1998 at age 38;
writer, teacher's aide; Texas

"I consider my tattoos badges of honor. I have survived. No one has ever asked me what they are—but should anyone ever do that, I would ask if they have had a mammogram this year."

Nancie Watson; diagnosed in 1995 at age 50;
social worker; Pennsylvania

"I have a suggestion. Instead of the black tattoo dots, why not use a small rose or a butterfly? At least then people wouldn't think you had a spot of dirt on your neck."

Kathleen Griffith; diagnosed in 1976 at age 42;
bookkeeper; Arizona

"My radiation oncologist didn't use tattoos. Instead, I got marked up daily with a purple marker. On my days off from therapy, I had to be careful not to wash off the marks or smear them off with the skin creams I used to condition my skin. I ended up wearing a man's tee-shirt under my clothing to protect it from being ruined."

Sharon Irons Strempski; diagnosed in 1997 at age 52;
registered nurse; Connecticut

"I bought inexpensive sports bras without underwires for radiation. The indelible ink that they use to mark your tattoos ruins good bras, and, at the end, when your skin is sore, the lack of underwires helped. I still wear bras without underwires."

Suzanne Pollock; diagnosed in 1995 at age 50;
stationer; North Carolina

"I brought black bras and a camisole, so that marks painted on me for radiation would not destroy good clothes."

Pauline Hughes; diagnosed in 1997 at age 61;
retired registered nurse; Florida

NUTS AND BOLTS

"Usually, as I would lie in the radiation room, watching the lights of the radiation equipment, I was visualizing a good sparkling 'rain' coming into my body, washing its way through, with the 'bad' cells flowing out through my feet and far, far away. Visualization will speed up the healing, removing the stress of the moment and bringing you peace!"

Deb Haney; diagnosed in 1996 at age 48;
administrative assistant, artist; Massachusetts

"Early in radiation, the sound of the machine released the floodgate of fear I was trying to sit on. Knowing I could not get through the radiation crying, I began talking to friends who were not there . . . or singing. These sounds diverted my thoughts and enabled me to put the sound of the radiation machine in the background."

Jeanne Sturdevant; diagnosed in 1990 at age 45;
artist; Texas

"Radiation is tiring. When I asked why, I was told that since the treatment was killing cells, the good cells have to work overtime. That makes sense to me."

Sharon Daniels; diagnosed in 2000 at age 49;
hairstylist, wig store owner; Massachusetts

"While I was taking radiation, a friend of mine suggested having a glass of red wine once a day to keep my blood up. It was wonderful and worked beautifully. Also, a small glass of sherry about one half hour before meals helped the appetite."

Barbara C. Sumner; diagnosed in 1982 at age 59;
homemaker; New Hampshire

"Talking and opening up to others in the radiation waiting room was very important. I made a fast friend there. We all felt pain for one woman who resisted passing the time of day with anyone. Holding completely back is so harmful. Everyone needs the concern and compassion of those who are going through what they are."

Sheila Roper; diagnosed in 1995 at age 57;
homemaker; New Hampshire

DEODORANT

"I put pure cornstarch in a beautiful shaker (for powdered sugar really) and used that for deodorant under the affected arm."

Suzanne Pollock; diagnosed in 1995 at age 50;
stationer; North Carolina

"My mother's radiologist recommended that she use Tom's of Maine deodorant and unscented Dove soap while she was undergoing radiation treatments."

Barbara Keiler;
daughter of survivor; Massachusetts

"A good deodorant to use is Naturally Fresh Deodorant Crystal. It can be found in General Nutrition Stores."

Irene Louise; diagnosed in 1995 at age 41;
retired executive secretary; Pennsylvania

"My radiation doctor approved of a metal-free deodorant from Mennen. It's called Crystal Clean (Caribbean Cool) by Lady Speed Stick."

Lauren Nichols; diagnosed in 2000 at age 53;
writer; Pennsylvania

"When you need a deodorant that doesn't have aluminum in it, use Arm & Hammer with Baking Soda."

Jennie Isbell; diagnosed in 1999 at age 76;
housewife, retired; New York

"One deodorant to use that contains no aluminum salts is something I get at Walgreens called Crystal Stick, a 4.25-ounce stick of 100 percent natural mineral salts. You simply wet the stick and rub it on. On the container it says that it lasts over a year. Mine lasted more than three years—and yes, I do use deodorant every day."

Gracie Schwingel; diagnosed in 1998 at age 51;
secretary; Wisconsin

"During radiation, my doctor approved the use of Jason Aloe Vera Gel Natural Deodorant. I still use it to this day."

Linda Perkins; diagnosed in 1999 at age 35; project manager; New Jersey

"When you go for radiation, take a zip-lock bag with a moist washcloth and a shaker of pure cornstarch. Use them in the changing room after treatment."

Rayna Ragonetti; diagnosed in 1993 at age 52; executive; New York

"I was afraid of getting an infection in the arm where the few lymph nodes were removed. So I was very careful and did not shave my underarms or use deodorant for a while. I washed the area several times a day. When healed, I carefully shaved and used a baking soda–based deodorant."

Carol Hattler; diagnosed in 1999 at age 65; retired nurse; Virginia

TOO MUCH SUN . . .

"Lubriderm and one of those clear 100 percent aloe vera gels are very soothing for skin burnt from the radiation treatment."

Sharon Irons Strempski; diagnosed in 1997 at age 52; registered nurse; Connecticut

"I used liquid vitamin E on my skin to help the dryness."

Therese Gunty; diagnosed in 1997 at age 70; homemaker; Illinois

"When I was going through radiation, my aloe plant was my best friend. Every morning I broke off a leaf, put it in my little Tupperware container, and carried it to treatment. When I finished that day's treatment, I slit the leaf open and slathered it over the radiation site. Most of the health care professionals laughed, or at least tolerated this. They told me to wait until I had skin symptoms. My reply was, "When do you put sunscreen on . . . before you go out in the sun, or after you get a sunburn?" I am happy to report that I had no skin reaction at all! And, if you want to hear something spooky, after the plant had been used thirty-two times, just when my radiation was done, she stopped growing! Guess she figured her work was done! I have since given friends aloe plants when they undergo radiation treatment, and no one complains. I even passed along the Tupperware container to a friend when she was newly diagnosed, as apparently it had such good vibes."

Sheilah Musselman; diagnosed in 1997 at age 56; registered nurse; Virginia

"My radiation oncologist suggested that I use Bag Balm on my skin after radiation treatments. It really helped reduce the amount of burning and discomfort that I had. Bag Balm can be found in many pharmacies and farm stores. It is the same stuff that farmers use on cows' udders. It was a bit greasy, but it definitely did the trick!"

Gail Dorfman; diagnosed in 1995 at age 34; stay-at-home mom; Massachusetts

"One of my radiation techs recommended Carrington Gel. I put it on my breast immediately after treatment, usually before I left the table, and it was wonderful. It is clear and goes on with no friction, which is the best part when the skin is sensitive and red, and it dries within seconds. It soothes and cools, taking the heat out of the breast and helping to prevent burning. It must be purchased from a pharmacy but does not need a script. It isn't inexpensive—costs about $20 for a 4-ounce tube—but it is well worth it."

Nancie Watson; diagnosed in 1995 at age 50; social worker; Pennsylvania

"During my radiation, I used mild Dove soap. A week after my last treatment, I got really burned and peeled. I smothered 100 percent (clear) aloe on my breast and put a medical pad over it so it did not stick to my clothes. I also did the Domeboro soaks when I was able to. It cleared up in a week."

Candice Jaeger; diagnosed in 2000 at age 24;
wife, mother; Illinois

"I used Biafine cream for radiation burns. It's not a prescription and can be ordered from a pharmacy or direct from the distributor in Tampa, Florida. Unbelievable. In twenty-four hours, the skin was repairing itself."

Phyllis Jezequel; diagnosed in 1999 at age 66;
missionary—personnel; Florida

"My breast started to shrink! Fourteen months after my radiation was complete, my affected breast suddenly looked markedly smaller than the other one. I was sure that it would shrink to just a nipple! The truth is that it can take about that long for the fluid to be reabsorbed postoperatively. Yeah, that breast will be smaller . . . but I can live with it!"

Donna Barnett; diagnosed in 1999 at age 40;
registered nurse; California

"When I had radiation, I used pure aloe gel on the area that became burned. Because the area under my arm was sensitive and the edge of my bra rubbed it, I sewed a small piece of new blanket material over the offending edge. When the last few treatments zeroed in on the area around my nipple, where the cancer had been, I coated a square of gauze with petroleum jelly and placed it there after each treatment. That gave much relief."

Lela Quimby; diagnosed in 1985 at age 56;
retired teacher; California

COMFORT CLOTHES

"During radiation, when your skin is most sensitive, wear over-sized white cotton tee-shirts cut off at the waist, and cut the sleeves out. Then turn them inside out so the seams do not rub."

Caroline C. Hudnall; diagnosed in 1992 at age 55;
retired legal tech of the Supreme Court of Alaska; Montana

"I went to Victoria's Secret—but primarily because I could not wear a bra and had to have very soft cotton next to my skin. So I purchased matching cotton teddies and sexy panties. What a boost!"

Nancie Watson; diagnosed in 1995 at age 50;
social worker; Pennsylvania

"I wore soft clothes like polar fleece almost constantly. Also, treatment areas can be pretty frosty, so taking a soft shawl with you can be a comfort."

Christine Foutris; diagnosed in 1999 at age 49;
teacher; Illinois

"Buy soft cotton undershirts. This will help after the operation, since your skin will be sensitive, and it provides a place to attach drains."

Alexandra Koffman; diagnosed in 1997 at age 40;
registered nurse; Massachusetts

"Feel like a kid again. Wear cotton bras, no underwire during radiation. Wear baseball caps in bright colors and comical characters, such as Tweety Bird. I bought a wraparound shirt in a stretch material that I could wear during radiation treatments. This saved me time in undressing and dressing. I had very early morning appointments, then went directly to my office from the hospital."

Ellen Beth Simon; diagnosed in 1998 at age 41;
lawyer; New Jersey

"As for favorite clothing during treatment, I bought a two-piece velvet-velour lounge suit that is as comfortable as a pair of pajamas and elegant enough to entertain visitors. It is also very soft against my skin."

Carrie Drake; diagnosed in 1998 at age 42;
administrative assistant; Colorado

"During radiation, breast tissue can become very tender. A simple support garment can be made by using 'tube' material, which can be purchased at most yard goods stores. This material comes in a wide variety of colors. Measure enough material to reach just past your waist. Stitch ¼ inch of elastic to the top, zigzag-stitch the bottom to prevent the fabric from raveling, and this makes a most comfortable strapless bra that can be used by both large- and small-breasted women. It goes on easily, comes off easily, does not bind sensitive shoulders, and can be washed and dried using regular washing and drying cycles. It surely provides non-binding relief to sensitive skin areas."

Florence Wade; diagnosed in 1999 at age 63;
retired school teacher, retired property manager; Texas

STORIES

"When my doctor advised me to undergo radiation, I told him that I didn't want to. He told me that it would increase my survival rate, and still I said no. With this, he looked me straight in the eye and said, 'Then I'd advise you to go over to Chernobyl in the Ukraine and stand in the middle of the town with all that radioactive material that leaked from the reactor!' I burst out laughing at such a ridiculous picture. Then I decided that radiation wouldn't be so bad after all if I did it the American way. At another point, this same doctor snapped me out of a dark mood by saying, 'Brenda, you are going to die, but not from this.' That was in 1986."

Brenda M. Kraft; diagnosed in 1986 at age 60;
retired school teacher, New Hampshire

"When I learned that I would have thirty-five days of radiation, I wrote to the thirty-five most important women in my life and asked them to send tee-shirts in lieu of flowers. The shirts, I explained, would be helpful in eliminating the minutia in my life—like "Whatever shall I wear to radiation for thirty-five days?" Over sixty shirts arrived—some new, some old and familiar. I felt closer to these friends in their shirts, and they knew that they had done something for me that we would both remember. Someone else's cotton shirt against your skin brings them close to your heart."

Betsy Ellis Bowles; diagnosed in 2000 at age 57;
private mortgage banker; Massachusetts

"Sometimes I would lie there wondering how the radiation technicians felt, knowing they were helping people heal but also causing damage in the process. Since it was Christmas, I wanted to do something to lighten the atmosphere. So I got an art book from the library and copied a large photo of one of the beautiful Roman lady statues with her arm up over her head and her bare breast hanging out of her tunic—a pose that I and dozens of others assumed every day. I made a holiday card, almost like a small poster, that said, 'Happy Holidays—To a great gang to "hang out" with.' The next time I went in for treatment, it was hanging on the wall in the cubicle where the technicians stood!"

Deb Haney; diagnosed in 1996 at age 48;
administrative assistant, artist; Massachusetts

"What do we need from our caregivers and significant others? I needed to be heard in a holistic way. I needed my doctor to acknowledge my mental needs as well as my medical ones. My oncologist stood still and listened; it was an amazing gift."

Jeanne Sturdevant; diagnosed in 1990 at age 45;
artist; Texas

"I argued with the radiologist every time I had my yearly mammogram because they would charge full price, though I had only one breast. I tried different hospitals and clinics and found the same thing. I won my fight when one hospital finally sent me a letter saying that they would never again charge a patient with only one breast for a bilateral test. I always have my mammogram there now."

Earlene Smith; diagnosed in 1985 at age 52;
part-time postal worker; New Hampshire

"When my friend started her thirty-five radiation treatments, I made a big calendar, and we counted down the seven weeks. When it was done, we celebrated with a dinner. I sent her flowers with a card that read, 'Congratulations to a survivor. You did it!' "

Grace Trocco;
friend of two survivors; New York

4 • Chemo and Hair

Mane Matters

L osing her hair is every woman's fear. You don't have to face chemotherapy to know this. Take a look at any magazine. Right up there with skin-and-bones in the beauty department is hair. There are products promoting healthy hair, swingy hair, shiny hair, and thick hair. There are ones promoting curls, ones that make hair straight and sleek, ones that color it here and there, or all over. Okay. So you can avoid magazines. But you have to buy food at the market, and hair care products are advertised there, too. Walk outside the market, and there's the side of a bus emblazoned with a gorgeous face surrounded by a riot of wonderful hair. It doesn't have to be long hair. It can be short, but it's always shiny and sexy.

So, what if you don't *have* hair. What then? How do you feel? How do those around you feel? How do you go places without thinking that everyone is staring at you? How do you maintain a semblance of femininity?

The devastation of losing hair to chemotherapy is a major issue for women. This came through loud and clear in the earliest submissions to *UPLIFT*. In fact, the subject generated enough response from the sisterhood of survivors to earn a chapter of its own.

Now, everything in *UPLIFT* is meant to be upbeat. By way of setting the scene, though, I'd like to quote Lori Bartz. Lori is a survivor from Wisconsin, who was diagnosed in 2000 at the age of forty-one. She had sent an early submission, which opened, "It seems weird to say that breast cancer could in any way improve my life, but it has." Later, though, she sent another note. I share this one with you in part because I sense that it echoes what many of you are feeling, in part because the people around us need to know that as upbeat as we are, we sometimes have to air our gripes, and in part because it illustrates one woman's ability to feel lousy but still rebound.

"The worst part of this entire experience," Lori wrote, "is losing my hair. I *hate* wigs, though I have had many, many compliments, some from people who don't know it's a wig. The chemotherapy would be so much easier if I had my own hair. I appreciate that the drugs are killing my cancer, but I still want my hair. I can finally look at my head, but it still seriously upsets me. I feel selfish that this 'hair issue' is so important to me. I can hide the mastectomy, but it's not so easy to hide a bald head. Thanks for the opportunity to vent on this issue."

You're welcome, Lori. Even beyond the need to vent, I would wager that women all over the country are nodding in agreement with your complaint—and it isn't that researchers aren't working their tails off to find chemo drugs that don't cause hair loss. In fact, many of the newer "targeted" therapies involve such drugs, but these are usually given following a few months of standard chemo, meaning that though we still lose our hair, the damage is less prolonged. Alas, for a little while at least, we're stuck with bald heads.

Listen to Deborah Schur. A sales rep from Massachusetts, she was diagnosed in 1994 at the age of forty-three. She wrote, "I remember saying to one of the men I work with that if I lost all my hair, I would be ugly. His reply was that even without hair, I would be beautiful. He also reminded me, sternly and realistically, that my hair would grow back."

A final word from Lori again, who concluded her note this way. "Thank God for my husband. He says I look 'cute' with no hair, hence the saying 'love is blind.' "

Take "love" in its broadest sense, and you have the heart of this chapter.

LOSING IT

"Don't let the drugs call the shots. When your hair first starts to fall out, cut it all off. You now have the control. And remember, the sooner it falls out, the sooner it grows back!"

Susan Schultz; diagnosed in 1990 at age 41; special education teacher's aide; New York

"My friend Meg came to see me with her hair cut shorter and shorter each time. One day when she came over, she was smiling and took off her hat. She had shaved her head. Right behind her came her husband, who whipped off his hat to show he had shaved *his* head, too. What a team!"

Betty Schulte; friend of a survivor; Michigan

"My twenty-seven-year-old daughter, Karen, came to visit at the time when my hair was coming out daily in clumps. I kept saying to her that I just wished it would all fall out and be done. Taking my hand, she led me into the bathroom, and we shaved my head. It was a great moment. She finally felt there was something she could do to help, and I realized that I wasn't alone."

Carol Englund; diagnosed in 1994 at age 58; retired administrative assistant; New Jersey

"I'll never forget the day we shaved my head. My best friend, Susan, who normally styles my hair, insisted on doing it. My son Mike, who always has a smart remark, took one look at me and asked Susan how much she charged for that haircut! Then when my other son, Matt, approached me, we could see the shock. So Susan said, 'Look at this cute little baldini.' From that day on, Matt kissed my bald head every single day and asked how his cute little baldini was. I'll never forget it. He made my day!"

Anita Leuzzi; diagnosed in 1997 at age 45;
legal secretary; New York

"I had a hair-cutting party to which I invited fifteen of my friends. They took turns chopping off sections of my long hair and tying them with pink ribbons. The party was a way for me to feel more in control of the situation. It also involved my friends in the process, so that they didn't feel as helpless."

Asha Mevlana; diagnosed in 1999 at age 24;
musician; New York

"When my extremely thick hair began falling out fast and furious, leaving unsightly bald spots, my husband shaved my head. That reduced the 'fallout' considerably but left me with an itchy, irritated scalp. What helped me the most was taking long, hot showers every morning and night (boy, all that water rushing over my shaved head felt good!), then rubbing vitamin E oil all over the scalp. I put a towel over my pillow at night so I didn't leak oil onto the pillowcase. My scalp got healthier and less itchy by the very next day. Any extra oil can be rubbed onto the scar tissue on the breast, which will help it heal faster."

Margaret Blair; diagnosed in 2000 at age 49;
writer; Maryland

"When my hair started falling out, I didn't know what to expect. Would it all come out at once? What does a forty-four-year-old woman look like with no hair? I sat outside, and pulled and pulled until I couldn't pull any more. It took me longer to get up enough nerve to look in the mirror than to do all the pulling. Then, because I looked like Bozo the Clown on a really bad hair day, I went to the beauty shop, where they shaved my head. But what about all those little stubs that kept falling out? My solution? The really strong tape that you use to mail packages. I wrapped this around my hand and kept applying it until my head was as smooth as a pool ball."

Denise Judy; diagnosed in 1999 at age 43;
sign language specialist; West Virginia

"When I reached the point where I could pull my hair out in clumps, I asked my partner to accompany me to a local nature sanctuary. We went to one of my favorite meadows, where the grasses and wildflowers grow tall, and the forest surrounded us. I pulled out handfuls of hair and scattered it in the wind, hoping the birds and mice would use it to make warm, soft nests. For me, this simple spiritual act transformed the trauma of chemo-induced hair loss into a connection with the earth and with life."

Dorian Solot; diagnosed in 2000 at age 26;
Massachusetts

"My hair started falling out after my first treatment. I got tired of waking up with hair all over my pillowcase and looking down at the shower drain and seeing lost hair. I decided to take matters into my own hands. My fabulous hairdresser Lori decided to take a day off from work and drive me to an upscale wig salon that had come highly recommended. Well, I don't know how many of these salons you have ever visited, but this was my first experience. They ushered us into a private room complete with salon chair, mirrors, and wig products galore. Lori put one wig on after another . . . nothing felt right. Too dark, too light, too curly, too itchy. We then started trying on the hats . . . now we were having some fun! I realized that wigs were not for me and that wigs or hats, my head would still be bald! We left the salon that day with a few hats and drove home hatching another plan. The next evening with a glass of wine in my hand and my husband standing nervously outside the door of my hairdresser's salon, Lori proceeded to shave my head. She cried as she did it, but said that I had courage. For me, taking matters into my own hands was important. That day, I also learned that a good hairdresser does not just cut hair."

Cindy Fiedler; diagnosed in 1998 at age 40;
registered nurse, mom; Massachusetts

"The worst was when I started losing my hair, but when that happened, at the suggestion of my hairdresser, I had my head shaved. I put on a wig immediately, and it made it much easier. When my hair started to grow back, it was like peach fuzz, so I felt like I was right in style! When it started getting long, I could tell it was thicker than it had been, and soft as a baby's."

Barbara Moro; diagnosed in 1999 at age 57;
law secretary; New Jersey

"If you're going to lose your hair, cut it short before you begin the therapy. Long hair can clog sink and bathtub drains when it falls out. Who needs a plumbing hassle when you're undergoing chemo?"

Barbara Keiler; daughter of a survivor;
Massachusetts

"Early on after my neighbor was diagnosed, she chose to shave her head rather than watch her very long, thick, braided hair fall out clumps at a time. As she is a statuesque, dark-skinned lady, it was actually quite becoming."

Nancy Summersong;
friend of a survivor; Tennessee

"When my hair started falling out, I had my husband shave it off. As horrifying as that was, I felt it was better to have it off quickly, than have a mess coming out in your hands, comb and brush, on your pillow, and so forth."

Rhonda Sorrell; diagnosed in 1998 at age 43;
special education teacher; Michigan

"My hair started to fall out on April 1st. Yes, April Fools Day. Some joke! People told me that it was a good sign, that it meant the chemotherapy had started working. I don't know if that's true or not, but it sure did help. At first I cried a little, but then I took control. I decided that looking at my thinning hair every day would be more difficult than looking at a bald head. So I called my hairdresser and had the remainder of my hair buzzed off. I felt much better. The thinning hair represented what the disease could do to my body. My buzzed head represented strength and control. I was in charge."

Val Long; diagnosed in 1999 at age 47;
administrative assistant; Massachusetts

"When I knew I would lose my hair, I cut it short into a style that I wasn't particularly crazy about. It wasn't so hard to lose a 'bad' short hair style as it would have been to lose my longer hair. I have to say that I found it fascinating to just run my fingers through my hair and come away with a handful. I thought that if the drugs are powerful enough to take my hair, what a job they must be doing on those cancer cells! When it got to the point where there wasn't much hair left, I took a scissors and cut it down to the scalp. That much I had control over!"

Gwen Loverink; diagnosed in 1994 at age 34;
police dispatcher; California

"I was strangely intrigued and curious by the thought of my hair falling out. Would I just wake up bald some morning, or would it come out gradually for days? I was told to expect it to fall out be-tween Days Fourteen and Twenty-two following my first treatment, so every day beginning on about Day Ten, I'd wake up, tug on my hair, and assure myself that it was still firmly attached to my head. On Day Sixteen, we had an unusually warm March day, and I decided to enjoy the fresh air as I drove along the highway. Bad idea! I almost choked to death with the hair flying all around the car. Since I hadn't been shedding up until that point, at first I couldn't decide what it was that kept blowing into my mouth. When I realized it was my hair, I pulled the car over to the side of the road to inspect my head in the mirror. There was no noticeable change yet, but I knew the process had begun. I soon learned that there's nothing gradual at all about the hair-falling-out phase. It is just not fun to vacuum your own hair from the bathroom floor or change the sheets and pillowcases as soon as you get up in the morning. By Day Nineteen, I was more than ready for the 'buzz party' that my husband and I had planned. We went out to the back porch, and he lovingly and silently buzzed my head. When he was finished, we collected all the hair and left a pile on the porch for the birds that were nesting in the eaves. For some reason, that pleased me. When we were finished and back in the house, my husband gave me a big hug and assured me that I looked 'just great.' I found that hard to believe, since I didn't look so terrific WITH hair, but I appreciated the sentiment. It didn't take me long to put the whole hair issue into perspective. OK, I was an overweight, middle-aged, fuzzy-headed woman. I was also on the road to recovery from a life-threatening illness, and I began to view my hair loss as a testimony to this struggle—sort of like a 'badge of courage.'"

Nancy Lane; diagnosed in 2000 at age 53;
teacher; Massachusetts

"I cut Judi's hair all off yesterday. She called, wondering if I would be comfortable enough to do this, then arranging a time. She appeared around noon, beach towel and kitchen scissors in hand. Not the tools of a trained hairdresser to be sure, but the best we could come up with. We spread the towel on the kitchen floor, put a chair on the towel, snapped a 'before' picture, and she sat down. I picked up her short blonde waves and cut them off. They went into the waste can in handfuls, the blonde sun-bleached top, then the brown locks from underneath. We saved a handful, a mixture of both colors, in a plastic bag for posterity. Judi is my good friend who shares my name and neighborhood. I can back out of my driveway and right into hers. I about took her mailbox out doing just that last week. We are both fifty. We were both diagnosed with breast cancer in the last four months and have both had mastectomies. Now, Judi is dealing with chemical warfare. She has a lot to live for. Her oldest son, LJ, is a sophomore in high school. He just got his Eagle badge. LJ plays football and is an excellent student. He is old enough and sensi-tive enough to her needs and hurts to be wonderful and com-forting. Jay is twelve, also a wonderful son. Jay plays soccer, a violin, and with many people. He is a busy kid and gets busier as Judi goes through surgery and treatment, which is his own way of dealing with the situation. Judi is taking control of everything she can, and that's a lot. That's why the hair was all cut off—it had started migrating from head to pillow, which was depressing for her to see. No hair is an adjustment, but she looks at its demise as evidence that the chemo is working. She regards the chemo as guerilla warfare—a powerful gun shooting into a for-est, hitting the good and bad alike. Once the enemy is gone, the good can regenerate and flourish again. We will both be thank-ful at our respective Thanksgiving tables this Thursday. Thank-ful for our lives . . . our families . . . the health care system . . . good friends. We'll be looking forward to next spring when I take the 'after' photo of Judi with new hair and new health. In the meantime life is good, with or without our hair, and we will live it to the fullest."

From the journal of Judy Von Bergen; diagnosed in 1997 at age 50; store owner; Wisconsin

HATS AND SCARVES

"The chemo that I needed was going to cause all my hair to fall out, so I decided to cut a lot off first. It was too short to donate for wigs for kids. So I saved it, and a friend gave me a baseball cap, and we stitched a ponytail coming out the back and wisps of my hair out around the rest of the hat. We put matching scrunchies around the ponytail, and *voilà!* Too real looking to believe!"

Cindy Ferus; diagnosed in 2000 at age 57;
circuit board technician, former school teacher; Massachusetts

"Wear a denim baseball cap—soft, smooth, stylish, and sold in youth sizes."

Mary Raffol; diagnosed in 1998 at age 44;
teacher; Massachusetts

"I had quite a collection of hats, both for spring and winter. My co-workers actually gave me a hat and scarf party! I really enjoyed wearing my spring hats. I would dress them up with scarves that matched my outfits. People at work looked forward to seeing what hat and scarf I would wear each day. Everyone from the president to the security guards commented. It was great fun."

Val Long; diagnosed in 1999 at age 47;
administrative assistant; Massachusetts

"A friend of mine gave me a small, fitted hat that was made of 100% cotton and felt like tee-shirt material. It's called the Headliner and can be purchased at many cancer boutiques. I did purchase a wig but found that it felt like a heavy, itchy swim cap. I wore the Headliner around the house and to bed. Amazing how cold your head gets without any hair! When I went out,

I mainly wore scarves. A friend made some for me, and I purchased a few. My aunt also made some headcoverings that fit and felt perfect. The American Cancer Society has a pattern for them."

Gwen Loverink; diagnosed in 1994 at age 34;
police dispatcher; California

"I bought many of my caps through the American Cancer Society catalogue. They have many styles and designs, reasonably priced, too!"

Rhonda Sorrell; diagnosed in 1998 at age 43;
special education teacher; Michigan

"Losing my hair didn't bother me. I took to wearing a baseball cap. Never bothered with a wig."

Carleen Muniz; diagnosed in 1998 at age 51;
artist; Massachusetts

"My single best purchase was a funky, charcoal gray hat. It went with everything. I bought it at a hat and wig boutique owned by a cancer survivor. I credit Carol with my lack of self-consciousness with my 'no hair' look."

Rosamary Amiet; diagnosed in 2000 at age 48;
program manager; Ohio

"Hats made it hard to hear, but I thought my wigs looked fake. Now, though, looking at pictures of me wearing my wigs, I think I looked pretty good. One advantage of the wigs: my hair was always perfect. But my hats were cool. I bought a dozen and wore a different one every day. I also bought big clip-on earrings and wore them every chance I got."

Betsy Goree; diagnosed in 1998 at age 40;
magazine publisher/editor; North Carolina

"Two breast cancer survivors loaned me their collection of hats for those long 'no hair' months. I accumulated a wardrobe of about three dozen hats—a veritable fashion show every day!"

Betty Harris; diagnosed in 1999 at age 64;
homemaker; South Carolina

"I wore hip children's hats from Target. I also bought a wig, but did not care for that in the summer."

Candice Jaeger; diagnosed in 2000 at age 24;
wife, mother; Illinois

"I bought a wig, which I came to name the 'rat.' But it was just never comfortable—I decided that the distance from the top of my ears to the top of my head was too short—and it itched terribly. So I switched to scarves. A friend made me several scarves and also lent me tons of others. They were large—thirty-four inches square—so I could wrap them around my head twice."

Robin Smith; diagnosed in 2000 at age 53;
microbiologist, homemaker; New York

"During the time when I had no hair and while it was beginning to grow back, I wore turbans and scarves. It was summer, and I was visiting my sister at the beach. Her seven-year-old grandson, Scott, was visiting also. Although he knew I was sick, he didn't know the details. He came over, sat next to me, and asked why I was wearing a hat (actually, a turban). I told him it was hot, and I just wanted to keep my hair out of the way. He said, 'Well, Aunt Carol, I think it looks really nice.' What a wonderful feeling came over me. I had often worried that the way I looked made the people around me uncomfortable."

Carol Englund; diagnosed in 1994 at age 58;
retired administrative assistant; New Jersey

"I sometimes wore scarves, but most often wore a stretchy, black velvet cap and then decorated it with colorful scarves to match my clothes or my mood. Once, when I was out to lunch with a friend, I wore a rather elaborately tied scarf on my head. The fabric matched my skirt and was rather chic. A woman at the table next to us complimented me on my 'hat' and wanted to know where she could buy one just like it."

Carrie Drake; diagnosed in 1998 at age 42;
administrative assistant; Colorado

"The best beach look? I always carried a scarf, so I wouldn't 'flip my wig' in an unexpected breeze. I did a great Jackie Onassis impression with big sunglasses and a scarf."

Sharon Carr; diagnosed in 1997 at age 42;
hospice grief counselor; Rhode Island

"Some of us are confident or have a pretty enough shaped head to just go bald. But if you must go through chemotherapy in the winter and you live anyplace the least bit chilly, even these gals will want to cover their heads. If you're lucky and really love your wig, then getting dressed will be easy. But if you're like me, your wig may not agree with you. Not only did my head itch and sweat, but the mirror reflected a strange and always crooked image. So scarves became my choice of cover-up. Once I learned how to tie them and adjust my wardrobe to match them, they actually became kind of fun."

Sallie Burdine; diagnosed in 1998 at age 44;
author; Florida

"One day, I invited friends for dinner. They came dressed with bandanas on their heads, plus one for each of us. They even brought one for the dog! For Christmas and Chanukah, my partner's mom knit the most outrageous hats, one for each day of the week. The entire family sat around the dinner table wearing some sort of head covering in pinks, reds, purples, and greens. The men in the family looked absolutely smashing."

Carol Snyder; diagnosed in 1992 at age 47;
special education teacher; New York

WIGS

"When my hair came out, I was a basket case. I thought I was prepared, but I was not. 'Hysterical' is how I would describe myself, but that was only for a few hours. Then I went home, put on my wig, and no one really noticed that it *was* a wig. I got questions like 'Did you get a new hair cut?' Not having hair is really no big deal. I'd just throw on a wig or one of my favorite ball caps and go out."

Michele Marks; diagnosed in 1996 at age 33;
CAD operator; Ohio

"The very best thing about losing my hair during chemotherapy was the realization that I could become a blonde, redhead, or brunette by purchasing wigs from a catalogue. This pleased me, since my natural brown color was never to my liking. Also, with a wig, my 'hair' was always ready to go, so turning down an invitation was not an option. Getting out of the house was important."

Jean La Frombois; diagnosed in 1996 at age 57;
homemaker, part-time bookseller; Wisconsin

"I most dreaded the whole experience of losing my hair and living bald in a world driven by cosmetic beauty. Little did I know what an experience it would become. I had gone shopping for a wig on my own once, and it was a terrible experience, so I decided I needed help. One Saturday, my daughters and I set out on our wig-finding adventure. We all tried on wigs and laughed at ourselves. It was hard to find a wig that resembled my own curly hair and looked nice, so my daughters convinced me to try a new style. It was a color my hair was when I was younger, and much straighter than my hair has ever been. After scrunching it around on my still hairy scalp a few minutes, I turned around, holding my breath, waiting for their reaction. The girls smiled approvingly and convinced me it was beautiful and made me look younger. Well, how could I resist looking younger?"

Ann Hurd; diagnosed in 1999 at age 57;
dental office manager; Colorado

"Buy your wig while you still have your own hair. When your hair starts to go, cut it, then shave your head. It makes you feel empowered."

Susan Rothstein; diagnosed in 1997 at age 49;
travel agent; Massachusetts

"Choose a wig that most flatters you, rather than one that closely replicates your current hairdo. The two may not be the same. Have an open mind, and don't be afraid to be daring. My wig was more glamorous than my own mop of hair, and my husband loved it. When not wearing a wig, try a baseball cap over a small scarf. No one looks at baseball caps anymore, whereas turbans often attract attention."

Patricia Baker; diagnosed in 1993 at age 49;
at home; Massachusetts

"My sister went with me to get a wig, and we laughed at the names of the wigs and those associations. Finally, I got two to have a choice."

Joanne Tutschek; diagnosed in 1998 at age 55;
research communications director; New Jersey

"I went wig shopping with three of my friends and tried on all the hairdos that I never would have thought of wearing. I figured this was a great time to try out a new style. Before chemo, I had long, straight black hair. Instead of buying a wig like that, I got a platinum blonde wig for going out; a red shag for work; and a pink, purple, and blue one to wear when I got bored with the other two. When my friends and I went out, I would let them borrow whichever wigs I wasn't wearing myself. This way, I didn't feel as self-conscious. They were happy to help."

Asha Mevlana; diagnosed in 1999 at age 24;
musician; New York

"Getting a good wig can really boost your self-confidence. In the beginning, I couldn't imagine spending six or seven hundred dollars on a hairpiece, especially if I was going to be sick and in the house a lot. Also, some people told me that wigs were itchy and uncomfortable. Well, mine wasn't. I felt pretty good after my first treatment and began to think that I shouldn't be stuck in the house because of the way I looked. I'm not a vain person, but I'd previously had so much hair that I had to cut it twice before it came out. So I bought a $625 wig, and it made such a difference. Most people thought it was my natural hair, just straight now."

Donna Troiani; diagnosed in 2000 at age 42;
part-time waitress, full-time mom; New York

"Buy a more expensive wig, not a cheap one. It needs to look good for you to feel good. Also, have your wig fitted before you lose your hair. You will get a better fit for your head and will be able to match your natural color."

Rhonda Sorrell; diagnosed in 1998 at age 43;
special education teacher; Michigan

"Though hair loss will be temporary, even simple, matter-of-fact comments about its growing back offer no consolation. Give yourself time, and shop seriously for a wig. It will be 'you' for the next year. Take a friend along, and you'll share some laughter and gain a valued opinion."

Mary Raffol; diagnosed in 1998 at age 44;
teacher; Massachusetts

"A friend who had gone through this a year before told me she had gone to a wig shop while her hair was the color and style she liked. They made a wig to match exactly. I did as she suggested, and even though I didn't go through chemo, I felt prepared and in control. The wig has come in handy several times and is nice to have."

Carol Hattler; diagnosed in 1999 at age 65;
retired nurse; Virginia

"The wig problem was very stressful for me. I have a large head, so the majority of wigs didn't fit. A friend suggested the Paula Young catalogue. This is a very nice and very private way to try on wigs!"

Sara Fallgren; diagnosed in 1978 at age 45;
retired teacher; California

"How does a person who never really knew what to do with her 'original' hair prepare for the loss of hair that follows chemotherapy? First, I had my hairdresser help me match a color swatch to my current hair color. Then, with her help I ordered a wig in a simple hairstyle that I felt I could keep in decent shape. The wig arrived, and I put it away until the day that I would need it. During this time, I was working as a manager of a retirement apartment community. When I first noticed large quantities of my hair falling out, I called the local beauty shop that was affiliated with the 'Look Good . . . Feel Better' program sponsored by the American Cancer Society. They suggested that I come in within the hour so that they could shave off the hair that I had left. Off I went, in such a rush that I forgot my wig. But there was no turning back. The ladies got out the hair clippers and before I knew it I was completely bald. As quickly as the hair was brushed away, these same two angels placed a short, blonde, pixie-cut wig on my sixty-four-year-old head. What fun! I had no time to whine or moan, as I had to get back to work. Well, the blonde wig was a huge success. It certainly didn't match my old hair color, but it didn't make a bit of difference. My residents loved the new look, and so did I. Maybe it really is true that blondes have more fun!"

Florence Wade; diagnosed in 1999 at age 63;
retired school teacher, retired property manager; Texas

"A little brown eye shadow applied to the area around the hairline of your face helps when wearing your wig."

Nan Comstock; diagnosed in 1988 at age 39;
self-employed; California

"Rub Sea Breeze astringent on your scalp before putting on your wig. It will prevent itching."

Cheryl Cavallo; diagnosed in 1997 at age 35;
homemaker; Massachusetts

"I wore a short wig in my usual hairstyle, so most people didn't know."

Becky Honeycutt; diagnosed in 1995 at age 53;
licensed practical nurse; Indiana

"I loved my wigs! Everyone complimented me on my hairstyle, I never had to fuss about having a good hair day, and being bald didn't bother me. I tried not to look in the mirror when the wig was removed, so it was not a concern."

Alyce Feinstein; diagnosed in 1993 at age 58;
administrative assistant; Massachusetts

"I had two wigs. One was a pageboy with bangs, and the other was short, straight, and layered. When my son, a senior in high school, was dressing up for Halloween, he needed a wig, so I gave him his choice. He wore the pageboy, and looked so good! The next day, I wore it myself, and when I drove up to the school to pick up my younger son, both boys' friends came up to me to tell me that they thought the wig looked better on Micah than on me!"

Jane Royal-Davidson; diagnosed in 1996 at age 47;
educator; North Carolina

"What got me through the difficult months of chemotherapy was making sure I always looked my best. I had purchased a great wig in a style very similar to my own hairdo. I went to each treatment wearing my beautiful wig, full face of makeup, and a favorite pantsuit. The nurses constantly told me how healthy I looked, which was extremely uplifting. For me, looking my best was key for maintaining a positive outlook!"

Gail Rice; diagnosed in 1999 at age 48;
teacher; Massachusetts

"Here's a tip. Hold on to your wig when getting out of the back seat of a car or taxi, lest the wig catch on the clothing hook and you emerge bald by surprise."

Mindy Greenside; diagnosed in 2000 at age 48;
midwife; Maryland

"When wearing a wig, watch out for the oven. Pulling that pie out could melt your hair. Don't try to layer with sweatshirts that go over your head, and forget dressing rooms if you are trying on clothes that go over your head."

Ann Hurd; diagnosed in 1999 at age 57;
dental office manager; Colorado

THERE IS SOMETHING TO BE SAID FOR . . .

"I lost my hair on Mother's Day with twenty people coming to brunch. I really knew that the chemo was working—the hair loss proved it."

Debbie MacLean; diagnosed in 1991 at age 47;
volunteer, hospital gift shop and hospice; Massachusetts

"It was not so bad losing my hair. Oh, it was emotional at first. But then, look how much time we women spend doing our hair. This was great. Toss on a wig or a hat, and that was that. And, oh, how my hair has grown back! It is great. Thick and curly. No more perms!"

Dee Pobjoy; diagnosed in 1999 at age 41;
sales clerk; Wisconsin

"There is something to be said for not having to shave our legs or pluck our eyebrows any more. I did have to learn how to draw eyebrows, and if I had to pick, I would certainly pick 'plucking' over 'drawing.' But hey, I enjoyed the break."

Sallie Burdine; diagnosed in 1998 at age 44;
author; Florida

"There were some good things about hair falling out. First, my son learned he really wasn't adopted, since his hair growth pattern and mine match. Second, the hair on my legs grows less quickly now. Third, the hair under my arms never grew back, which is *not* a bad thing. Fourth, my son's wrestling team would rub my head for luck before a match; it felt good, and since I was comfortable, they were, too."

Jane Royal-Davidson; diagnosed in 1996 at age 47;
educator; North Carolina

"One week after my first chemo, my hair started falling out. I was so amazed that I could just pull it right out, and it didn't even hurt. I didn't cry. I kept reminding myself that it was only temporary and that it would grow back. I thought to myself, 'Gee, think of all the money you'll save on shampoo! And you won't have to shave your legs or underarms.' I laughed about that, and it made me feel better. I got a wig that was the exact same color as my own hair. In fact, everyone thought the wig *was* my own hair! One day a friend stopped by. She said, 'You look so good! You haven't even lost your hair!' I took off the wig, and the look on her face was priceless. A few weeks after my last chemo, my hair started growing back. My head felt like a giant peach!"

Paula Porter; diagnosed in 2000 at age 47; telephone operator; New York

"Rather than feel bad about my hair loss, I decided to sleep the extra hour in the morning. I did not need to blow-dry my hair or put mascara on, as I had no eyelashes—and I actually needed the extra sleep."

Jacki Anthony; diagnosed in 1998 at age 48; nurse; Massachusetts

"After my treatments, our family took its annual July trip to the beach. Walking on the hot sand with my wig proved to be miserable. I traded my wig in for a cute ball cap, and continued on with my vacation. When we went out for dinner, I would again doll up with my wig and makeup, but I did not allow myself to become a prisoner of the situation. This was my vacation, and I was determined to enjoy it."

Jean Joyce; diagnosed in 1999 at age 51; hairdresser, salon owner; Virginia

"Funny thing about hair. They told me I would lose it, and I wanted to. That way, I wouldn't have to hear my husband say, 'When are you going to let your hair grow long?' But, guess what? It didn't fall out! It stopped growing and got a bit thin, but it stayed."

Pam Waddell; diagnosed in 1998 at age 38; writer, teacher's aide; Texas

"When I was assured by the oncologist that my long blonde hair would fall out during chemo, I had it cut 'punk' and let my daughter dye it blue. When my scalp started to ache as the hair started to thin, I asked my son to buzz it with the clippers. We laughed together and cried together. After my hair was gone, I wore a mid-length fall with a scarf, bandana, or hat. Friends gave me scarves that they had collected, and I discovered that twenty-two-inch dinner napkins from April Cornell were not only the perfect size, soft (100% cotton), and washable, but they came in colorful prints that really lifted my spirits. Now that my hair is long enough to go without, I am making a quilt with all of the scarves. It gives new meaning to the word 'comforter.' "

Linda Jones Burns; diagnosed in 2000 at age 40;
high school registrar; New Hampshire

"I think about my friend in Arkansas. She sent me a card saying that she would like a picture of me in my 'wig.' My thought is that I don't have a 'wig,' I have 'hair,' and it's mine any way I figure it. I don't call it a 'wig.' I'm really attached to my hair. In fact, I need to wash it in Woolite again."

Sandy Williams; diagnosed in 1999 at age 51;
children's public services librarian; Texas

"When my hair started falling out, I did not want my grandchildren to see me because I was afraid of what they would think. But they said they had friends who had lost their hair because of cancer, and it was okay."

Wahnita Hawk; diagnosed in 1999 at age 56;
licensed practical nurse; Pennsylvania

"I had my hair buzzed right before Easter. My daughter, Wendy, brought Brittany, my six-year-old granddaughter, up to visit. Brittany told her mom that I looked like an alien. I became her 'Alien Grandmother.' My other granddaughter, Sarah, who is four, didn't want to see me without my wig. I spent many hours with her just talking about my hair and wig, but she was adamant about it. One day, when we stopped by to visit, Brittany and Sarah were playing in the garage. As we left I pulled off my wig and said, 'Your Alien Grandmother says goodbye.' Sarah looked at me with her eyes and mouth open wide, unsure of what to do until she heard Brittany laughing. After that, it was all right to see me without my wig. Summer came, and I started to wear a baseball hat, which she always wanted me to take off so she could feel my hair."

Nancy Ellis; diagnosed in 2000 at age 53;
quality technician; New York

"You may lose your pubic hair with chemo. But it, too, grows back."

Monica May; diagnosed in 1997 at age 40;
organizing consultant; New Mexico

"I chose to be bald most of the time, rather than wearing a wig or scarf. When I went out, people would often ask me questions about my bald head. I gave my favorite response to a woman in a store who asked me if I'd lost my hair. 'No,' I told her matter-of-factly. 'It's invisible.' She had nothing more to say."

Dorian Solot; diagnosed in 2000 at age 26;
Massachusetts

"During the time that I was wearing a wig because of chemotherapy, I had to tell a precious little third-grader that she did not test into the gifted program at school. It had been so important to her to be in this program, and I used every ploy, explanation, and example I knew to have her understand that she was not a failure because of one test. But I couldn't get through to her. She was so sad, and the tears were still flowing. Finally, I said that she needed to count her blessings and be happy for the things she did have. When she still questioned herself, I pulled off my wig with a flourish and said, 'Look, you could be bald like me!' She collapsed into laughter and promised not to say anything to the other students, because it might upset them. Today, that young lady is a very successful college student who graduated from high school with honors. Although we had moved away from that state when she graduated, I received an invitation to her graduation party with an enclosed note thanking me for loving and encouraging her when she was a little girl."

Brenda Carr; diagnosed in 1988 at age 40;
wife, mother, retired school counselor; Texas

"Following my chemo treatments, I joined with some other volunteer hairdressers to work with cancer victims. While giving classroom tips one day, I took a volunteer from the class. She got a complete makeover. After marveling at her appearance, she presented another wig on a foam head for me to style. I told her to put it on. She was a little embarrassed and did not want the class to see her switch wigs. I said, 'We will all turn our heads for you to make the switch.' While everyone was turning their heads, I reached up and pulled my wig off, laying it on the table beside hers. You can image the surprise in the classroom when the women looked back up. They had only known me as 'Jean the Volunteer Beautician,' not 'Jean the Cancer Survivor.' This was truly the icebreaker for my class. They immediately started opening up to me. One asked when I became comfortable taking my wig off in front of others. I told them, 'When I came to realize that there was so much more to life than a pretty head of hair.' "

Jean Joyce; diagnosed in 1999 at age 51;
hairdresser, salon owner; Virginia

HAIR AGAIN

"When my hair started coming in, random people on the street started commenting on how much they loved my haircut. They all thought I had such guts to cut it so short. Most of them said they had always wanted to try it but couldn't get the courage to do it."

Asha Mevlana; diagnosed in 1999 at age 24;
musician; New York

"What a relief it was when my hair began to grow in. At first, I thought I'd go mad with the itching of my scalp. At times, wearing my wig was unbearable because of the itching. By Christmas, my hair resembled my son-in-law's buzz cut. As the family was gathering for the holiday festivities I relaxed and took the itchy wig off. My seven-year-old granddaughter walked over and tried it on. She turned around, looking for all the world like Tina Turner, and, cocking her head to the side, announced, 'I don't think this is my style.' Today, my hair is thicker and less gray than it was before treatment. I will never complain about a 'bad hair day' again."

> Ann Hurd; diagnosed in 1999 at age 57;
> dental office manager; Colorado

"I didn't lose all of my hair, but it was thin and so dry that it was three shades lighter. I made sure I got a good wash-and-wear haircut so I could stop blow-drying it, and it was back to its normal brown curly mop within a month of my last chemo treatment!"

> Lynne Rutenberg; diagnosed in 1980 at age 35;
> retired teacher; New Jersey

"There was a time when my greatest fear was that my hair would never grow back. That was six years ago now, and any complaint about a 'bad hair day' will never again be truly sincere."

> Kathi Ward; diagnosed in 1994 at age 47;
> merchandiser; South Carolina

"When my treatment ended, my hair began to grow back. And you know what? I look great in short hair. I've always had long hair and never would have considered cutting it."

> Linda Perkins; diagnosed in 1999 at age 35;
> project manager; New Jersey

"I am convinced that Mane 'N Tail Shampoo helped my hair grow back fast."

Kathy Rabassa; diagnosed in 1999 at age 34;
administrative assistant; South Carolina

"My beautician told me that when my hair started growing back in, I shouldn't wear a wig or scarf when I was at home. She said that if you wear nothing on your head, your hair will grow back faster. She also said that massaging your head makes the hair grow in faster."

Paula Porter; diagnosed in 2000 at age 47;
telephone operator; New York

"I loved the first bit of fuzz when my hair started growing back. I felt like I was being given a chance to experience what I had gone through as a baby. It was incredible. My hair was so soft. If you haven't gone through this, it may sound a bit weird, but it was great. Like having been reborn and being allowed to experience it with all your senses. I loved it."

Val Long; diagnosed in 1999 at age 47;
administrative assistant; Massachusetts

"I liked my new curly hair so much, I have been having body waves ever since. My hair came in white, after having always been dark and dyed. My husband said, 'Well, at least we know what the real color is!' "

Joanne Tutschek; diagnosed in 1998 at age 55;
research communications director; New Jersey

"It's been a year and a half since I completed chemo for breast cancer. I had straight hair for forty-five years, and now I have wonderful curly hair. It took nine months for my hair to grow in enough so that I didn't have to wear my wig."

A survivor; diagnosed in 1998 at age 45;
dentist; Indiana

"The second my hair had grown back enough to cover my head, I did away with the head coverings. It felt so good to feel the breeze on my hair! It came in much thicker and curlier. Hardly takes me any time at all to style it—just fluff and go!"

Gwen Loverink; diagnosed in 1994 at age 34;
police dispatcher; California

"When my hair was gone, I didn't like wearing my wig and only did so when I was wearing 'grown-up' clothes. Other times I wore floppy-brimmed hats or went bare-headed. As soon as I had enough hair to cover my head—and look like a really chic 'do'—I left the hats at home. My hair came in evenly and, as it grew longer, began to curl. The best part, though, was when friends and family who had watched me go through this would rub my new hair and curls. I knew that they were as thrilled to have that hair back as I was. And, of course, the hair only represented what we all wanted back and were thankful for—my health."

Faye Hardiman; diagnosed in 1998 at age 50;
wife, mother, teacher; Georgia

"When the hair started to fall out in clumps a couple of weeks after the first round of chemo, my husband used his beard trimming kit to shave off the rest of my hair. I wore a cute wig when I went out or to work and a bandanna (often under a baseball cap) around the house and in the yard. The new hair came in really curly, which was a wonderful surprise, and I quit wearing the wig and bandanna for our first wedding anniversary weekend getaway!"

Beth Compton; diagnosed in 1995 at age 27;
civil engineer; South Carolina

"I wore one of the little soft cotton stocking caps to sleep in. They can be purchased at a wig shop. That kept my head warm at night, and I felt 'protected' from the baldness. I didn't look at myself in the mirror much without my wig. I can't tell you how many people asked me where I got my hair cut. I actually grew so attached to my wig that it was hard for me to give it up. I was a redhead before the chemotherapy. Now my hair is a dark, dark brown. Before, my hair was limp and straight. Now I have waves and body. Sometimes I look in the mirror and wonder who I am!"

Sandy Williams; diagnosed in 1999 at age 51;
children's public services librarian; Texas

5 • Chemo and Everything Else

A Smorgasbord

Side effects. They're the pits. On one hand, you need the drugs to kill the cancer. On the other, the drugs kill some good stuff in the process. The result is tantamount to adding insult to the injury of a breast cancer diagnosis. What's the old saw—if the cancer doesn't get 'em, the cure will? I certainly don't believe that. I wouldn't be bothering with this book if I did. No, I do believe in the cure. But I also believe that we need to get a handle on those unfortunate side effects.

The last chapter talked about hair loss. This chapter deals with the rest—a broad group that includes stomach upset, fatigue, and a couple of other little things that are totally annoying. For starters, there's *nothing* worse than taking a medication and experiencing side effects that may be perfectly normal but that no one has warned you about! Lauren Nichols, a writer from Pennsylvania, who was diagnosed in 2000 at the age of fifty-three, had that experience during chemotherapy.

"The anti-nausea meds I was given before my first treatment not only made me sick, but wired me so badly that deep inside my-

self, I was bouncing off the walls. The awful thing is, I didn't realize I wasn't supposed to feel that way, so I did the 'stiff upper lip'
thing and said nothing until my followup check-up. That's when
the nurse told me that some people have what amounts to an al-
lergic reaction to certain drugs. They put me on something else,
and it worked well."

In this instance, as in others mentioned later in this chapter, a simple switch in anti-nausea medication solved the problem. Unfortunately, the chemo itself can't be switched. There just aren't enough
drugs with the same ability to cure without those side effects. And
it's not that all women experience them. Every woman's body is different. Some of what you'll read here is common, some less so.
Moreover, chemo regimens change over time. Suffice it to say here
that one woman's body may experience a side effect that another
woman's never will. That said, there's no harm keeping UPLIFT
nearby just in case—because while the medical community
searches for antidotes to side effects, the sisterhood has its own
ideas. Call them folk remedies, but, hey, if they work . . .

So. The most common side effects of chemo are well known—
namely, hair loss and nausea. But there is another one that takes
people by surprise. Michele Marks, from Ohio, who was diagnosed
in 1996 at the age of thirty-three, broached it first. "When I went
through chemo, no one told me I might have trouble remembering things or get distracted easily. It's chemo-brain, and it explains
a lot. I found half-finished notes and longer papers that I started
but didn't finish, and I couldn't think of words or remember things.
For a while, I thought I was going crazy. It was chemo-brain. But
nobody told me then."

Betsy Goree, from North Carolina, who was diagnosed in 1998
at the age of forty, elaborated on that with a certain Southern
charm. "Simply put, chemo-brain is the way your brain reacts to
the chemo drugs. Chemo-brain makes you forgetful. You might
feel like you are coming down with Alzheimer's (don't worry, it's
only cancer) because you can't recall a song title or your next-

door-neighbor's name. You may have a hard time finishing a sentence, or remembering your dog's name or a trip to the store. This is annoying. It is especially bad when your loved ones give you the look that says 'chemo-brain' (so try not to do that, y'all). This look used to upset me because I would realize that I had (again) forgotten something. I don't forget near as much anymore, but if I do, I just say to myself, 'Chemo-brain is a real thing. You have it because you had cancer and you went to great lengths to kill the cancer. How important is that 1940s movie star's name anyway?' Sometimes when I am alone in my car, I say this out loud, then look at myself—and all my hair—in the rearview mirror and ask a disbelieving, 'You had cancer?' "

Betsy skips a line, then adds, "The good thing about chemo-brain is that it goes away."

This sentiment is shared by Linda Perkins, from New Jersey, who was diagnosed in 1999 at the age of thirty-five. "The gradual end of chemo-brain and the return of my short-term memory reminds me daily of my good fortune and the light at the end of the tunnel."

Which just goes to show that the glass can be half full even when you can't remember putting any water in it at all!

Which has absolutely nothing to do with smoking pot.

Though I've heard that that does help curb nausea . . .

KEEPING IT DOWN

"Always eat before going to chemo. Nausea is more acute with an empty stomach, and it is often difficult to eat after the treatment. For that reason, eat whatever you want whenever you can. Nutrition is important, but your regular diet may not be palatable. Comfort foods that line the stomach make a difference—rice, potatoes, pasta."

Patricia Baker; diagnosed in 1993 at age 49;
at home; Massachusetts

"What works best for me in the nausea department is keeping my stomach full just before treatment and for two days after it. I also drink plenty of water before treatment. I eat a light breakfast, and if I have to wait long, I bring dry crackers to munch on before I go in. The carbs seem to do it for me at this time. Lots of bread is not good for the waistline, but . . ."

Donna Troiani; diagnosed in 2000 at age 42;
part-time waitress, full-time mom; New York

"The Christmas after my surgery, my Christmas card to my college roommate crossed paths with hers to me. Both contained the same message—that we had had mastectomies that year. Her advice to me was to keep my stomach full. I ate blueberry muffins by the dozen, and it helped."

Jane Vaughan; diagnosed in 1991 at age 53;
writer; Texas

"Morinda noni juice was very helpful during my chemo time. After I began taking it, I had no nausea at all. A friend told me to drink two liters of tonic water over two days following the chemo infusion. The quinine in the water was like a miracle. No more leg and foot pains. I mixed it with orange juice and sipped it. What a difference!"

Phyllis Jezequel; diagnosed in 1999 at age 66;
missionary—personnel; Florida

"What helped me get through my diagnosis, five surgeries, and nine months of treatment for breast cancer, at the age of thirty-five? The three G's—God and plenty of faith, Ginger (crystallized) and Ginger Brew (both available in health food stores) to help the nausea from treatment, and Garlic. And Graham Crackers. And, of course, Jewish Penicillin (Chicken Soup) on a regular basis."

Linda Perkins; diagnosed in 1999 at age 35;
project manager; New Jersey

"My absolute standby for food when I felt nauseated was saltine crackers. The fat-free ones seemed lighter and were my favorite. I also always kept packets of instant oatmeal on hand to pop into the microwave. Oatmeal is bland and filling, and the packets were great to take to work. Popsicles were good, also. I was always thirsty!"

Deborah Lambert; diagnosed in 2000 at age 47;
medical secretary; Massachusetts

"Of everything my friend Tammy tried on chemo days, Funyuns worked best to keep the metal taste out of her mouth. They have an oniony flavor and lots of crunch. She would wash them down with Mountain Dew. Also, she was told to drink lots of water. This gives you beautiful skin, which is important, since people are more apt to notice your skin when you have no hair."

Nanette Carter;
friend of Tammy Blackwell; Arkansas

"I had read in a book that eating an ice pop during treatment helps with the gum soreness that I had after my first treatment. So I went to the second treatment, ice pops in hand, but they melted. I had a very cold ginger ale and resorted to swishing that in my mouth, and the truth is it did help."

Donna Troiani; diagnosed in 2000 at age 42;
part-time waitress, full-time mom; New York

"During chemotherapy, suck on ice chips for a few minutes while the solution is first entering your veins. This actually works to eliminate mouth sores."

Cheryl Cavallo; diagnosed in 1997 at age 35;
homemaker; Massachusetts

"Ice pops immediately before my chemotherapy froze the cells in my mouth and prevented me from getting mouth sores. Treatment also resulted in vaginal dryness, which can be very painful for a young woman. Thank goodness for Replens vaginal moisturizer!"

> Linda Perkins; diagnosed in 1999 at 35;
> project manager; New Jersey

"A great anti-nausea technique used by friends of mine who've had breast cancer is to drink Gatorade (no ice) through a straw. Also, aromatherapy helps, especially Vicks Vaporub under the nose and on the throat."

> Elaine Raco Chase;
> friend of many survivors; Virginia

"For chemo, I would always bring an extra-large iced coffee and sip away. It is important to have lots of liquids. If possible, bring someone with a great sense of humor—a good friend or family member to share the time with."

> Rayna Ragonetti; diagnosed in 1993 at age 52;
> executive; New York

"Chicken soup was the only meal I ever ate after chemo treatment, and I never got ill from it."

> Penny Trosterman; diagnosed in 1996 at age 45;
> English teacher; New York

"My favorite food during chemo was Mexican food. It had spice in it that I could taste through the 'metal' mouth that chemo causes. I also ate a lot of ice cream. It felt good to have something cold in my mouth, especially when I had mouth sores. Overall, though, I pretty much ate whatever I could whenever I could. On the good days, I tried to make up for the bad days, so my goal was to get as many calories into my system as I could."

> Gwen Loverink; diagnosed in 1994 at age 34;
> police dispatcher; California

"Eat cold, raw foods during chemo treatment times. Carrot sticks, celery, ham sandwiches—anything that doesn't have a strong odor. Hot foods with a strong smell can make nausea seem worse. Also, breathe through your mouth if odors begin to bother you. The clinic where I had chemo treatments always had coffee going in the lobby. I couldn't stand the smell of it after two treatments. I started breathing through my mouth so the smell wouldn't bother me. When I had a funny taste in my mouth, I sucked on peppermint candy."

Jennifer Wersal; diagnosed in 2000 at age 30;
marketing; Texas

"During chemo, eat light. After my first treatment, I ate spaghetti, and that did not work. Drink lots of juices and ice-cold tea."

Mary Ann Lee; diagnosed in 1988 at age 46;
tax collector; North Carolina

"For a while, nothing at all tasted good, and I could only stomach Popsicles. Then there was a period when grilled cheese sandwiches and Jell-O were all I could eat. Then Stouffer's frozen macaroni and cheese and pudding cups tasted good. It was months before I could enjoy a good steak, a nice salad, and a glass of red wine—but when I did, I savored every mouthful."

Carrie Drake; diagnosed in 1998 at age 42;
administrative assistant; Colorado

"Eating tofu during my recovery gave me a wonderful boost. I could actually feel healing after a tofu milkshake. It eased the tissues. Most people douse tofu with soy sauce and fry it until it tastes horrible. I invented putting a slice of tofu (as thick as a slice of bread) in a blender along with a half cup of pineapple, a banana, and a glass of milk or juice. Beat it, and it comes out thick and creamy and delicious. That was usually my breakfast or lunch."

Lorraine J. Pakkala-Lintala; diagnosed in 1992 at age 62;
editor, author; Florida, New York

"A neighbor had breast cancer. While going through chemo, she was able to keep organic oatmeal down, cooked on the thin side. It's soothing to the stomach and strengthens the body—vital when it's being zapped by chemo and radiation. I also noticed that she gained some weight during the break between her chemo and radiation treatments. I thought she looked great and told her so. She said she'd been purposely eating more in order to gain weight, so when she had the inevitable weight loss, she'd be pretty much at her normal weight. Very clever. She never had an emaciated look—never looked like a patient at all!"

Nancy Summersong;
friend of a survivor; Tennessee

"I was surprised that my appetite was so good. I expected to lose weight during chemotherapy. In fact, I was sort of counting on it. Big disappointment. The first week after I recovered from chemo, I wanted to eat everything in sight, and usually did. The first food I craved was a McDonald's fish fillet sandwich. Talk about weird. After my fourth and fifth chemos, I wanted Shaw's potato salad, which was even *more* weird, since I had never tasted it before. The foods I wanted and could eat seemed to change during the course of the chemo. My rule of thumb was that if my brain and my stomach agreed on a food, I would eat it."

Val Long; diagnosed in 1999 at age 47;
administrative assistant; Massachusetts

"The biggest surprise: despite heavy-duty chemo, surgery, and radiation, nothing was as bad as I thought it might be. I never even threw up once! The new medications are wonderful, and ginger tea helped my stomach before it even thought of acting up."

Sharon Carr; diagnosed in 1997 at age 42;
hospice grief counselor; Rhode Island

"Being one of the lucky people who did not become nauseated from chemotherapy, I was determined to keep up my strength with lots of protein and dairy products. When the hospital dietitian said to me during one of my chemo treatments, 'Jean, I really don't think you need all those cheeseburgers and shakes—you weigh a little too much,' I knew I wasn't wasting away!"

Jean La Frombois; diagnosed in 1996 at age 57;
homemaker, part-time bookseller; Wisconsin

"After my first chemo, I went home and threw up for three days straight. A girlfriend had come to be with me after the chemo, and we joked that this was the way to lose those extra twenty pounds I'd been trying desperately to lose. For the remaining chemo sessions, I asked for more anti-nausea medication and didn't throw up another time."

Patti R. Martinez; diagnosed in 1999 at age 54;
realtor; California

"What helped most for the nausea was walking, breathing cool clean air, making myself move. I'd have a treatment, and my husband would come home and say, 'Hey! You need a walk.' And out the door he would pull me, but I did feel much better."

Pam Waddell; diagnosed in 1998 at age 38;
writer, teacher's aide; Texas

MAGIC BULLETS

"I had my water bottle and a baggie of animal crackers (the Wal-Mart brand was my favorite.) Animal crackers are just dry enough and just sweet enough. They became my best friends."

Michele Marks; diagnosed in 1996 at age 33;
CAD operator; Ohio

"The only foods that tasted good to me when I was on chemo were spaghetti and pudding. I ate them every day."

Paula Porter; diagnosed in 2000 at age 47;
telephone operator; New York

"Tuna fish and chicken noodle soup were great feel-better foods for me after a round of chemo. Chocolate chip cookies were a great soother, too."

Kathy Rabassa; diagnosed in 1999 at age 34;
administrative assistant; South Carolina

"Having crackers to chew on and a bottle of flat coke under my desk at work kept me going during chemo."

Alysa Cummings; diagnosed in 1998 at age 45;
educational trainer; New Jersey

"A glass of chocolate milk helped me during chemo."

Pam Waddell; diagnosed in 1998 at age 38;
writer, teacher's aide; Texas

"I craved cottage cheese. It made me feel good to eat it, and eat it I did. It did not nauseate me when I was having chemo. I ate it by the gallon."

Judy Komitee; diagnosed in 1998 at age 52;
secretary; New Jersey

"I swear by my Chinese tea and believe it is a huge contributing factor to my not having nausea at all during chemo."

Sandy Rodgers; diagnosed in 1999 at age 44;
homemaker, mom, registered nurse, Reiki master; Massachusetts

"Someone told me my symptoms sounded like a really bad hangover! Their suggestion that Gatorade was good for hangovers led to my drinking gallons of it, which helped steady that queasy shakiness."

                                         Jane Vaughan; diagnosed in 1991 at age 53;
                                                                  writer; Texas

"For me, it helped to eat a big lunch before chemo and to drink pop or my favorite Grapefruit Twister juice during chemo."

                                         A survivor; diagnosed in 1998 at age 45;
                                                               dentist; Indiana

"My favorite food was a donut. I'm not sure why, but it helped my stomach. Crackers helped if I felt sick."

                                    Mary Ann Budnick; diagnosed in 1991 at age 44;
                                                      school bus driver; Michigan

"Sucking on hard candy during treatment helped me minimize the nausea of chemotherapy."

                                      Nan Comstock; diagnosed in 1988 at age 39;
                                                       self-employed; California

"Soda crackers and mint ginger ale worked best for me for nausea."

                                       Irene Louise; diagnosed in 1995 at age 41;
                                         retired executive secretary; Pennsylvania

"My favorite food was a boiled potato. It helped with the nausea."

                                     Frances Gallello; diagnosed in 2000 at age 51;
                                          mental health assistant; New York

"For nausea, Life Savers really are life savers!"

                                   Mitzi Scarborough; diagnosed in 1999 at age 37;
                                              childcare provider; Arkansas

"Orange Gatorade tasted best to me during chemo. I drank it by the gallon."

Becky Honeycutt; diagnosed in 1995 at age 53;
licensed practical nurse; Indiana

"I ate lots of applesauce, and actually gained ten pounds during my last three months of chemo!"

Rosamary Amiet; diagnosed in 2000 at age 48;
program manager; Ohio

"When my cousin was going through chemo, she only wanted thick chocolate shakes."

Donna Krol;
cousin of survivor; Massachusetts

"I had a cup of coffee and a donut with my treatments, and I drank lots and lots of water."

Susan Schultz; diagnosed in 1990 at age 41;
special education teacher's aide; New York

"Lots of ginger, ginger tea, cookies, and nuts all help with nausea."

Mindy Greenside; diagnosed in 2000 at age 48;
midwife; Maryland

"My favorite things to eat and drink during treatment were ginger ale and Lorna Doone cookies. I ate yogurt every day to combat mouth sores and diarrhea, neither of which I ever got."

Deborah J.P. Schur; diagnosed in 1994 at age 43;
sales rep; Massachusetts

"With chemo, I gained so much water weight—once it was eleven pounds. So I ate watermelon, which is a natural diuretic, and I lost all the weight in two days."

Judith Ormond; diagnosed in 1996 at age 49;
symphony musician—piccolo; Wisconsin

STAYING UPBEAT

"Think positive. Chemo is something they do *for* you, not *to* you. Chemo is a weapon in a war. You are taking control by submitting to chemo. You are now the aggressor. Each treatment is a bombardment of the enemy. When you really feel lousy, then you know the weapon is doing a good job attacking that enemy."

Patricia Baker; diagnosed in 1993 at age 49;
at home; Massachusetts

"I used Pac Man as imagery to eat up any errant cancer cells during chemo. When I walked, which I did most every day (I think that really helped with fatigue also), I would picture those little guys gobbling up all those bad growing cells in and around lots of my organs and bones."

Robin Smith; diagnosed in 2000 at age 53;
microbiologist, homemaker; New York

"My friends came to all my treatments and helped pass the time. We ordered food and watched movies, which made everything much more tolerable."

Asha Mevlana; diagnosed in 1999 at age 24;
musician; New York

"If you have to spend a prolonged stretch in the hospital, bring music with you. Most hospitals have TVs available, but no radios. Music can be a tonic or a tranquilizer. It's an effective, healthy mood enhancer with no bad side effects."

Barbara Keiler;
sister, and daughter of a survivor; Massachusetts

"I felt a hundred years old after eight rounds of chemo. No one could explain why. Finally, a doctor at another medical center said that about a quarter of his patients felt like this for no known reason after the completion of chemo."

Monica May; diagnosed in 1997 at age 40;
organizing consultant; New Mexico

"I always applied skin care products and makeup daily, so I never looked sick. Friends would always comment on how good I looked, and before long I started feeling that way."

Cheryl Cavallo; diagnosed in 1997 at age 35;
homemaker; Massachusetts

"Makeup, makeup, makeup! Nothing helps to restore your sense of femininity more than a face that looks better than people expect it to. Eyeliner disguises the loss of your eyelashes, and bangs on a wig hide disappearing eyebrows. Do anything not to feel like a patient. Always get dressed and groomed in the morning, even on the bad days. With the greatly improved anti-nausea medication, life can go on. I never missed a party. Even if I couldn't eat the hors d'oeuvres, festive company took me out of myself, and my family and I were better for it."

Patricia Baker; diagnosed in 1993 at age 49;
at home; Massachusetts

"I put on makeup every day. A good eyeliner pencil does wonders when the eyelashes are gone. Draw on eyebrows, then use a brow brush to make them look real. Don't do what I did several times—accidentally rub one of your brows off! I still laugh about that. Remember to smile every day. It feels good!"

Sherry Ann Wells; diagnosed in 1997 at age 45;
homemaker; Missouri

"My first round of chemo, the nausea drug worked okay *if* I could take it and keep it down. I took an immediate dislike to the look of the pill, and I'd never been very good at taking pills anyway. I'm a gagger, and just the thought of taking something four times a day would get me started. The second round of chemo, they gave me a new drug. This was like a miracle. First, I liked the way it looked. Second, I only had to take it twice a day."

Val Long; diagnosed in 1999 at age 47; administrative assistant; Massachusetts

"I did not tolerate chemo well. When you get sick from drugs and nothing helps, you just want to end the suffering. Then I looked at the faces of my two Corgi dogs, and I knew I could not leave my husband and them. I decided that I could beat this. Sure enough, we found an anti-nausea drug that helped."

Kathy Rabassa; diagnosed in 1999 at age 34; administrative assistant; South Carolina

"For hot flashes brought on by chemo, invest in a powerful air conditioner and wear cotton clothing."

Penny Trosterman; diagnosed in 1996 at age 45; English teacher; New York

"I gained weight during treatment; now I've lost it again. What a great feeling!"

Linda Perkins; diagnosed in 1999 at 35; project manager; New Jersey

"Camisole tops made of a nice silk were my favorites during treatment. I bought several loose jackets and blouses like jackets, and wore them over the tops or a dress."

Carol Hattler; diagnosed in 1999 at age 65; retired nurse; Virginia

"It's important to have really comfortable jammies. I did a lot of lounging around my apartment, and my purple flannel pj's almost never came off my body."

Asha Mevlana; diagnosed in 1999 at age 24; musician; New York

"For chemo sessions, I wore tee-shirts from exciting events or trips. They were a sort of talisman."

Judith Ormond; diagnosed in 1996 at age 49;
symphony musician—piccolo; Wisconsin

"I covered my baldness with a funny baseball hat. For each day of treatment I wore different cartoon tee-shirts. My favorite was Goofy with a high sign! At the last treatment, I gave cartoon tee-shirts to all the staff."

Carol Snyder; diagnosed in 1992 at age 47;
special education teacher; New York

"On the days of chemotherapy, I would finish my treatment; have lunch with family, friends, or co-workers; and then go home and catch a quick nap. On that weekend, we always planned a fun trip or event. This way the attention was taken away from me and placed on a fun family outing. Not only did it entertain the kids, but I enjoyed these outings. Also, on the night before most of my chemotherapy treatments, I would have a full-body massage to help relax and renew me. Later, I learned that Reiki is very helpful before treatments. I have since become a Reiki practitioner and help other women before they have their chemotherapy."

Deborah J.P. Schur; diagnosed in 1994 at age 43;
sales rep; Massachusetts

"During chemo, you'd be better not using fingers for makeup application. Instead, use a sponge or disposable applicator. Discard makeup that you used before chemotherapy, as it may contain bacteria that your body can no longer ward off because of the drop in white blood count. When defenses are down, it is also a good idea to open a new mascara every three months."

Jean Joyce; diagnosed in 1999 at age 51;
hairdresser, salon owner; Virginia

"Three days after completing chemotherapy, I served as a team captain for the local Race for the Cure, just as I had for the three years before my diagnosis. Though I didn't attempt running or walking, my participation let everyone know I was okay."

Ellen Beth Simon; diagnosed in 1998 at age 41;

lawyer; New Jersey

"Can someone tell me how to lose weight while I'm taking tamoxifen? I have two more years to take it. But then, needing to lose weight isn't so bad. I'm alive and plan to stay that way for many years to come."

Penny Trosterman; diagnosed in 1996 at age 45;

English teacher; New York

6 • Taking the Reins

Regaining Control

Loss of control is a major issue for those with breast cancer. It starts early on, when a problem is first suspected, and suddenly we're taken over by fear, not to mention mammography machines, localization needles, hospital release forms, and biopsies. Then a positive diagnosis comes, and we're *really* hit for a loop. We're swamped by new information, confused by choices, intimidated by sterile rooms. We worry enough to lose sleep; we're hurting from surgery, weak from anesthesia, and stressed over family demands; and we are *not* looking forward to the treatment ahead. There's this big . . . big C looming over us, pressing us under its weight, threatening to dominate our daily lives for the next however-long.

But stop. Take a breath. Tell yourself that you *have* to be positive, because you're the one in the driver's seat here. Oh, you may have to work at it a little, and the change may not take place overnight. Being positive can take practice. More than anyone else, though, you can make it happen.

"You need to set the tone," wrote Anne Jacobs, managing part-

ner of a Massachusetts real estate firm. "I found that being upbeat, coming to therapy with a smile on my face, being interested,
and communicating that interest to the people around me had an
uplifting effect on everyone. I remember feeling down one day in
the elevator on the way to therapy. As the doors opened I forced a
big smile. My whole body responded, and I bounced into the waiting area. I felt in control."

Jane Royal-Davidson, an educator from North Carolina, came
at it a different way. "I was more frightened by the chemo than the
cancer, but I had been told by my friend, a doctor, that I was the
driver of the train. I had complete control. So I let only those people who were supportive on the train, and left those who were uncomfortable off. I could control cancer, or it would control me. I
chose to have control."

Cathleen D'Antonio, a Connecticut survivor who learned she
had breast cancer in 1994, was 28 at the time. "My being diagnosed was a huge shock," she wrote. "But instead of dwelling on
the 'why me' factor, I saved my energies for tackling the disease.
One of the things that has helped me over the years is accepting
that there are going to be some dark days. The light at the end of
the tunnel comes from knowing that I have nephews, nieces, parents, and other family members who are always there to give me a
laugh, a shoulder to cry on, or a good ear to listen. I was just going
through a rough breakup when I was diagnosed. Even in my sadness, I learned that I was a great person, that I could enjoy being
myself."

Someone else learned it, too. In his own contribution to UPLIFT,
Cathleen's husband, Mark D'Antonio, writes, "I fell in love with my
wife one year after her diagnosis . . . ."

Which is proof that having a positive attitude does more than
beat cancer.

So. There's determination, imagery, and love. There are also
some more concrete things that we can do. Cornelia Doherty, a
sixteen-year survivor from Massachusetts, recalls, "I needed to

have some control in a situation over which I had no control. So I decided that I would drive myself to every one of my chemo treatments and to every day of radiation. Many, many people wanted to help me, but it gave me great strength to do it myself."

Florence Wade, a Texan who was diagnosed in 1999, regained control by keeping busy with things that made her happy. "I read two or three novels each week, kept a journal now and then, and put together a grandmother's memory book, which I had duplicated and bound for each of my four grandchildren."

Helaine Hemingway, who was diagnosed at the age of forty-one, tells how she regained control. "Long-term goals were helpful. I continued to teach and work on my masters degree."

What did I do to regain control? I've been thinking about that a lot. I mean, I told you that I got my own tattoo, which satisfied my need to thumb my nose at those other little blue ones. And the convertible. . . . Oh. I didn't mention that? Well, I needed a new car anyway, and the boys were grown and had cars of their own, and I'd always wanted a convertible but had never thought they were safe enough. Then it struck me that I'd had cancer. I could do what I wanted to do. So I bought the convertible, and these many years later I still own it, even over the objections of our oldest son, who never tires of arguing that my convertible would be much happier in balmy Washington, D. C. (with his wife and him), than in the cold and stormy Northeast.

Sorry, Eric. That baby's mine. For me, that convertible is a symbol of health, strength, and freedom from fear. It also represents the broader tactic that helped me regain control when cancer tried to rob me of it—defiance.

Oops. Is "defiance" too strong a word? Okay. Try boldness. Boldness enabled me to say, *Yes, I want a convertible!* It also allowed me to do a slew of smaller things that really helped—like finding a tailor with whom I was comfortable enough to be able to say, *I've had breast cancer and reconstruction, so I'd like you to alter the darts on the front of this dress to fit my new breasts,* and like looking a pushy saleswoman in the eye and saying, Yes, I know that I'm young enough to wear that barely-there bathing suit you're holding, but I've had breast cancer and reconstruction, and I'm not quite comfortable with that particular upper half. That shut her up fast! Actually, my speaking up worked like a charm in both cases; both women were understanding and solicitous. Quite frankly, I cannot imagine another woman being anything but understanding and solicitous when we tell them something like that.

In an attempt to remember other things that I'd done during those months that helped on the issue of control, I went through my stash of old calendars and pulled out the ones that had hung on the kitchen wall during the years of my surgeries and treatment. Well, we went to dinner with friends, and we went to family events. We went to parents' weekends at the kids' colleges and to Florida weekends for my husband's law firm. I gave some local speeches, plus one in San Antonio. I went to cousins' lunches, to the dentist, to the eye doctor. I had my car serviced. I went with son No.1 when he had his wisdom teeth pulled, and son No. 2 when he needed clothes, and son No. 3 on a date for Thai food. I had my hair cut. I had my hair highlighted. I had my nails done— actually had them done every week during that whole time and still do—and I make no apologies for the indulgence. With my hands on a keyboard all day long, I see my fingernails more than any other part of my body!

So. No clues to coping with cancer on my calendars. They were filled with the normal day-to-day workings of my life, not particularly different from the years before and since.

Of course . . . you guessed it. The remarkable thing was the absence of cancer on those pages. I actually had to struggle to reconstruct that journey—dates of biopsies, surgery planning sessions, start of radiation. The only note on my calendar that marked my mastectomy was a large squiggle over the day. Two days after that, the twins turned twenty-one. They were in col-

lege, one in Connecticut and one in Pennsylvania. I remember
sending them gift baskets of crackers, cheese, and microbrewery
beer to mark their being old enough to drink. Not that beer took
precedence over cancer, but my sons' twenty-first birthday certainly did!

Studying those calendars, I realized that my method of coping
with cancer had been to continue on with the rest of my life. Oh,
yeah, I did figure out that "2 P.M. with Dr. Y" meant an appointment
with my plastic surgeon for saline injections. But notes like that
weren't prominent. They were entered on those calendars in the
same small print that I used to mark the time when the exterminator
was due for his quarterly visit. *Everything looks good, Mrs. D. A few
mice in the garage, comin' in from the cold, but we can live with that.*

I sure can.

FEELING GOOD ABOUT OURSELVES

"What made me feel feminine again? Aromatherapy—scented
candles and a nice, hot bath sprinkled with scented salts and oils.
Also, sexy lingerie worn under lace or velvet tops."

Carrie Drake; diagnosed in 1998 at age 42;
administrative assistant; Colorado

"The best thing that I do for myself right now is to use a foamy
body wash in the shower so that those bubbles of foam cover my
body. I love that feeling."

Susan Smith; diagnosed in 2000 at age 53;
medical library technician; Pennsylvania

"After my surgery, I learned to enjoy the luxury of a long hot
shower. I had always been in too big of a hurry to allow myself to
stay in the shower for ten to fifteen minutes!"

Wanda Null; diagnosed in 1986 at age 41;
librarian; Massachusetts

"Never underestimate the value of a good shopping spree—by catalogue from home, if necessary."

Susan Rothstein; diagnosed in 1997 at age 49;
travel agent; Massachusetts

"One of my fondest memories was strutting into Victoria's Secret to find the sexiest black lace bra they had . . . the more expensive the better."

Kathi Ward; diagnosed in 1994 at age 47;
merchandiser; South Carolina

"The main thing we all need to remember is to rest and eat. I was always one to go, go, go, and now this is the time to relax and enjoy life. That is how I feel to this day. Life is precious."

Candice Jaeger; diagnosed in 2000 at age 24;
wife, mother; Illinois

"Get a massage or a pedicure or both. I did, and it really gave me something to look forward to. If you've just had surgery, you might consider reflexology. It is a massage of the feet that lasts an hour and relaxes the entire body. You will be very comfortable and not have to worry about the surgery site."

Rhonda Sorrell; diagnosed in 1998 at age 43;
special education teacher; Michigan

"I bought several beautiful nightgowns, a fabulous wig, great hats, and new makeup. I always wore the wig, and I always dressed impeccably, no matter how awful I felt. It was important to me that no one think of me as sick."

Cornelia Doherty; diagnosed in 1985 at age 45;
mother, widow, speaker; Massachusetts

"My advice? Do not sit back feeling sorry for yourself. Take one day at a time, and do all you can to live as normally as possible. For me, that meant looking my best every day. I wore a nice wig and made sure that my makeup was on the minute I was out of the shower. I felt very special when I did this."

Carol Downer; diagnosed in 1997 at age 48;
legal secretary; New York

"When I left the hospital, I was determined to look my best—and I succeeded, although I crawled into bed when I got home and slept for four hours! I knew that if I felt good about my appearance, it would go a long way toward speeding my recovery. When I became tired or my incision hurt, I learned to take care of myself by lessening physical activity until I felt stronger. The long-term effect was that my house isn't as clean as it used to be, and there is definitely more clutter, but I am comfortable with that."

Wanda Null; diagnosed in 1986 at age 41;
librarian; Massachusetts

"Hire a housekeeper once a week. Save your strength for your family."

Rhonda Sorrell; diagnosed in 1998 at age 43;
special education teacher; Michigan

"The most practical thing that I've done for myself since last year is to have my house cleaned professionally every two weeks. The two hours that it takes two women to do an excellent job saves me the stress of wanting a clean house while juggling the need to have fun and still working full time."

Christine Foutris; diagnosed in 1999 at age 49;
teacher; Illinois

"The advice that I would give to a friend? Clean house. Clean up your inner and outer house, meaning your mind and your body, to make room for new positive thoughts and actions."

Carol Pasternak; diagnosed in 1986 at age 47;
artist; Ontario, Canada

"Acupuncture helped me overcome fatigue. I also tried heal-touch therapy and had massages. It's good to feel cared for."

Judith Ormond; diagnosed in 1996 at age 49;
symphony musician—piccolo; Wisconsin

"Walking and meditation helped me a lot. There was a great group meditation in my ten-week mind-body class, and they gave us individual tapes for meditation, since it was difficult to get my mind to concentrate enough to do it myself. Also, to help feel in control, I attended discussion groups, swim therapy, and yoga for cancer patients, plus a wonderful support group that I still attend at the cancer center."

Joanne Tutschek; diagnosed in 1998 at age 55;
research communications director; New Jersey

"I read a book that opened my eyes to the connection between diet and cancer. I changed my diet completely after reading it. I used to be a junk food junkie, eating whatever I wanted whenever I wanted. Now, I am almost a total vegetarian—eating only organic turkey on occasion, and organic eggs and raw goat milk cheese. I don't eat out anymore, and I cook everything from scratch. In spite of the cancer, I feel better than I have in the last ten years. I wouldn't change this for anything."

A survivor; diagnosed in 2000 at age 43;
teacher; Illinois

"During my hospital stay, I was quite a health nut. I took vitamins E and C daily, ate garlic regularly, and believed that tofu was a food of the gods. I watched my hospital roommates down potato chips and Coke for breakfast. They were always awake in the night complaining of indigestion and restlessness."

Lorraine J. Pakkala-Lintala; diagnosed in 1992 at age 62;
editor, author; Florida, New York

"I had a need to control something, and walking helped. That was 'my' time. An hour with earphones and music helped reduce anxiety. I focused on eating healthier. That was something else I could control. I also made a decision to smile every time I looked in a mirror, and I soon found that I smiled a lot and that the reflection looking back at me no longer seemed so frightened."

Pauline Hughes; diagnosed in 1997 at age 61;
retired registered nurse; Florida

"I felt most in control when I was pulling weeds in my front yard. This 'therapy' was mindless but productive work that allowed for much daydreaming. I likened the pulling of weeds to the killing of cancer cells. I still love to weed."

Beth Compton; diagnosed in 1995 at age 27;
civil engineer; South Carolina

"These days the sun seems brighter and the sky bluer. I continue to plan ahead, as it helps me to have something to look forward to. We live in Colorado, and the mountains are truly healing for me. Hiking and four-wheeling to see the backcountry is the best medicine around!"

Judy Peterson; diagnosed in 2000 at age 58;
registered nurse; Colorado

"Being a couch potato is okay, too! You don't have to do anything—fighting cancer is enough."

Linda Perkins; diagnosed in 1999 at age 35;
project manager; New Jersey

"I continued to work, write letters, and shop even though I did feel tired sometimes. Good food, good friends, and a loving family made it all worthwhile."

Marge Fuller; diagnosed in 1994 at age 63;
Yakima school district, retired; Washington

"I think the best thing you can do to regain control is to live your life as you did before. Go to church, go to weddings, visit family, play with your children or grandchildren, take drives to the mountains. Read or walk. My husband would take me for ice cream frequently during chemotherapy. I know one woman whose husband took her dancing every week when she was undergoing cobalt treatments many, many years ago."

Faye Hardiman; diagnosed in 1998 at age 50;
wife, mother, teacher; Georgia

"After having a mastectomy, I was devastated to learn that I would have to go through months of chemotherapy. So I found a project to do. My closet shelves were lined with boxes of my two daughters' memorabilia, from their first drawings through their college scrapbooks. My husband, Fred, joined in to write special messages of our memories of different events. These were albums of love and hope for me, my own special therapy, and it worked! I realized that there were still so many memories to make with my family, and it made me strong."

Carol Merrill; diagnosed in 1996 at age 48;
housewife; Missouri

"What kept my friends and relatives so supportive was their seeing me out doing things and not feeling down. I was determined not to put my life on hold. Four days after my first chemo treatment, my husband and I went camping. Three days after coming home from the hospital after my mastectomy, I went to dinner with the Ladies Auxiliary of the VFW. People were surprised to see me out, but I felt good. A positive attitude helps the healing process."

Diane Zellar; diagnosed in 2000 at age 51;
homemaker; New York

READING, WRITING, AND REASONING

"What helped pass time in lieu of worrying? For me it was reading. I read tons of books. It was a great escape."

Gwen Loverink; diagnosed in 1994 at age 34;
police dispatcher; California

"I often felt saddest at bedtime, when my mind would fill with fear. I found it helped to read before bed each night to help replace the terror with other thoughts and images. My favorite reads turned out to be what I called 'comfort food books'—novels I'd read before and loved. Although usually I rarely reread books, during this time it felt too overwhelming to focus on new books, particularly since so many plots involve tragedy and death, either of which would have made me feel worse. Returning to the pages of old friends was comforting and safe, often evoking warm memories of the first time I'd enjoyed the book. A five-minute reading dose each night made a noticeable decrease in the number of nightly tears on my pillow and panic-filled cancer dreams."

Dorian Solot; diagnosed in 2000 at age 26;
Massachusetts

"Having a creative project that doesn't give you time to feel sorry for yourself after surgery is a wonderful help. I write a mystery series about an absent-minded sleuth, and the deadline for the fifth book in the series was six months after the mastectomy. So I immersed myself in my writing."

Elizabeth Daniels Squire; diagnosed in 1998 at age 71;
author; North Carolina

"Writing has always helped me through tough times. I began keeping a journal about my experience. It helped to get thoughts—both good and bad—out of my head. Often it let me see that something wasn't as bad as I thought, or it simply organized the thoughts that kept running randomly through my head."

Val Long; diagnosed in 1999 at age 47;
administrative assistant; Massachusetts

"I started writing in my journal an hour every day. I call it 'My Healing Journal.' I also meditate and take long walks. I started acupuncture and acupressure treatments to balance my energy and unclog any stagnant areas, and I take Chinese herbs twice daily in the form of tea."

Sandy Rodgers; diagnosed in 1999 at age 44;
homemaker, mom, registered nurse, Reiki master; Massachusetts

"A friend gave me a 'grateful journal' to write down my thoughts. I began to write three things I was grateful for each night. I would drift off to sleep thinking of those things, rather than of the fear that I felt."

Cheryl Cavallo; diagnosed in 1997 at age 35;
homemaker; Massachusetts

"I joined a memoir writing class specifically for breast cancer survivors. That has helped me deal with the emotional impact of having breast cancer."

Judith Ormond; diagnosed in 1996 at age 49;
symphony musician—piccolo; Wisconsin

"I continued to work, and since I am involved in a helping profession, it was great for me to not have time to dwell on my own problem too much. I did contact a professional colleague and went back into short-term counseling. Of course, I am a three- to five-book-a-week romance reader, which also helped!"

Nancie Watson; diagnosed in 1995 at age 50;
social worker; Pennsylvania

"I found that a wonderful aid was a pillow speaker, so that I could hear the radio when I woke up startled, remembering that the cancer was real. The small speaker, which can be bought at Radio Shack, rests on the pillow and is most distracting from frightening thoughts. The sound of the radio also helps put you to sleep."

Debbie MacLean; diagnosed in 1991 at age 47;
volunteer, hospital gift shop and hospice; Massachusetts

"My condo is my sanctuary. Being able to stay where I choose, at home in Telluride, means I'm in control."

Carrie Drake; diagnosed in 1998 at age 42;
administrative assistant; Colorado

"Take care of something. Buy some plants and keep them in good shape. Get a kitten and give it loving attention. The presence of living, growing things at a time of great stress helps decrease the stress and gives you realities outside yourself and your immediate situation. The same thing is true of art. Go to a theater, a museum, a concert, or ballet. Art can take us out of ourselves, lift us beyond our immediate environment, enrich us spiritually and aesthetically. Opening yourself to great beauty is always a life-enhancer. In times of crisis, it's also healing."

Susan Stamberg; diagnosed in 1986 at age 48;
broadcast journalist; Washington, D.C.

"I had two Siamese kitties at the time, and they certainly kept my spirits up. Always an animal lover, I feel that the love of a pet is something everyone should experience."

Barbara C. Sumner; diagnosed in 1982 at age 59;
homemaker; New Hampshire

"Before, during, and after my mastectomy and reconstruction, I used a series of audio tapes called the Surgical Support Series. I think it was due to these tapes that I was able to leave the hospital after a day and a half, rather than the five days predicted. Included in the series are recovery and recuperation tapes, which I later used to relax and program my body to heal and to handle pain. During chemo, I used another series of tapes, the Positive Immunity Program. Turning off the telephone, closing my bedroom door, and putting on my earphones was a wonderful escape from the stresses and anxieties of my life. I still use the Immunity tapes occasionally now to relax, boost my mood, and direct my energies toward healing. Since my diagnosis, I have cured myself of a lifelong eating disorder, quit a job that I hated, fulfilled a lifelong dream by buying a house on the coast, and learned an awful lot about love."

Sandra Miller; diagnosed in 1997 at age 50;
attorney; California

"It's important to feel positive and in control during chemo. Have projects to look forward to completing: take a computer class at a local college, do a cross-stitch sampler for a friend's new baby, keep a journal, take a watercolor class from a local park system. I redecorated my bathroom—I figured I was spending so much time in there, why not make it cheerful and fun!"

Sue Braun; diagnosed in 1988 at age 41;
homemaker; Ohio

"I was diagnosed with cancer in 1978. I had opened a gift and gourmet shop the previous year and was enjoying its success. I am glad I had the shop to keep me busy and my mind from dwelling on the negative."

Adelaide D. Key; diagnosed in 1978 at age 42;
community volunteer, philanthropist; North Carolina

"After you decide that you're going to live, it's time to make changes for yourself. Do things you want to do, and learn how to say 'no' to things you don't. I turned down a chance to be secretary of my local kennel club again. On the other hand, I've be-

come more active in the union at my job. I've also made changes
in my lifestyle. For example, I'm now a member of 'our lady of
perpetual diets,' and I've taken up the treadmill. I really hate this
stuff, but I've figured out a way to make it bearable. I'm rewarding myself for weight loss—with jewelry. I have rewards for each
weight goal. There's nothing like positive reinforcement to get
you to do what's good for you!"

Sharon Irons Strempski; diagnosed in 1997 at age 52;

registered nurse; Connecticut

"The best thing I did was decide to take off the rest of the school
year and use the time to enjoy my friends and do things for which
I normally didn't have time. I played with my dog's litter of pup-
pies, met friends for lunch, and generally enjoyed my 'vacation.'
As I see it, you have two choices: You can put your head under a
pillow and go 'Poor me!' or you can go on with your life. I guess
you know which I chose."

Lynne Rutenberg; diagnosed in 1980 at age 35;

retired teacher, New Jersey

WORKING AT IT

"At first, I just wanted to stay home and nurse my wounds, both
physical and mental, but I really couldn't. I was running a doctor's
office by myself, since my co-worker had just relocated. My daughter had become engaged a few months before, and we were smack
in the middle of planning a big wedding. And my husband and I
had bought a new house right before my diagnosis, so we had to
pack up the old house and move into the new one. All great
things, but horrible timing! The point of this is that everything
worked out fine, and the time went by quickly because I was so
busy. I was definitely distracted from thinking about cancer!"

Deborah Lambert; diagnosed in 2000 at age 47;

medical secretary; Massachusetts

"My treatment took place in October, November, and December—the most stressful time of year. I had to learn to let go of what wasn't important, and that included a lot of self-induced stress over the holiday preparations."

Deb Haney; diagnosed in 1996 at age 48;
administrative assistant, artist; Massachusetts

"To keep my spirits up when I wasn't feeling well, I had a quote hanging on my mirror. Muhammad Ali once said, 'I hated every minute of training, but I said to myself, *Suffer now and live the rest of your life as a champion.'* I changed it around to say, 'I hated every minute of chemo, but I said to myself, *Suffer now and live the rest of your life as a champion.'* "

Asha Mevlana; diagnosed in 1999 at age 24;
musician; New York

"Before my diagnosis, I had been discouraged by the prospect of turning fifty with my life not going the way I wanted it to. After my surgery, I lay on the couch feeling even worse! I don't know what it was—probably all the phone calls, flowers, and cards—but it suddenly hit me. I realized that I could either dwell on this and be miserable, or get on with my life. The things I was depressed about were not important. The things I was looking for were right in front of me, and I didn't know it! I had the love of family, friends, and co-workers, and most of all my boyfriend Jerry. I am greatly thankful."

Sharon Daniels; diagnosed in 2000 at age 49;
hairstylist, wig store owner; Massachusetts

* * *

"Because I wanted a full-length bathroom mirror
I had a shower door installed with one
Before I went somewhere, I could check my clothes
See if I looked OK.
Finally, the doctor said I could shower

All of my things gathered, I went in
Started to undress, suddenly, I felt sick
That huge mirror, I was standing in front of it
Without the bandage, I hadn't seen the scar
Didn't want to see it, never wanted to see
That area again. What to do?
A large towel, I hung it over the door,
Covered the mirror. For several months I did that
One day I felt I could look, slowly took the towel down
Crying, I stood there, but realized it didn't look so bad . . .
It has been seven years
I don't think about all these things much anymore
Alive, I'm just happy to be
Just to be happy, I'm alive."

Regina Vaughn; diagnosed in 1993 at age 45;
drapery shop owner; Ohio

* * *

"Hindsight can be harmful. Let go of the 'what ifs,' the 'maybes,' and the 'should haves.' Practice living life to the fullest."

Stella Norman; diagnosed in 1999 at age 64;
addictions counselor; Virginia

"My entire being seemed to change overnight. I was no longer the blonde, athletic, zestful, happy-go-lucky girl I'd once been. My past was over, my future looked grim, and my present seemed futile. I became so miserable that I was forced to live moment by moment instead of one day at a time. But those moments kept coming, and gradually, like a thousand dazzling lights slow-dancing toward me, I saw that life does go on for cancer patients. This revelation surprised me and filled me with a sense of relief the likes of which I've never felt before. It was as if a great big 'WHEW' blew through me. I began getting up every morning, putting on makeup, and getting dressed. One day I accepted an invitation to lunch. Another day I began to take regular walks. Before I knew it, I was back to my old self—except for one major difference. I took nothing for granted—not a star, not a song, not a smile—nothing. Life would never be the same for me. I could grieve or I could celebrate. The choice was mine."

Sallie Burdine; diagnosed in 1998 at age 44;
author; Florida

"I was the only person who could take control of my life. I knew that I was not ready to go anywhere, since I wanted to see my grandchildren grow up. So, after the upset of learning I had cancer, I decided that my humor, my faith, and most of all my attitude would be how I could take control."

Barbara Moro; diagnosed in 1999 at age 57;
law secretary; New Jersey

IMAGERY AND ART

"I like visualization and imagery. It's something that I always put in the category of don't-know-if-it-helps-but-it-can't-hurt! When I was undergoing radiation treatment, I visualized myself sitting under a waterfall in Hawaii and having the water flow over me and wash away all the cancer cells. It was peaceful and calm, and the scenery was beautiful. A couple of times, when the radiation therapist came back into the room and told me I could go, I said I wasn't finished with my visualization, so I couldn't leave just yet!"

Sheilah Musselman; diagnosed in 1997 at age 56;
registered nurse; Virginia

"Years ago, I had heard about the use of visualization in the treatment of cancer. So I started visualizing my healthy 'good' cells traveling through my body wearing 'headlights' like coal miners. Shining their light beams to identify 'bad' cancer cells, the 'good' cells used picks and shovels to dump the 'bad' cells outside of my body. I sent in as many 'good' cells as were needed, until all the 'bad' cancer cells were gone. I still periodically send in those 'good' cells, searching with their 'headlights' to keep my body cancer-free."

Joan Eldredge; diagnosed in 1998 at age 65;
motor home enthusiast and U.S. circumnavigator, retired psychotherapist;
Pennsylvania

"As an artist I have a vehicle through which I can transform my experiences into healing objects. For instance, when I was in pre-op for surgery, lying there with wires sticking out of my breast to mark the perimeter of my tumor, my surgeon stuck his head in and asked if I was picking up any good radio stations with my antenna. Later I used polymer clay to make a 'boob pin,' depicting the breast as an old-fashioned radio, with wire antennas and nipple knobs. I made a smaller 'A cup' size one for the surgeon and a slightly larger 'B cup' size one for myself. For years, I displayed this pin when I did art festivals as a reminder to women to have regular mammograms and to the men in their lives to see that they did."

Jeanne Sturdevant; diagnosed in 1990 at age 45;
artist; Texas

"I was first diagnosed in 1978, a divorced single mother of thirty-eight. For the better part of twenty-two years, I have lived with breast cancer, and life is joyful, precious, and peaceful. Because I am a collagist, I favor the 'collage approach' to coping. A collage is an art form in which diverse elements are arranged to form a new image. Collage is also an empowering metaphor for designing life. Each of us is the powerful creator of the work of art in progress—the masterpiece known as our life. The elements in my own personal collage include twice-daily meditation, regular yoga practice, a vegetarian diet, therapeutic massages, sessions with a hands-on energy healer, time spent in nature, reading reading reading, writing, journaling, and collaging. I coach people in using the latter: a simple tool for releasing stress and upsets, discovering one's true Self, and learning the pleasure of creative expression. My home is a sanctuary filled with delights for all my senses. I cultivate quiet, calm, contemplation, close friendships, and love. I consciously practice a 'gratitude attitude' daily, count my many blessings, and make certain that each day is as delicious as I can make it."

Susan Zimmerman; diagnosed in 1978 at age 38;
collagist; California

"THE WORRY BOX"

"I found that the most constructive thing I did was to say, 'I have cancer.' Like many people, I didn't want to say the word. It was like swearing in front of a priest! I also had to tell my family that it was okay to say 'cancer.' It is important to be able to say it freely. It is also important to let people know that you are not giving up on life. I was not going to let cancer get me down. I refused to worry about it. I knew that worrying wouldn't help and that positive thinking was important. Attitude has a lot to do with your recuperation."

Barbara Moro; diagnosed in 1999 at age 57;
law secretary; New Jersey

"I think one of the very best things I did was to talk about what I was going through. I told everyone I could. Saying the words 'I've been diagnosed with breast cancer' helped me accept my situation. I didn't want people to feel weird talking to me after they found out from others. By my telling them myself, they were able to see that I was okay. I think that my honesty and openness gave me strength and had a big impact on my friends and family. I tried to keep the tone light, positive, and upbeat when I talked to people, and this made them want to stay connected to me. I needed this connection, and I needed it on a daily basis. I needed to hear myself sounding okay."

Julie Crandall; diagnosed in 1998 at age 31;
stay-at-home mom; North Carolina

"Talk, talk, talk. The more you talk about your problems, the more people around you will understand what you're going through. They are going through this with you, too."

Tammi Keller; diagnosed in 2000 at age 30;
mom; Pennsylvania

"One of the things that helped me get through this was talking to friends and family about my feelings and concerns. One friend advised me to take charge of my illness, not to leave it up to other people. I truly believe this is one reason why I have been cancer-free for thirteen years."

Polly Briggs; diagnosed in 1987 at age 41;
secretary; Mississippi

"When I felt depressed, I went for counseling. It was the best thing I could have done. I learned to love myself—a very important part of the healing process."

E. Mary Lou Clauss; diagnosed in 1991 at age 55;
homemaker, retired registered nurse; Pennsylvania

"See a counselor. I did, and it helped relieve my anxiety and my feeling of hopelessness. It was a very positive experience."

Rhonda Sorrell; diagnosed in 1998 at age 43;
special education teacher; Michigan

"Plan a trip now for a post-treatment celebration. It will give you something to look forward to."

Alexandra Koffman; diagnosed in 1997 at age 40;
registered nurse; Massachusetts

"The best advice I got was from a good friend who said, 'Pamper yourself! If it feels good, do it!' That sometimes meant a good cry and a long nap."

Sharon Carr; diagnosed in 1997 at age 42;
hospice grief counselor; Rhode Island

"Allow yourself life's little indulgences. It feels good. Indulge in a good cry when you need it."

Susan Rothstein; diagnosed in 1997 at age 49;
travel agent; Massachusetts

"The Worry Box. In the winter of 1992, when I was forty-two, I was diagnosed with breast cancer. I was immediately focused. I knew what I had to do, and I did it. I researched my disease, and my family and I made decisions. After the mastectomy, though, I began to worry. I worried about our decisions and the impact of all that had happened on my family. I worried about the future. I worried about a recurrence. I worried about my daughter. I worried about *everything*. A counselor suggested a strategy that helped me more than anything. I found a box and glued colorful scraps of wrapping paper on the top. Inside it, each morning, I tucked handwritten notes about my worries and fears. Then I closed the lid and went on with the rest of the day, whether it was walking in the woods, listening to music, grocery shopping, paying bills, or cuddling up with my daughter to read a book. The Worry Box also provided me with a concrete way of saying 'Enough! I want to live

my life and make the most of each and every day!' I have the
box to this day."

Nancy Burgess; diagnosed in 1992 at age 42;
teacher, mother, wife; New Hampshire

"Do for others. There are always some who are in deeper trouble
than you are. It takes your mind off yourself."

Betty Pollom;
daughter of Frances Davis; California

7 • Family

Our Inheritance

F amily members come with the territory. We don't ask to have them. We're born, and they're there. In the old days, we lived on the same block, if not in the same house with them, even into adulthood—and in some instances that hasn't changed. More often, though, they now live across town, across the state, even across the country. They may not be involved in our lives on a daily basis, until something like breast cancer hits. Then they gather 'round in person, on the phone, or over the Web.

How many times have we said—or overheard others say—what a shame it is that it takes a crisis to bring families together? So why does that happen? Is it because of a shared past, shared memories? Is it because of a shared gene pool, which makes other family members immediately invested in the disease? Is it because, deep down, when we move past extreme expectations and consequent disappointments, sibling rivalry, and petty grievances, we feel a primal link?

Family is a support group. The sisterhood makes no bones

about that. It isn't necessarily the kind of support group that gives you answers, but rather the kind that is there to help. But here we go again with those extreme expectations. We assume that family being family, its members know just what we need. Unfortunately, that isn't always true. This may be their first experience with breast cancer, and watching us go through it may be harder than if they were going through it themselves. We need to tell them what we need, but that is sometimes easier said than done.

"There are times when I feel that no one wants to talk to me about my cancer," writes Glenda Chance, an Ohio wife and mother who was diagnosed in 2000 at the age of thirty-eight. "How do I get my loved ones to understand that even though it is a painful subject, it is a subject that I need to talk about? I am not looking for them to give me the right answers or even say all the right things. They just need to know that just because my body has healed from surgery, my mind and heart have not. But . . . it's me. I'm at fault, too. I've created a silence and used it to push them away. It's up to me to involve them in my life and tell them how I feel inside. They, too, are survivors in this, and they need to know from us what they can do to make our lives easier."

Yes, they need to know what they can do, but they also need to know that we want their help. Carol Englund, a New Jerseyite who was diagnosed in 1994 at the age of fifty-eight, writes, "I truly believe that without family, I would not have come as easily to the place where I am now. As important as it is for us to be able to accept the help of others, it is also important for them to know that they can help."

This chapter is a step in that direction. It's a small step, a tentative one, given that one woman's family situation may be very different from another's. But it's a starting point. Members of the sisterhood tell you what relatives did to help and what it meant to both sides. So listen good. Just as family has a disproportionate power to disappoint, it can also boost us in wondrous ways.

And the boosting can go on for years. As Massachusetts survivor Debbie MacLean wrote, "Where did I hear about *UPLIFT?* My son Douglas sent me an info-card on the tenth anniversary of my being diagnosed!"

WHEN I FIRST LEARNED . . .

"The most difficult person to tell about my diagnosis was my mother. She lives in Kentucky, and we only see each other once or twice a year. Fortunately, she had planned to come for Thanksgiving (I was diagnosed in mid-November), so I was able to tell her in person and she could see that I was doing all right. She did not come for the surgery, which was my family's choice. The day of my surgery, my sister-in-law's mother showed up unannounced at Mother's with a huge picnic lunch (in January!), and she spent the day with my mother until my husband called to say everything had gone smoothly. I always felt that was one of the most generous gifts anyone could have given my mother that day. Isabelle knew my mother would be worried, and she did her best to provide company and cheer her up."

Wanda Null; diagnosed in 1986 at age 41;
librarian; Massachusetts

"It was hardest to tell my mom. She has gone through some great sadness in her life, and she has always been a pillar of strength. I needed her in my corner for that very reason. The news spread through my family quickly, and I went on to tell my children's teachers, and my friends and co-workers. Telling all these people helped me to be in charge."

Cindy Fiedler; diagnosed in 1998 at age 40;
registered nurse, mom; Massachusetts

"Telling my mom, who lived eight hundred miles away, was tough. My dad died eighteen years ago from brain cancer, and now I had to tell her I had cancer. That was a very hard phone call, but she was there for me and came to be by my side."

Kathy Rabassa; diagnosed in 1999 at age 34;
administrative assistant; South Carolina

"When I first found out I had breast cancer, my in-laws were in Florida. My mother-in-law was so supportive. She told me that if I needed to talk, just to call her. She might not understand a word I was saying, but she was there to listen. My brother-in-law called me after each treatment just to ask 'how ya'all are.' That meant so much to me. As a special thank you, I baked him a raspberry pie (his favorite).".

Nancy Ellis; diagnosed in 2000 at age 53;
quality technician; New York

"I feared most telling my parents that their oldest daughter had cancer. We don't live in the same state, and I couldn't break the news on the phone, so I wrote them a letter. I made it clear that what I needed most was their love, support, and optimism. They called within a day of receiving my letter and were very positive."

Carrie Drake; diagnosed in 1998 at age 42;
administrative assistant; Colorado

"I most feared telling my parents, so I told them last. I went to their home early in the morning, sat at the kitchen table with them, and spoke in reference to my father's mother. 'You know how Nana had varicose veins, and I have them, too. And you know how Nana had bunions, and I have them, too. I seem to have her breast cancer as well.' As always, my father took control. He wanted to make arrangements for the two of us to fly to California to take advantage of the latest treatments. I declined. I hate flying."

Deborah J.P. Schur; diagnosed in 1994 at age 43;
sales rep; Massachusetts

"My daughter and I did not get along well before this, but when I had cancer, she changed dramatically. She said, 'I will be here to take care of you,' and she was. There was nothing I needed that she was not right there for."

Barbara Moro; diagnosed in 1999 at age 57;
law secretary; New Jersey

"When I first learned I had breast cancer, I only told two people: my husband and my best friend. My three sons were in college and in the midst of final exams. I didn't want to give them any news that would distract them from their studying. Then, on the last day of radiation, they and their girlfriends sent me a large bouquet of flowers. The poor delivery man had to wait until I stopped crying before he could leave."

Fran Hegarty; diagnosed in 2000 at age 47;
librarian; Massachusetts

"The best thing I did after learning of my diagnosis was to keep the news between my husband and myself. We did the Christmas holidays as planned, so that they could be enjoyed before the family knew of my upcoming surgery."

Irene Louise; diagnosed in 1995 at age 41;
retired executive secretary; Pennsylvania

"A cancer diagnosis can bring out of people an openness and honesty that is so genuine. One of the most touching moments I experienced after I was diagnosed was when my brother called me to talk. He said that he had been thinking about me and crying, which in itself was a shocker, because I hadn't seen him cry since we were kids. We were talking about the cancer, and he said, 'I love you, Jules . . .' Although we have always been very close, we had never said 'I love you' to each other before. It was a very special moment. I still get a little choked up when I think about it. When there is a cancer diagnosis, there is an urgency to express our feelings, and that is how it should be. It is important to help everyone realize how special they are. When someone is facing a serious illness, there is no greater gift than those simple words, 'I love you, Jules . . .' "

Julie Crandall; diagnosed in 1998 at age 31;
stay-at-home mom; North Carolina

TELLING THE KIDS

"When I was diagnosed with breast cancer, the hardest thing for me was to tell my son, who was ten at the time. In the three preceding years, we had lost several family members to cancer. He didn't know anyone who had survived, or so he thought. I pointed out to him that his grandmother and an aunt had breast cancer many years ago, and here they are today."

Tammy Delin; diagnosed in 1997 at age 33;
teacher's aide; California

"My family had bad feelings about radiation because of my father's illness. There was tension and fear. So I insisted that my children, their spouses, and my two grandchildren come with me to radiation to see what it was about. As they did I could feel the tension leave their bodies. What the mind imagines is far worse than reality. My eight-year-old granddaughter said, 'Grandma, what's the big deal? We see you lying that way on your bed!' My daughter, Karen, who was thirty-four when I went through my treatment, says that the more open I was with my feelings, the better it was for her. She lives near me and appreciated going to see where the radiation took place. That gave her a visual, and wasn't the gloomy thing she had imagined."

Anne Jacobs; diagnosed in 1999 at age 62;
managing partner, real estate; Massachusetts

"I was concerned about my grandson seeing my without any hair. He was just turning two, and had always held onto the side of our hair to fall asleep. One afternoon, it was so hot that I took my wig off and laid it on the back of the couch. He came in, sat beside me, and pointed to the wig. 'Is that your hair?' he asked. I told him that it was, and he told me to put it back on and laughed. After that I knew I didn't have to wear that wig all day long."

Carol Keen; diagnosed in 1999 at age 48;
office clerk; West Virginia

"My daughter was fifteen, frightened and depressed. She had a wonderful history teacher, who took her aside and disclosed that she was a survivor and shared her and her family's experiences. It made all the difference."

Barbara Jentis; diagnosed in 1983 at age 41;
attorney; New Jersey

"Allow your children to help you. My sixteen-year-old daughter blossomed right before my eyes. She thrived on helping me with the house and the cooking, and mostly with her younger sister, with whom she became very close. She grew tremendously in self-confidence and self-esteem."

Cornelia Doherty; diagnosed in 1985 at age 45;
mother, widow, speaker; Massachusetts

"My children were eight and fourteen at the time, and the younger one handled it much better than the older one. My oldest daughter was concerned that we had not told her all the details. So we invited her to accompany us to the hospital when we went for a second opinion. The day of my surgery she missed school and kept her father company at the hospital."

Wanda Null; diagnosed in 1986 at age 41;
librarian; Massachusetts

"The most humbling experience I had with breast cancer was having my son, a registered nurse, take care of my incision and drains after my surgery."

Rosamary Amiet; diagnosed in 2000 at age 48;
program manager; Ohio

"My husband and son were very, very good to me. My son used to joke around and keep me laughing, even though he was scared himself. One day, when he wanted me to go somewhere with him, he said, 'Put your wig on, sister, and let's go!' He told me that I didn't need to go to a support group, that I had a support group right at home, and he was right. My son is twenty."

Paula Porter; diagnosed in 2000 at age 47;
telephone operator; New York

"My son, who was fourteen when I was diagnosed, remembers feeling disbelief. He says that what gave him the most comfort was my keeping him informed of the status of my health and treatments. My twelve-year-old son understood my need to rest on the day of a treatment and kept his friends quiet while they played in the house. The day the dressing came off my incision, he ran into the house and asked to see it. I held up my shirt. He took a long hard look, and went back outdoors to play, seemingly content that everything looked fine. My daughter, who was not quite nine when I was diagnosed, went to school the next day and quite matter-of-factly told her art teacher that I had breast cancer. I think the teacher was floored!"

Deborah J.P. Schur; diagnosed in 1994 at age 43;
sales rep; Massachusetts

"My diagnosis of breast cancer was the most shocking experience of my life. My husband's mom had died of breast cancer when he was thirty, and it brought up many emotions for both of us. But he said to me, 'It looks as if we have a battle to fight, honey, and we are going to win.' He was my 'knight in shining armor'—there for me, supporting me, taking care of me and the kids every step of the way. We have three children. Our girl was fourteen, and our boys were eight and two-and-a-half. We told them the truth from the beginning and answered all of their questions honestly. I made sure that our daughter knew that my responsibilities around the house were not expected to be accomplished by her. We had friends help me, so that she didn't feel any added burdens to her already busy high school life. She also made a positive affirmation about her breasts growing, so that her fear wouldn't affect it. As for me, I got a nutritionist and cleaned up my already fairly healthy, predominantly organic food diet as much as I could. I went on a cleansing diet first, which helped a lot before my surgery and chemo."

Sandy Rodgers; diagnosed in 1999 at age 44; homemaker, mom, registered nurse, Reiki master; Massachusetts

WITH ME EVERY STEP OF THE WAY

"My son and his wife made arrangements to have my house cleaned during my recovery from surgery. It wasn't that the cleaning itself was so important to me, but that they had thought beyond my diagnosis to do this for me."

Susan Smith; diagnosed in 2000 at age 53; medical library technician; Pennsylvania

"My mother, grandmother, Aunt Dee, and Aunt Judy (my godmother, who flew cross-country to be here) cleaned my house from top to bottom and then polished all of the leaves on my house plants with mayonnaise!!"

Beth Compton; diagnosed in 1995 at age 27; civil engineer; South Carolina

"My grandmother sent me a check with the instruction that I was to have fresh flowers in the house at all times. I love flowers, but usually splurge on them only for special occasions, so having them around for months on end felt like a special treat. It was a soul-nourishing gift, especially since I was diagnosed in the middle of a long, bleak New England winter."

Dorian Solot; diagnosed in 2000 at age 26;
Massachusetts

"My family helped me considerably, financially as well as physically. They even bought me a new sofa and chair, so that I could be comfortable on those days when I didn't feel well. My mom and two sisters flew out several times to spend time with me. It was wonderful having them there as a support system and also, during my surgery, knowing that they were at my home taking care of everything and my two cats. It was one less thing I had to think about."

Gwen Loverink; diagnosed in 1994 at age 34;
police dispatcher; California

"The most special thing that was done for me was that my older brother wrote me a check for the amount of money I made before my diagnosis for the entire year. He didn't want me to think about losing money from not working. All he wanted me to do was to concentrate on getting better!"

Cathy Hanlon; diagnosed in 2000 at age 42;
school researcher; New York

"The most practical things my family did to help? Several family members sent money. Others had a stackable washer/dryer installed in my condo."

Carrie Drake; diagnosed in 1998 at age 42;
administrative assistant; Colorado

"One of my daughters made a countdown calendar for me, starting with 6 and going down to 0. I thumbtacked it to my bathroom door and, after each chemo treatment, tore off a page. What a sense of triumph it was to tear off those pages one at a time until finally reaching the last one."

Faye Hardiman; diagnosed in 1998 at age 50;

wife, mother, teacher; Georgia

"Friends or family members can help by taping videos of great upbeat romantic movies—e.g., *Sleepless in Seattle, When Harry Met Sally*—to watch while recovering from treatment. They can also prepare meals and freeze them for future consumption. Receiving phone calls from friends and family is the best medicine."

Ellen Beth Simon; diagnosed in 1998 at age 41;

lawyer; New Jersey

"The most practical thing done for me by a family member was when my mother-in-law did my laundry."

Frances Gallello; diagnosed in 2000 at age 51;

mental health assistant; New York

"My son, Michael, brought me a Cabbage Patch doll. The doll went with me to all doctor appointments. My surgeon's comment when he saw the doll was, 'You pull out all the stops, don't you!' "

Jeryl Abelmann; diagnosed in 1986 at age 46;

elementary school teacher; California

"My one niece, Suzanne, knew the right questions to ask the surgeon to be sure that I would be all right. Questions, questions, questions. Do not be afraid to ask!"

Barbara Moro; diagnosed in 1999 at age 57;

law secretary; New Jersey

"My sister, Vel, who lives on the West Coast, was calling all the time, sending cards daily, plus surprise goody packages. She may have lived far away, but Vel made every effort to let me know that she was there for me. She's a true blessing in my life."

Sherry Ann Wells; diagnosed in 1997 at age 45;
homemaker; Missouri

"I felt empowered by the goodness of people. My sister came from Ohio, sixteen hours by train. She did not come alone but brought her infant son, and she made the ride numerous times. She cleaned my house, did my laundry, and talked with me for long hours about the things only sisters can talk about. She gave me hope. My mother insisted on driving me to every session of chemotherapy and radiation. Not that I was not perfectly capable of doing so myself, but she indicated that this was not optional. My Aunt Chris provided me with endless homemade chicken soup. This helped me do battle with the nausea that I felt during chemotherapy. Friends and family members called and sent flowers, candy, and even money."

Cindy Fiedler; diagnosed in 1998 at age 40;
registered nurse, mom; Massachusetts

"Above all else, I was fortunate to have my husband sitting next to me for eleven months during my treatments."

Susan Schultz; diagnosed in 1990 at age 41;
special education teacher's aide; New York

"When my husband and I purchased a new home in the middle of my chemotherapy treatments, my cousin and brother-in-law packed us up and moved us, and my sister unpacked and organized my kitchen and bedroom when I couldn't get off the couch."

Linda Perkins; diagnosed in 1999 at age 35;
project manager; New Jersey

"I knew I would be recovering from my surgery for four to six weeks. My husband, who is the absolute greatest, cannot cook. He only defrosts. So I spent a couple of days before surgery cooking our favorite meals and putting them in single-serve-size cartons and freezing them. The cooking was therapeutic for me, and we ate well for quite a while!"

Jennifer Wersal; diagnosed in 2000 at age 30;
marketing; Texas

"My family has been there for me every step of the way, making sure that the everyday chores are taken care of, that I am properly nourished, and just being very supportive in everything they do and say. Since my diagnosis, my youngest daughter has even undertaken to do breast cancer research at her high school!"

Carol Downer; diagnosed in 1997 at age 48;
legal secretary; New York

WHEN MY MOM WAS DIAGNOSED . . .

"Having my mom diagnosed with breast cancer was a life-defining event for me. I was twenty-nine at the time and filled with my life's happenings, and I had taken her presence for granted. I attended every doctor's appointment with her, and when she had a mastectomy, I was blessed to be able to give back a small fraction of the care and love that she had given me for so many years. We were together on the day she received the news that her cancer had not spread. Before she was diagnosed, we had started planning a cruise to the Bahamas with friends. That cruise became her celebration of life—even though she worried that she would lose her prosthesis in the ocean. This past year, during Breast Cancer Awareness Month, I sent her a gift every week to remind her that I love her and that she is a survivor. I don't think that I have ever told her, but her strength and positive attitude through it all blew me away."

Jennifer Schuster;
daughter of a survivor; Michigan

"Breast cancer can devastate a person's health, yet all the while encourage the soul to bloom. When my family was told of my mother's diagnosis, our hearts seemed to stop. I cried more tears then I had in my lifetime. Yet, my mother's touch was peaceful and accepting. Over the past nine months, she has experienced pain, but she remains strong. She is determined to conquer this cancer—not with shouts of anger, but by providing unconditional love to hurting friends and family and gentle words of hope to those who support her. In my mind, she has already won."

Heather Marie Zielke;
daughter of a survivor; Virginia

"I remember getting a call from my mom, and her giving me the bad news that she had just been diagnosed with breast cancer. She was so upbeat that I remember thinking she must be in shock. As the months passed and she went through chemo treatments, she paid close attention to her diet and exercised on a regular basis. She still seemed too happy to me. I kept wondering how I'd feel if I were in her shoes, and the only word that came to mind was 'devastated.' Yet, there Mom was, laughing and checking to see how everyone else was doing. Never once did I see her cry. Well, she won! She has now been cancer-free for a while. To this day, she has neither cried nor shown self-pity. The main thing this has shown me is that my mother has an inner strength the likes of which I never knew existed. That strength, along with faith and the grace of God, can lead us through anything in life."

Bec Wiget;
daughter of a survivor; California

"In the busy times we live in, we don't always have the ability to see our family members every day. My mother's chemotherapy treatment required injections for ten consecutive days after each treatment. For those ten days, over a period of months, I would inject my mom, sit at the kitchen table, and chat with my mom and grandmother. The positive side was a retreat back to times when families visited each other every day!"

Regina R. Young;
daughter of Claire E. Reber; New Jersey

"On a visit to my mom when she was having chemo, I did her nails. She enjoyed that so much. My massaging her hands and filing and polishing her nails was very relaxing to her. I think it's important for women going through this to be good to them-selves—whether it's having their nails done or their hair washed, or doing something else that is relaxing and fun."

Laura Thomas;
daughter of Roberta Price Wilcox; Iowa

"My sister, Cathleen, is my best friend. We are fourteen months apart in age and have always been close. She was diagnosed, against all statistics, before she was thirty. To say that we were shocked is an understatement. I am doing as much as I can do by supporting her and offering an ear or a shoulder whenever she needs it. And her two littlest angels, my sons Seth and Benjamin, are two of her strongest lifelines."

Angela Thompson;
sister of Cathleen D'Antonio; Connecticut

"How do you comfort someone you love who has been told she has breast cancer? What words can ease the fear? How can you help her sleep at night? Reading! Books have a way of taking you into another world, time, and place. I gave Nan one of my favorite books and told her that even if she just read a few pages at night, it would help her. Today, my sister reads about eight books a month. She also belongs to a book group. She says that I've given her the gift of reading, and what a pot of gold that is!"

Maybelle Timm Eley;
sister of Nan Comstock; California

"Humor and a strong faith in God were two of the most important tools that helped our family make it through a terrifying time. My mother-in-law is a breast cancer survivor today, and we are so very grateful. We constantly teased her about her bald head and even about her lopsided chest. I know that might seem distasteful to some, but we chose to smile rather than walk about looking stricken. The loss of her breast was traumatic, but it was such a small part of a wonderful woman who is so much more than any breast can be!"

Judi Scally;
daughter-in-law of Marian Scally; Michigan

"I was totally untouched by breast cancer until my favorite aunt developed it two years ago, shortly before my son's wedding. She wanted to make sure that she had the necessary surgery in time to enjoy the wedding, so that her absence didn't put a damper on the festivities. Because of a bad cold and several other mishaps, the date of her surgery kept being delayed. She finally had it just two weeks before the wedding, but still she was determined to be with us. Though she'd had options to stay in private homes, she insisted on staying at the hotel so that everyone got to see her at the big open house my husband and I held there the night before the wedding. She wanted to make sure that she would see everyone then and answer all their questions, so the focus the next night would be on the bride and groom alone. Well, on the night of the wedding, everybody was in a party mood, and there was my Aunt Jean, up on the dance floor celebrating with everyone else! I know she was in pain, but she let nothing stop her or *any* of us from enjoying a very special event!"

Marilyn Eichner;
niece of Jean Firkser; Massachusetts

AMONG MY CANCER BLESSINGS . . .

"Among my cancer blessings were spending a great deal of cherished time with my husband as he took time off from work, finding out that I look pretty good with very short hair, and realizing the amazing trust my two teens had in me when I said, 'The doctors are going to take care of me. I'm going to be okay.' "

Diane Bongiorno; diagnosed in 1998 at age 43;
instructional aide; New Jersey

"My kids were great; they did a million things to bolster my spirits, as did my husband. My daughter did the Avon 3 Day Breast Cancer Walk in my honor. The sight of her crossing the finish line will always be a cherished moment."

Suzanne Pollock; diagnosed in 1995 at age 50;
stationer; North Carolina

"Support and love and laughter from the Ablemenn in my life brought me the strength I needed to get through this time of my life."

Jeryl Abelmann; diagnosed in 1986 at age 46;
elementary school teacher; California

"Friends and family need to keep panic and emotions in check. When my close cousin in Israel e-mailed me her hysteria, I told her that I couldn't correspond that way. And it stopped."

Anne Jacobs; diagnosed in 1999 at age 62;
managing partner, real estate; Massachusetts

"I became twins with my bald dad. We had numerous photos taken like that."

Asha Mevlana; diagnosed in 1999 at age 24;
musician; New York

"During chemotherapy treatments, some weekends I felt much better than others. My husband and I always made simple plans for those weekends, apple picking or taking a walk on the beach. On my bad weekends, our family took comfort just talking and being together. Thanksgiving fell during one of my more difficult chemotherapy treatments. As a family, we decided to move the holiday to a different date. It gave us something to plan for and look forward to."

Helaine Hemingway; diagnosed in 1988 at age 41;
teacher; New Hampshire

"My daughter-in-law cooked her first Thanksgiving dinner at our home after I had begun chemo. What a treat!"

Betty Harris; diagnosed in 1999 at age 64;
homemaker; South Carolina

"I just celebrated my two-year survivor anniversary. I was diagnosed when my daughter was four months old and had bilateral mastectomies by the time she turned five months old. It was an eye-opening experience for my husband and me, particularly since we had been married only a year and a half when this occurred. We are expecting our second child this summer, and truly feel that our children are miracles. Our first child was a miracle because if I hadn't had her I would have never found the cancer as quickly as I did. Our second is a miracle because we have overcome so much. We didn't know if I would be able to have any more children because I'd had cancer, but when I had my yearly visit with my oncologist, she gave me a clean bill of health."

Tresa Johnson; diagnosed in 1999 at age 23;
executive secretary; Oklahoma

"We booked a trip to Las Vegas. Then I was diagnosed with breast cancer. I kept telling Jerry I couldn't go because of how I would feel after treatments, but he wouldn't hear of our not going. He said he would carry me if he had to, so I could see my son, who had recently moved there. Well, we had the best time! A whole bunch of us went—family and friends, even my ex—and there was a big surprise. My daughter and her boyfriend got married in a small chapel in Vegas. I wish for her to be happy and healthy!"

Sharon Daniels; diagnosed in 2000 at age 49;
hairstylist, wig store owner; Massachusetts

"My birthday was eight weeks after my diagnosis, and my family wanted to take me out to dinner. This was my first real night out since D-day (diagnosis day), and I remember feeling reasonably good and a bit excited about dressing up and going out. I'll never forget going to my bedroom with hopes of finding something pretty to wear. Instead I came out in tears. Nothing in my new beautiful scarf collection matched any of my old not-so-beautiful clothes. All of my scarves were printed and therefore clashed with the majority of my clothes, which were also of printed fabric. I needed a new wardrobe. My husband was taken aback when I announced this to him—bald, crying on my birthday, and in front of my parents. But he said, 'Sure, sweetheart, anything you need.' After that, getting dressed became a breeze. Almost as easy as . . . the drop of a hat (had to say it)!"

Sallie Burdine; diagnosed in 1998 at age 44;
author; Florida

"After countless compositions in my head, when I finally sat down to write something that I thought would be profound, I discovered that everything I thought I had to say was totally bland. How could I be an inspiration to anyone? Then I remembered that despite the fact that I was not near family members during my surgery and subsequent treatment and recovery period, I was constantly in touch with them through the magic of e-mail. This is such a wonderful way to keep in touch with the outside world. I received and sent letters on a daily basis, documented my true feelings to family members who I knew would care, wrote short stories and poems for personal satisfaction, and found joy in the many inspirational poems and essays that family members forwarded to me."

Florence Wade; diagnosed in 1999 at age 63;
retired school teacher, retired property manager; Texas

"I was twenty-six, and I had breast cancer. I didn't know how, but I knew why. I got breast cancer because God wanted me to be able to share my experience with other women. Up to this point I still wasn't sure what I wanted to do with my life. My kids were now in school, so I had time to do anything I wanted, but I had no idea what that was. The first thing on my agenda was to kick this cancer's butt. Luckily, I had nothing but the best medical care. I went through eight sessions of chemo in six months. I lost my hair, lost weight, and gained a whole new respect for myself. I couldn't get over how strong and how happy I was. I grew to love my husband and children more and more every day. I thought I loved them all that I could. How wrong I was. If you've never stared death in the face and won, then you haven't lived. Every day when I wake up and see my kids' smiling faces and hear those precious words, 'I love you, Mommy,' I get chills. I fell in love with my husband all over again. There I was, feeling as if I looked like something that the cat dragged in, and he would tell me how beautiful I was and how much he thanked God that I came into his life."

Kimberlee Richardson; diagnosed in 2000 at age 26;
mother, Air Force wife, student; Mississippi

8 · Friends

We Pick 'Em

Not all of us have family. Breast cancer hits women who are single and divorced, who have no siblings and whose parents are no longer alive, who live too far away for their family to help with the mechanics of juggling cancer and life, or who simply . . . don't get along with family. For these women, friends *are* family.

I am fortunate enough to have family *and* friends. No, my problem wasn't having people who would have helped if I'd asked. My problem was asking. Members of the sisterhood warn against this. They point out, time and again, that people really do want to help and that their help makes all the difference. Another of my problems, of course, was that many friends didn't *know* I had breast cancer. If they didn't know, how could they cook for me? Or send cards? Or call just to let me vent?

Lest you start feeling sorry for me, let me say that I wasn't suffering. In addition to my family and those few close friends in the loop, I had the characters I was writing about at the time. They were wonderfully solicitous, waiting patiently while I took time out for a treatment, a lunch date, a manicure, or a nap. They took me outside of myself and my own problems, helped me put things in perspective—because they were dealing with Alzheimer's disease. By comparison, I had it easy.

But this chapter isn't about imaginary friends; it's about real ones. If I were to single out the nicest thing that a friend did for me during this period, it would have to be the generosity of Jane.

Months before my mastectomy, I had agreed to speak at a national conference of the American Library Association. The conference was being held in San Antonio, which I had never seen but which sounded like a perfectly delightful place to visit during the pits of a Northeast winter. Then breast cancer came along, and my mastectomy took place a mere six weeks before the conference. I was fine. I could go. My luggage was the problem. It was heavy.

I was into the saline expansion phase of my reconstruction, and my chest and upper arms were weak. So I brought Jane with me as my own personal porter, and we had a ball. We toured the Alamo, explored the Riverwalk, toasted each other at every possible meal. As far as anyone else ever knew, she had come along just to keep me company—a reasonable excuse, given how lonely business travel is. Bless him, my husband came through even then. When we checked into our hotel in San Antonio, there waiting for us were roses and chocolate-dipped strawberries from Steve! He knew that I'd been apprehensive about the mechanics of the trip and, unable to get away himself, was as grateful to Jane as I was.

This chapter has two purposes. First, I want women who are newly diagnosed to take a deep breath and realize that they aren't alone, that friends do come through. Second, I want friends to be able to glance through these pages, gain a better understanding of our needs, and thereby have more of an idea how they can help.

Sometimes that simply means showing up and not doing a thing, which brings me to a quick word about the term "friends." I take it in its broadest sense. Hence, I give you Bear.

"To help me pass the time," wrote Barbara Moro, a law secretary from New Jersey, "I went to work, slept when I was really tired, and spent time with my best friend, my dog Bear. I know it sounds strange, but he was very soothing to me when I was feeling bad. He was most attentive to me during this time."

I find that humbling. As arrogant as we humans are—as cocksure that we are a higher species—our pets do sense what we need. In a pinch, without a word of instruction from us, they come through. If they were able to speak or to write, I would have solicited their help with this chapter. Absent of that, I rely on the following very human words.

BREAKING THE ICE

"As soon as I found out I had breast cancer, I called everyone I knew so that they would hear it from me directly and not feel weird talking about it with me. I also created a website to document my experiences, so that people who weren't comfortable talking to me about it could learn what I was going through on their own terms. I had so many people calling on the phone that I couldn't keep up with it all. So I changed my answering machine to say, 'If you want to know what happened to Asha, press 1. If you want to know her treatment plan, press 2. If you want to know how she's doing, press 3.' "

Asha Mevlana; diagnosed in 1999 at age 24;
musician; New York

"I told everyone that I had breast cancer. I didn't want people talking behind my back. Some people didn't know what to say to me, but I hadn't changed. I was the same person I'd always been."

Judy Peterson; diagnosed in 2000 at age 58;
registered nurse; Colorado

"Actually, I think going out in public helps to break the ice for others. I learned from my experience that others were more frightened than I was about encountering me back in the 'real' world. Once the initial hello and/or hug and/or acknowledgment was over with, so was the awkwardness."

Sallie Burdine; diagnosed in 1998 at age 44;
author; Florida

"During recovery, people were hesitant toward me, not knowing how to react. I quickly realized that they were taking their cue from me. They calmed down when they saw that my reaction was positive."

Carol Pasternak; diagnosed in 1986 at age 47;
artist; Ontario, Canada

"People often just don't know what to say to you. They try to put emotions into words, and that can't always be done. I always appreciated a simple, 'Good luck, we're thinking of you.' "

Kim Vermeire; diagnosed in 1992 at age 18;
computer consultant; Illinois

"It is important to understand that some people are *afraid* to speak to you about breast cancer."

Eleanor Anbinder; diagnosed in 1991 at age 50;
sales manager; Massachusetts

"Let people hug you. It warms your sad heart!"

Sarah Stuart; diagnosed in 1999 at age 52;
banking human resources assistant; Vermont

"I had always been a very private person who dealt with my own problems and didn't burden others. I opened up to people and discovered how caring others can be when you give them the chance. I am much more open now about things."

Sue Watson; diagnosed in 1996 at age 53;
teacher; Texas

"People were trying to protect me and second-guess me. I think others were more frightened than I was. Of course, I was doing too much and was tired, so I was possibly sending the wrong message."

Sandy Williams; diagnosed in 1999 at age 51;
children's public services librarian; Texas

"The best thing I did for myself was to go shopping with my girl-friend. She insisted I buy myself something pretty and comfortable for the hospital. We spent all day at the shopping center. She was wonderfully patient with me."

Fran Hegarty; diagnosed in 2000 at age 47;
librarian; Massachusetts

"What most raised my spirits when my hair started falling out were the friends—both male and female—who told me I was beautiful often."

Carrie Drake; diagnosed in 1998 at age 42;
administrative assistant; Colorado

"I cried a lot. I appreciated the people who just listened to me cry."

Suzanne Pollock; diagnosed in 1995 at age 50;
stationer; North Carolina

"My husband had a business dinner, so I went out with a friend. We talked about her marriage. It was therapy to listen to someone else's challenges in life."

Sandy Williams; diagnosed in 1999 at age 51;
children's public services librarian; Texas

"My advice to friends? Listen, listen, listen. Sometimes we need to talk. But talk about your own life, too. We need to be as involved as we ever were with the rest of our lives."

Anne Jacobs; diagnosed in 1999 at age 62;
managing partner, real estate; Massachusetts

"The most helpful thing others did for me after my diagnosis was to hug me. There were no words that would comfort me, but anyone's arms enfolding me were comforting. In turn, I learned to give freely of my hugs to friends and strangers. It's the best!"

Deborah J.P. Schur; diagnosed in 1994 at age 43;
sales rep; Massachusetts

"What I remember most about the first week of diagnosis was the outpouring of support from family and friends. I could have opened up a card shop, florist shop, and restaurant with all the cards, flowers, and food that was sent. One of the most touching things that week was returning home from several hours of medical tests to find that my next-door neighbors had cut our grass!"

Beth Compton; diagnosed in 1995 at age 27;
civil engineer; South Carolina

"Just one day after surgery, I was discharged from the hospital. The dark dismal morning mirrored my spirits. I brought my hand up to the bandages that covered my chest, and a nurse instructed me on the care of my alien breast. My husband arrived to take me home, and we drove in silence. The rain became a steady drizzle as grief tightened its grip. When we pulled into the driveway, though, a splash of color exploded before my eyes. Two newly planted gardens framed the walkway to my house. Pansies, salvia, petunias, and impatiens created a kaleidoscope of color. 'Who?' I asked my husband, but I already knew. 'Eileen, Kate, and Cathy,' he said, adding with a smile, 'and in the pouring rain, too.' The next morning, I awoke to sun and went to the window. The color was even more vibrant than the day before. I smiled. My garden was a gift from dear friends, who knew that words alone weren't adequate to convey encouragement and hope. As spring slipped into summer and I moved from radiation to chemo, this magnificent display greeted me daily. Tenderly nur-

tured and cared for by loved ones, my garden and I thrived and
grew strong."

Jacqueline Hickey; diagnosed in 1993 at age 39;
secretary, aspiring writer; Massachusetts

THEY REALLY WANT TO

"Surround yourself with good people and let them do things for
you. My neighbor came over to sit with me one day after surgery
and was so insistent upon helping around the house that she
washed an entire basket of clean clothes. We still laugh about that
today."

Jennifer Wersal; diagnosed in 2000 at age 30;
marketing; Texas

"A nurse friend came to stay with me for a week following
surgery. I didn't actually need the physical help as much as someone to talk to. She had a little surprise gift every morning to get
us started on a happy note."

Carol Hattler; diagnosed in 1999 at age 65;
retired nurse; Virginia

"If your friends want to take you to your treatments, accept their
kind offer to help. They want to participate in your healing. Besides, it makes the trip more pleasant, and sometimes you are
more exhausted than you realize."

Helen Wilker; diagnosed in 1999 at age 58;
assistant teacher; Massachusetts

"A simple thing such as a phone call to say 'hello' or 'how are
you?' means so much during treatment. A brief note saying
'thinking of you' is never out of place."

Susan Clemente; diagnosed in 1990 at age 46;
retired registered nurse; New York

"My friends helped a lot. One of them called me every day. I looked forward to our talks. Other friends sent me cards, flowers, and food. It made me feel so good to know how much they cared."

Paula Porter; diagnosed in 2000 at age 47;

telephone operator; New York

"I was always a caregiver and never allowed anyone to help me. After hearing my diagnosis, though, I didn't know how I was going to get through it. So, I learned during this time of surgery and treatments that I had to let go and allow others to help me. That was very hard for me to do. My best friend told me to practice doing it, and it would get easier."

Carol Keen; diagnosed in 1999 at age 48;

office clerk; West Virginia

"One of my dearest, oldest friends drove two hours in a snowstorm for just one night to help me blow-dry my hair . . . and my sister-in-law and husband took turns sleeping with me the first few nights, until we were all so tired that we woke up one morning, all three of us in bed!"

Bonnie Schneider; diagnosed in 1998 at age 45;

audiologist; Connecticut

"When I came home from the hospital, my best friend drove seven hundred miles to be there to take care of me. Boy, did I feel special."

E. Mary Lou Clauss; diagnosed in 1991 at age 55;

homemaker, retired registered nurse; Pennsylvania

"My best friend from high school quit her job and moved to New York from Boston to stay with me for the length of my treatments."

Asha Mevlana; diagnosed in 1999 at age 24;

musician; New York

"Accept help from others when offered, especially with meal preparation, childcare, and rides to medical appointments. It is not a sign of weakness. In fact, avoid thinking about how other people may judge you. You will be overwhelmed by the care and concern of others."

Mary Raffol; diagnosed in 1998 at age 44;
teacher; Massachusetts

"When I went into the hospital for my surgery, my friends got together and cleaned my house from top to bottom. When I came home from the hospital, they brought me dinner every night for a week."

Carleen Muniz; diagnosed in 1998 at age 51;
artist; Massachusetts

"I concentrated on trying to hang in there and let my friends do the praying, and I truly believe it worked. I still get emotional when I think about how good everyone was to me."

Virginia Danczak; diagnosed in 1995 at age 58;
phone company investigation center; Nebraska

"One of my friends had breast cancer surgery and treatment exactly a year before my diagnosis. When I called to tell her about my treatment plan, which included chemotherapy, she said, 'You can do this.' That simple—you can do this."

Faye Hardiman; diagnosed in 1998 at age 50;
wife, mother, teacher; Georgia

"Before surgery, each of my friends gave me the best of themselves in their individual ways. One told me to visualize his little finger and hold onto it as I went into surgery. Another talked to the deer about me and flew a kite while thinking of me. A third one, knowing I do not embrace his religious beliefs, asked if I minded if he prayed for me. I am someone who gives from the heart for my friends. This was the first time when I have been the one who needed that heartfelt embrace. Remembering their loving gestures still brings tears to my eyes."

Jeanne Sturdevant; diagnosed in 1990 at age 45;
artist; Texas

"It meant a lot to me to have someone take me to chemo treatments to talk with and keep me company. This often involved my husband or friends taking the day off from work. One friend took me to a full-day chemo treatment when she was nine months pregnant and about to give birth! When neither my husband nor my friends could do it, I was driven by wonderful volunteers from the American Cancer Society. As an added bonus, those volunteers often have positive personal experiences to share."

Linda Perkins; diagnosed in 1999 at age 35;
project manager; New Jersey

"Friends had special luncheons and parties for me. This was their way of showing me love and support. The radiation therapists even adjusted my 'time slot' a couple of times during the six weeks, when girlfriends and I wanted to go over to the Napa Valley for lunch or a wine tasting."

Patti R. Martinez; diagnosed in 1999 at age 54;
realtor; California

"I wrote down the names of everyone who called offering to help, and then called them when I needed them. I threw a big thank-you party later (on my fiftieth birthday)!"

Judith Ormond; diagnosed in 1996 at age 49;
symphony musician—piccolo; Wisconsin

GOODIES . . .

"One of the nicest things people can do for a cancer patient is to send food to the house, because it is so difficult and tiresome to have to cook. A meal sent in by caring friends tastes so much better!"

Susan Clemente; diagnosed in 1990 at age 46;
retired registered nurse; New York

"My friend Pat would call or stop over and see me often. She would always ask, 'What can I do for you?'—not realizing, I guess, that just stopping by and calling was more than enough. However, on one of her visits she brought a homemade dinner, cooked it, ate with me, and cleaned up afterwards. It was just wonderful."

Carol Englund; diagnosed in 1994 at age 58;
retired administrative assistant; New Jersey

"I have young children, and people brought over dinner meals, instead of gifts. It was the most thoughtful thing that can be given to a woman just home from major surgery. Friends also brought cookies and treats for the kids."

Rhonda Sorrell; diagnosed in 1998 at age 43;
special education teacher; Michigan

"Never take casseroles to families with teenagers. Take plain meat and potatoes, or, better yet, order pizza and ice cream cake. A casserole will only make their dog fat!"

Mitzi Scarborough; diagnosed in 1999 at age 37;
childcare provider; Arkansas

"Friends sent flowers and cards. I was bowled over by thoughts, prayers, and generosity. The most generous and most helpful gestures were made by the friends who either brought me dinner or took me out to dinner. They knew that I needed nourishment to fight the fatigue, and they were there for me."

Christine Foutris; diagnosed in 1999 at age 49;
teacher; Illinois

"The single most helpful thing done for me was the delivery of meals organized by our church. Since we have no family in the area for support, the collective generosity of those women relieved me of having to think about preparing meals."

Wanda Null; diagnosed in 1986 at age 41;
librarian; Massachusetts

"A friend packed her car with frozen homemade soups and casseroles and drove four hundred miles to help fill my freezer for those I-don't-feel-like-cooking days ahead. Another friend made a special effort to attend church that first Sunday after diagnosis, saying, 'I just didn't want you to sit by yourself today.' "

Betty Harris; diagnosed in 1999 at age 64;
homemaker; South Carolina

"Kathy, my incredible artist friend, hated to cook. So during her treatment, I took her to have a dinner of her favorite Mexican food. She had two of the largest margaritas we ever saw, and we laughed through the entire meal!"

Sandra Baldwin Brown;
friend of a survivor; Colorado

"I got flowers, candy, and presents, but the best thing was a gift certificate to my favorite restaurant."

Jill Gross; diagnosed in 2000 at age 51;
bank head teller; Massachusetts

MORE GOODIES . . .

"My daughter's fourteenth birthday was on the day I came home from the hospital. My friend Diane met us at home with balloons, a homemade birthday cake, and gifts. This was Diane's gift to me."

Aileen Pandapas; diagnosed in 1989 at age 41;
mom, volunteer, former secretary; Virginia

"I had a wonderful support system. My co-workers sent food to my home, starting the day I came home from the hospital, and continued for a couple weeks. My best friends came and did work around the house, sat with me during my treatments, and took me to lunch, shopping, or a movie."

Carol Keen; diagnosed in 1999 at age 48;
office clerk; West Virginia

"I live in an adult community called Concordia. The support that I received after diagnosis and surgery was beyond belief. I received more than a hundred get-well cards, and when I got home after my surgery, every night someone sent in dinner for my husband and myself."

Jean Firkser; diagnosed in 1998 at age 66;
housewife, retired receptionist; New Jersey

"Friends volunteered to drive me to appointments so that I never had to go anywhere alone. They volunteered to shop for groceries and pick up mail. They even took out the trash regularly—down three flights of stairs!"

Carrie Drake; diagnosed in 1998 at age 42;
administrative assistant; Colorado

"A housecleaner as a gift is really nice, even if only once."

Stephanie King;
friend of two survivors; New York

"A friend installed a detachable shower head, so I could wash my hair with all the bandages still on."

Judith Ormond; diagnosed in 1996 at age 49;
symphony musician—piccolo; Wisconsin

"Two gifts that meant a lot to me were very different: one was a pair of great-looking earrings for when I was better. The other was a small framed motto that says 'Tough times don't last. Tough people do.' I looked at it every day."

Suzanne Pollock; diagnosed in 1995 at age 50;
stationer; North Carolina

"My book club friends kept dropping by with favorite books for me to read. They were the best medicine for sleeplessness, nausea, or just spirit-lifting."

Betty Harris; diagnosed in 1999 at age 64;
homemaker; South Carolina

"When my friend Cathy was first diagnosed, I wrote her a short poem, since she loved poetry. Even when her treatment progressed, I continued to write and frame poems for her."

Nanette Thorsen-Snipes;
friend of two survivors; Georgia

"My friend's chemo treatments came during the summer, and she bemoaned the fact that she could not enjoy all the fresh summer fruit she loved so much, as it was something she was told to avoid. So I found these terrific fruit gel candles in peach, strawberry, watermelon, honeydew, and blueberry. I would light one for her as I read to her from some of her all-time favorite comfort books, like *Little Women* and *Anne of Green Gables*. The aroma was delicious and the next best thing to taking a bite. The house smelled like summer and put a smile on her face. It lifted her family's spirits as well. We are both avid readers, and going back to the stories of her childhood was comforting to her. It transported her to another time and place, and helped pass the time. The sound of my voice, the familiar words and summer smells gave us some special moments together. We still buy these candles and light them whenever we sit down to read."

Cheryl Brinker;
friend of Susan Thornton; Connecticut

"The most practical thing someone did for me was that my friend Linda came over and deadheaded my entire flower garden! She also sent me cards to celebrate the end of each chemo treatment."

Rosamary Amiet; diagnosed in 2000 at age 48;
program manager; Ohio

"A friend brought me a little gift every Friday to celebrate the end of the week of radiation treatment. The last day of radiation, my son came home from college to go with me. I took gifts to all of the technicians."

Sharon Erbe; diagnosed in 1999 at age 54;
nurse educator; New York

MORE GOODIES . . .

"I was overwhelmed by the number of cards, flowers, and visitors I received. I never realized so many friends were thinking of me. I made new friends, too. The young nurses would gather in my room and talk about their pets and hobbies, as most were away from home. A waitress who worked in one of the restaurants where we frequently ate came to visit and brought the fried shrimp that she knew I loved. Another friend was away on vacation, but she called and sent cards every day."

Barbara C. Sumner; diagnosed in 1982 at age 59;
homemaker; New Hampshire

"People's notes and gestures of support meant more than I could have imagined. Lesson learned—never pass up an opportunity to pick up the phone or send a card of encouragement. Better to make a mistake of commission than omission."

Patricia Baker; diagnosed in 1993 at age 49;
at home; Massachusetts

"I received cards constantly. Some friends sent them weekly, and they brought many chuckles. Frequent 'just to let you know I'm thinking about you' phone calls kept my spirits up, way up. These things helped me know that I had not been forgotten, and that no matter what I looked or felt like, my friends and family saw me as a valuable person."

Betty Harris; diagnosed in 1999 at age 64;
homemaker; South Carolina

"What helped me were the many, many cards and notes I received, but especially from those who were also cancer survivors. Some of the people I had known quite well and never even knew they had cancer. I surely don't agree with keeping this as a hush-hush situation, as by my knowing others who have survived for a long time, it gave me a much brighter outlook on my future."

Sally Martel; diagnosed in 1996 at age 60;
wife, mother, retired accountant; New Hampshire, Florida

"I hung every single card I received on the wall in our family room. They reminded me of all those who loved me and cared about me. And I loved seeing my 'wall of cards' grow. I can't tell you how much it meant to me to know so many people were thinking about me and praying for me. It gave me strength and a daily boost. When I finally took all my cards down, I had a feeling of closure on my experience."

Julie Crandall; diagnosed in 1998 at age 31;
stay-at-home mom; North Carolina

"My role as a friend was just to be there. When my friends finished radiation, I sent them both flowers to congratulate them
on a job well done. I put on their cards that they were truly examples of courage to all of us."

Grace Trocco;
friend of two survivors; New York

"When my friend Susan was going through her chemotherapy,
the three to four days after the treatments were the hardest for
her. She often complained of the soles of her feet feeling like
they were on fire. For those occasions, I found a wonderful lavender foot cream that I would put in the refrigerator at the start of
my visit. Then, the last thing I would do for her before I left was
to get her all comfy in bed and give her a gentle foot massage
with the cooled cream. I could almost immediately feel her body
relax, and the lavender scent helped her to relax enough to even
drift off, as sleep was also difficult for her at these times. To this
day, we both continue to use this product."

Cheryl Brinker; friend of Susan Thornton; Connecticut

"When I was newly diagnosed, unbenownst to me, a quilt friend
put out a notice on the local quilt e-mail directory asking folks to
make me a heart patch, a red heart on a white-on-white background, and write something on it. At that time, I didn't have a
computer, so was not aware of what was happening and was rather
confused when I started receiving these patches in the mail! I
spread them out on the dining room table, and every time I
walked by, I got a wonderfully positive feeling from seeing the
hearts and reading the messages. Then I extended the offer of
participation to various nonquilting friends and family. In the
end, I had over a hundred patches, no two alike, and put together
two quilts. They are not all red hearts on white-on-white background . . . quilters tend to be somewhat independent! However,

they all have a special place in my heart (pun intended), and I will always be thankful to those who gave of their hearts."

Sheilah Musselman; diagnosed in 1997 at age 56;
registered nurse; Virginia

RETURNING THE FAVOR

"A colleague and friend, who is also a breast cancer survivor, gave me wise advice. She told me what I should ask my doctors, what I should wear, and where I could buy what I needed. Every week for months she wrote me encouraging notes. 'Courage is fear with prayer' was my very favorite. When I asked how I could ever thank her enough, she answered that I should do for any others what she'd done for me. At the time I had hoped to be spared that, but two of my colleagues at school this year needed advice, and I was glad and proud to help them."

Christine Foutris; diagnosed in 1999 at age 49;
teacher; Illinois

"One of the most helpful things people in my neighborhood did was meals for our family. Twenty-five women from my small community signed up to prepare meals for us five days a week for six months!! It was wonderful, and I got visitors every day. Now, I have the opportunity to give back to another friend in our community recently diagnosed. It's great being on the receiving end, but I think the giving makes you feel even better."

Anita Leuzzi; diagnosed in 1997 at age 45;
legal secretary; New York

"Promise yourself that you will return the kindnesses that were offered to you. Someday it will be your turn to help, and you will feel good about reciprocating."

Mary Raffol; diagnosed in 1998 at age 44;
teacher; Massachusetts

"Women friends are more important to me since my surgery. It takes time to have friends—time and effort that we don't always have when we're raising families or working. But my priorities have changed."

Anne Jacobs; diagnosed in 1999 at age 62;
managing partner, real estate; Massachusetts

"When I went in for a mammogram, I saw a friend, Kim, sitting there. I talked to her and found that my experience had prompted her to get a mammogram."

Sandy Williams; diagnosed in 1999 at age 51;
children's public services librarian; Texas

9 · The Workplace

Making It User-Friendly

There's nothing like being your own boss. In that sense, I had the best possible scenario when it came to working through breast cancer treatment. Yes, I work on deadline, but the deadline that I set for myself is usually a month or more before the one that my publisher sets for me. This means I have leeway should something crop up. It sure took the pressure off when I was diagnosed.

Another bennie of being your own boss is being able to work at home. I wore sweatsuits. I wore big men's shirts. I sat with a heating pad between the chair and my back (no one *told* me my back would hurt when my chest wall was pushed out to make room for new breasts—but that does get better, ladies), and no one looked at me askance. I didn't have to apologize or explain when I took off for a couple of hours to have radiation or to take a nap.

Not everyone has this luxury. Occupation-wise, members of the *UPLIFT* sisterhood run the gamut from bus driver to musician to banker. We have dentists and dental assistants, lawyers and legal assistants, microbiologists, psychotherapists, and midwives. We have a lieutenant governor. We have a broadcast journalist. We have architects, sales clerks, and telephone operators. We have a symphony musician.

If I were to single out the occupation with the heaviest concentration of submitters, it would be teachers—but then, we do expect that teachers like to write. There are also a striking number of nurses in the group. Of course, they were in a prime position to learn about this project and care about passing on their advice. Lord knows, they've seen the downside of women who are in the dark.

And there were moms and wives galore—far more than are listed in the credits—and I'm sorry for that. When people were asked about their occupation, they often listed their outside-the-home job, when the content of their submissions clearly suggests that they juggle inside-the-home jobs as well.

Inside or outside, an amazing number of women said that they worked right through treatment. I can identify with these women. For me, work was an escape. It enabled me to minimize the impact of having breast cancer, and was a reminder that life went on.

Not every woman works right through, and remarks from these women are included here, too. They'll tell you about the flexibility of their bosses and about how taking time off worked for them. *Worked for them.* That's the key, here. What works for one woman may not work for another. What works in one job may not work in another. The thing is, you need to take a step back, think about yourself and your situation, then speak up about what may work for you. In every situation, you have choices, and the choices are all *good.* What pleases one woman may not please another.

Which is why they have menus in restaurants, as my dad used to say.

SPILLING THE BEANS

"I never made a secret of my diagnosis. My staff knew almost as soon as my family. I did try to choose carefully the time and circumstances when I told friends and acquaintances—I did not want to appear melodramatic, but I also didn't want people to find out from a source other than me. I felt strongly that I was the best source of information about my illness, and I knew I felt good and looked good."

Wanda Null; diagnosed in 1986 at age 41;
librarian; Massachusetts

"Talking about my diagnosis, my appointments, my procedures, and my observations was one of the best things I could have done. By sharing my experiences, I was able to reduce some of the fear that my friends, family, co-workers, and I were experiencing. Everyone at work has been supportive. I really believe that because I was open and honest, I was able to educate them. When people become educated about a subject, they become less fearful of it. I encourage everyone to ask whatever questions they might have."

Val Long; diagnosed in 1999 at age 47;
administrative assistant; Massachusetts

"I am a hairstylist, so I can make my own schedule, with chemo and all. Losing my hair was the worst, but I bought a wig that was close to my hair, so no one really knew. Customers of the salon who have heard I have cancer have come to me telling of their stories with the disease. I've found support everywhere!"

Sharon Daniels; diagnosed in 2000 at age 49;
hairstylist, wig store owner; Massachusetts

"How did I do it (juggle breast cancer and work)? I adopted a slight variation of the notorious 'don't ask, don't tell' policy. On the private side, only a few close friends and family members heard the news about my breast cancer diagnosis. On the professional side, I did not share details about my health crisis with any people outside my organization. When customers made comments (once I was wearing a wig), like 'Oh, you've changed your hair!' I responded with a simple, 'Yes, I have.' I acknowledged. I smiled. Nothing more. Good thing nobody asked, 'Hey, where are your eyebrows and eyelashes?' With practice, simple responses that revealed nothing became automatic. This worked for me; I could maintain my privacy and productivity level during treatment. I didn't have to drain my energies dealing with everyone else's level of discomfort with cancer. But most importantly, though, I could stay focused on work and address critical health issues at the same time."

Alysa Cummings; diagnosed in 1998 at age 45;

educational trainer; New Jersey

"I discovered my cancer three weeks before opening night of my favorite musical, *A Funny Thing Happened on the Way to the Forum.* The stress of that, plus a four-week cold, took its toll. I looked terrible. Fellow teachers asked me if my cough was going to kill me. Frightened that they were right, I would run away to cry. A simple 'How ya doing?' seemed inane; I wanted to answer 'I'm afraid I'm going to die from cancer. How are you?' I had always stressed honesty with my students, but I was not composed enough to tell them anything. Fearing what a crisis might do to a high school cast, and thinking this would be the last show I ever directed, I decided to enjoy Saturday's closing night and go in for surgery the following Monday. I also decided to write a letter to the students, and my musical director generously agreed to read it to them. In the letter, I stated the situation, my planned procedures, and my doctor's optimism for my total recovery. I reminded the students of their many resources, appealing to their sense of creativity in solving artistic and personal problems. I ended my letter with 'When I return, we will learn and produce art together.' Almost a decade later, I still communicate with many of these students, and we're all still learning and producing art."

Judy Thibault Klevins; diagnosed in 1992 at age 47;

arts educator; Maryland

"My most difficult task was telling my middle-school–age students that I had breast cancer. I would be absent for the remainder of the term, and I felt that they had a right to know why. I came to school on what was to be my last day, and had decided to tell the students right after morning assembly. I had no clue what I would say or how they would receive the news. Would they be glad to have me leave? Would the boys snicker at my condition? I don't exactly remember what I said, but I told the facts—that I had breast cancer, that I would need surgery, and that I was scared. I told them that they were approaching the best time of the academic year—the latter part of the spring term—and that I would miss sharing it with them. I'm not sure what else I said, but when I really looked at my kids, I was astonished to see crying, upset children. My classes that day began in a somber fashion, but as we discussed my condition and they shared stories about cancer in their own families, we came to a peaceable moment when they each hugged me as they left the classroom. I had an Arab student at the time who told me that he had never before prayed for a Christian, but he promised to pray for me. I think that being a teacher is special, but during a time of crisis, students can be your best ally. After the assembly, the teachers were greeted by crying kids entering their classrooms. It ended up being a school-wide occasion. All the faculty were helpful in discussing the problem of breast cancer, the librarian made books available, the head of the Science Department made materials available for all of his classes. By 9:00 the flowers started arriving in my classroom—my students and their parents were sending them. I was amazed that many of the boys, in particular, called their mothers to give them the news. At one point, the headmaster called me in to tell me that my students were sneaking off campus to go to the local flower shop and that he was going to let them continue to do so. The kids were so wonderful that I left school elated. Shortly after I arrived home, my surgeon called to inform me that the 'just in case' biopsy of my other breast showed cancer, and that I would need surgery on both breasts. My mood at that time had been so positively influenced by my students that I barely reacted. I took the news calmly and told her of my day. Although the day of surgery was one of the scariest days of my life, the experience with my students helped me face it with confidence."

Lee Williams; diagnosed in 1996 at age 56;
teacher; Massachusetts

A WORKPLACE MANUAL

"Here are the strategies that helped me maintain that crucial balance between cancer and work: (1) I scheduled doctors' appointments early in the day or at the beginning of their 'seeing patients' time block. This way I was in and out of the office nice and fast. Doctors' schedules seem to back up as the day wears on. (2) Since radiation treatments are scheduled daily at the same time for six weeks, I begged and groveled to get a time slot near the end of the business day. (3) I planned my surgeries (especially elective reconstruction procedures) for Fridays, vacation, or slow times for business. Weekends are great times to recuperate and get back on your feet without losing precious work time or sick days. (4) I got an understudy and trained her. When I knew that I would not be feeling my best, (i.e., the first three days after a chemo infusion), I scheduled the understudy to work side by side with me. That way I had a safety net."

Alysa Cummings; diagnosed in 1998 at age 45;
educational trainer; New Jersey

"My young third graders cherished me and took care of me. They wouldn't let me lift or carry anything because they knew I wasn't supposed to be using my arm at that time."

Sue Watson; diagnosed in 1996 at age 53;
teacher; Texas

"While I was having treatments, I worked every day, but I finally realized that it was okay to take naps. Once I figured this out, it helped me get through a hard week a little better. My body let me know what it needed."

Michele Marks; diagnosed in 1996 at age 33;
CAD operator; Ohio

"My boss got me a laptop so that I could work from home on the days I didn't feel well."

Asha Mevlana; diagnosed in 1999 at age 24;
musician; New York

"My boss at the time was my brother. He suggested I go for radiation treatment in the morning, work a few hours, then go home and rest in the afternoons. That is what I did, because even though I looked great, I was unbelievably tired. When illness comes, we need to listen to our bodies and give them the time to rest and recover. I hadn't anticipated it, but those afternoon hours became a truly peaceful, nurturing time to read and rest and enjoy quiet time."

Deb Haney; diagnosed in 1996 at age 48;
administrative assistant, artist; Massachusetts

"I work at a regional high school with over twelve hundred students. During chemo, I was concerned about being exposed to so many people and possibly getting sick. The school district was great. They purchased a telephone headset for me to use, so that I wouldn't be exposed to unnecessary germs."

Linda Jones Burns; diagnosed in 2000 at age 40;
high school registrar; New Hampshire

"In the workplace, it was helpful that people stayed away from me when they had colds. The owner of the company told me to work only when I was up to it, and my bosses were patient with my distraction and my distracting others. There were lots of questions and curiosity, and I answered them all. I wanted to educate everybody along with myself. Work was my salvation. My fellow employees were supportive and continue to be so in my efforts to raise funds for cancer research. On the flip side, I've become the company support person on breast health. I even had my surgeon come and give a talk."

Deborah J.P. Schur; diagnosed in 1994 at age 43;
sales rep; Massachusetts

"It was very important to me to show people that I was alive and well. I rested between patients at the office, scheduled lightly, and didn't work around the house. I saved my energy for the office. My husband accompanied me to many functions and meetings at our children's school. We would never stay long, but I wanted to show my face."

A survivor; diagnosed in 1998 at age 45;
dentist; Indiana

"I juggled cancer and work by just giving up some things, like housework. I discovered that the house could go for weeks without being vacuumed or dusted—and not only did the sky not fall, it didn't even crack!"

Rosamary Amiet; diagnosed in 2000 at age 48;
program manager; Ohio

"If you are a large-breasted woman who has a lumpectomy with radiation, and you're working during treatment, you face a dilemma. You don't want to go without a bra in the workplace, because you feel like a cow! You can't wear a bra with bones or underwires, because they cause pressure on the radiation area. You need wide straps so that nothing digs into your shoulders, and you need a fabric that doesn't irritate your skin. During radiation, sexy goes out the door, and comfort is the watchword! The full-figure Bali bra style 3821 fit the bill for me. Go to a shop that has a professional fitter, and try on everything. I'd suggest buying one of the most comfortable and trying it out for a week before buying another one. The bra can be washed out every night. That way you haven't wasted a fortune on bras, only to find that they don't go the distance."

Sharon Irons Strempski; diagnosed in 1997 at age 52;
registered nurse; Connecticut

"The company I work for was very supportive, giving me time off when needed and consoling me when I felt down. I was on disability for a few months and then returned to work while still getting chemo treatments."

Sandy Mark; diagnosed in 1998 at age 55;
administrative assistant; Connecticut

BETTER THAN A CHRISTMAS BONUS

"I always knew I enjoyed the people I work with. But I never knew that they loved me—that they would be there for me—that they would cheer me up, encourage me, make me laugh—that they would help me believe in myself, so that I would know that I'd get well!"

Carolyn Stein; diagnosed in 1998 at age 45;
medical secretary; New York

"The people I work with brought a meal for every night of the week for three weeks, so that my family didn't have to worry about any of it. These co-workers all gave days of sick leave to me so that I would not have to go a day without pay. I only missed work when I absolutely had to. If I sat around doing nothing, I felt worse! The best thing I did was go to work and walk . . . walk . . . walk."

Pam Waddell; diagnosed in 1998 at age 38;
writer, teacher's aide; Texas

"I missed work for my surgery and the six weeks after it. My boss brought an ice cream cake to the hospital as a gift. We had no knife or plates, but the nurses loved it. Later he brought work to my house for me."

Irene Louise; diagnosed in 1995 at age 41;
retired executive secretary; Pennsylvania

"I worked with some of the best people. They called to check up on me. One friend went to all of my appointments with me. The principals kept telling me not to worry about the time off, and they kept paying me."

Michele Marks; diagnosed in 1996 at age 33;
CAD operator; Ohio

"My co-workers organized and arranged a schedule whereby someone brought me home-cooked food at least once a week. A quiche or casserole lasted several days!"

Carrie Drake; diagnosed in 1998 at age 42;
administrative assistant; Colorado

"When I was first diagnosed, I was worried about losing my job. But everyone at work was very caring. They were always asking for updates on my progress. A co-worker offered to shave my head in increments so that it would not be so devastating all at once. We would cut a little each week until it was time to shave it all."

Kathy Rabassa; diagnosed in 1999 at age 34;
administrative assistant; South Carolina

"My surgery was in the summer break from school, and I resumed work the following fall. During this time, I underwent chemotherapy and radiation. My school friends did many small things to make my life easier. They formed a dinner 'brigade' and took turns making dinners for us on my 'sick from chemo' days. They were aware that I would have temporary memory loss from medications, so instead of just telling me about a problem with a certain child, they would write me 'love' notes and put them on my office door to gently remind me. My principal allowed me to take my usual lunch break to have radiation therapy. When this took longer than the allotted time, she reasoned that I had spent many breaks working with teachers or children, and had at least that much time earned to use for this purpose. Therefore, I didn't lose work time for those appointments. It was so important for me to be 'normal,' and these ladies and men provided that normalcy for me."

Brenda Carr; diagnosed in 1988 at age 40;
wife, mother, retired school counselor; Texas

"I work with a wonderful group of people. After learning of my breast cancer, I received gifts almost daily. This was better than Christmas or my birthday! The day before my surgery, they surprised me with breakfast . . . a going-away party for my breast!"

Rosamary Amiet; diagnosed in 2000 at age 48;
program manager; Ohio

"I had only been at my job less than a year, so I had not accumulated much leave time. The people there donated their sick and vacation time to me to use for the bad days during chemo, and for my surgery and recovery. Their kindness will always be appreciated and remembered."

Gwen Loverink; diagnosed in 1994 at age 34;
police dispatcher; California

"I was blessed to work in a school district personnel department with co-workers who were incredibly supportive and understanding. Every day for six weeks, I joked that I was actually going to the beach to work on my tan, rather than heading to the hospital for my daily dose of rays. On the morning of my last treatment day, I picked up a beach party feast for my 'office family.' We had bagels in a beach bucket, cream cheese on a sand shovel, and cool fruit smoothies from the blender, and I gave everyone a bright Hawaiian lei. In turn, they surprised me with a beautiful Estee Lauder heart-shaped compact. Later I engraved on it the words 'Beach Party, December 3, 1999.' It is a constant reminder to me of the love and support of very dear friends."

Paula Linman; diagnosed in 1999 at age 48; school district personnel secretary; South Carolina

"Since I had taken time off from work to focus on and get through treatments, that meant my husband had to work more. My girlfriends were worried that I was not having enough fun, so often we would meet for lunch. They would always pick up the tab, knowing that my husband and I were counting every penny to see that the bills got paid. One Sunday, my girlfriends called to say that they would be arriving to baby-sit my two boys and that they were ordering my husband and me to go out to eat. When they arrived, they handed my husband a gift certificate to the most romantic restaurant. Off we went and enjoyed a most delicious dinner. Later, when I entered my bedroom, I noticed a single rose on our pillows. Under the rose was a card, signed with the good wishes of all the people I worked with. Enclosed was also a check. The card read that the money was to be used for whatever I felt my family needed it for. While a trip to Disney sounded very appealing, the bills were mounting fast. There was no question. This gift allowed us to make two mortgage payments. It is a true friend who goes the extra mile to find what it is that you and your family really need."

Cindy Fiedler; diagnosed in 1998 at age 40; registered nurse, mom; Massachusetts

"I was stunned by the love and support I received from friends and co-workers during my illness. When I returned to work, I wrote this Top Ten list and read it at a department gathering.

Top Ten Reasons Why Having Cancer Is Not *Completely* **Horrible**

No. 10   I lost ten pounds.
No. 9   I read several books.
No. 8   I got lots of e-mail, cards, and presents.
No. 7   I had eight months off with disability income.
No. 6   I saved a lot of money on haircuts and shampoo.
No. 5   I learned to appreciate nose hair.
No. 4   I could watch the daytime talk shows.
No. 3   I met strong, inspiring women.
No. 2   My husband and I are even closer.
And the No. 1 reason why having cancer is not *completely* horrible is . . . that the people who love me have told me so."

Lisette; diagnosed in 1999 at age 47;
business analyst; Connecticut

KEEP ON TRUCKIN'

"I was out of law school one year when diagnosed. Work was my salvation. I went back to it ten weeks after my mastectomy and only remember missing two days during my six months of chemo."

Barbara Jentis; diagnosed in 1983 at age 41;
attorney; New Jersey

"Thank goodness for children. I have a group that comes before the library opens to the public. They are bright and alert. As I do their story time I get lost with their expressions and responses."

Sandy Williams; diagnosed in 1999 at age 51;
children's public services librarian; Texas

"I was told by the people at work to take all the time I needed for anything I needed. But I didn't miss work. Keeping busy was my salvation. Each day, I put on makeup and a smile. When my hair fell out, I put on a great wig. It cost a fortune, but it was money well spent. No one knew it was not my hair."

Frances Gallello; diagnosed in 2000 at age 51;
mental health assistant; New York

"I worked through the whole thing. I think that my having breast cancer bothered others more than it bothered me."

Carleen Muniz; diagnosed in 1998 at age 51;
artist; Massachusetts

"I learned to do things differently at work as a school bus driver to help take the pressure off just one arm."

Mary Ann Budnick; diagnosed in 1991 at age 44;
school bus driver; Michigan

"When my sister was diagnosed with breast cancer, I thought it would only strike one sister. Boy, was I wrong. Three years later, I was diagnosed, and had a lumpectomy, chemotherapy, and six weeks of radiation. I've been selling real estate on commission for twenty-two years—I'm divorced and support myself—so having to go into the hospital wasn't exactly what I wanted. The good news is, I was home for two days resting, then went out and listed two homes with one side of my chest bound and aching!"

Patti R. Martinez; diagnosed in 1999 at age 54;
realtor; California

"I worked with twenty women at the office. They were loving, caring, and devoted to me, and my boss was extremely generous and giving of herself. Work helped to bridge the gap for me, and I resumed as much of my lifestyle as I could without any alterations."

Alyce Feinstein; diagnosed in 1993 at age 58;
administrative assistant; Massachusetts

"Stay busy. I was fortunate to work for a bank that allowed me to work with flexible hours."

Jill Gross; diagnosed in 2000 at age 51;
bank head teller; Massachusetts

"The only work I missed was during my surgery. I worked every day while I went through chemo, even though I was tired. It made me feel like there was some semblance of normalcy in my life."

Barbara Moro; diagnosed in 1999 at age 57;
law secretary; New Jersey

AFTER THE STORM

"I showed up to work every day and had a smile for everyone. I still do. You smile, and everyone around you knows you're okay."

Pam Waddell; diagnosed in 1998 at age 38;
writer, teacher's aide; Texas

"I felt feminine once I had my new prosthesis, as I had lost fifteen pounds and wore a new dress on my return to work. I felt they would all look and think, 'Which side was it?' However, when they saw me, they were so glad, they hugged me and kissed me, and we all laughed. I felt good from then on."

Irene Louise; diagnosed in 1995 at age 41;
retired executive secretary; Pennsylvania

"I sent out a company-wide e-mail where I work, urging younger female employees to schedule mammograms and practice self-exams. Twelve women in my office scheduled exams that week. The company now plans to bring a mobile mammogram unit to its parking lot."

Joy West; diagnosed in 2000 at age 34; advertising account coordinator; South Carolina

"How did I juggle breast cancer and work? I was determined to maintain an appearance of normalcy as I scheduled surgeries, chemotherapy infusions, radiation treatments, and doctor's appointments while operating a small business. Two years after diagnosis, I am pleased to report that my business is thriving, and (knock on wood) according to my oncologist, so am I."

Alysa Cummings; diagnosed in 1998 at age 45; educational trainer; New Jersey

10 • Support Groups

From Traditional to Offbeat

"A breast cancer diagnosis puts you into an exclusive club. You wouldn't choose to join it, but once you do, you find a sisterhood like no other." This thought was sent in by Stephanie King, an oncology nurse from New York who passed it along second-hand, but the sentiment was too good not to pass on again. Indeed, one of the most meaningful parts of my experience with this book has been meeting survivors. Yes, there's an instant rapport. Regardless of how old we are, where we live, or what treatment choices we made, having gone through breast cancer gives us a connection. Never having joined a support group, I'm experiencing this bond for the very first time.

Why didn't I join a support group? There are several reasons, not the least of which had to do with time. Between family, career, and cancer treatment, I was busy enough; attending a weekly support group meeting would have been one commitment too many. There was also the privacy issue; even back then, my name was recognizable, and I was trying to keep word of my cancer quiet. I was also afraid of joining a support group, because there was a chance that someone in the group might die, and I didn't think I could handle that.

No, a traditional support group didn't appeal to me, but, looking back, I would have liked to have had a cancer buddy. I did try once. On a recommendation, I phoned the friend of a friend, but the woman so depressed me that I hung up the phone and cried. She was clearly the wrong person for me, not upbeat at all. But many members of the sisterhood have found the right person, and the experience sounds wonderful.

For the purposes of this chapter, I use the term 'group' in its loosest form. There can be a 'group' of thirty, a 'group' of eight, or a 'group' of two. Indeed, in the course of organizing UPLIFT, I learned about the many different sizes of groups. I've organized this chapter along those lines. There are traditional support groups that meet at regular times, often in a hospital setting. Some are defined by age, some by the time from diagnosis. There are one-on-one support pairings—some set up by a hospital, some by a friend, some by a fluke. There are *unusual* support vehicles, one of the most promising being cyberspace.

And then, of course, there's UPLIFT. It is definitely a support group and just the kind that would have worked for me. I could have availed myself of it from the privacy of my bedroom, could have spent five minutes with it or an hour, could have picked up bits of advice and gotten the encouragement that I wanted, could have been absolutely, positively assured of an optimistic response from hundreds of women. In the course of compiling this book, I corresponded with many of its contributors. We shared theories and compared stories, to the extent that I do now consider them friends. So here is another kind of support group. If I had to fit UPLIFT into one of the slots in this chapter, it would be "Off the Beaten Path."

Now, you—you can have UPLIFT and another support group, too! Remember, though: what works for one woman may not work for another. As in so many other aspects of breast cancer survival, there are choices. Here are the different kinds of support groups. Pick yours.

TRIED AND TRUE

"A friend of mine was going through her illness at the same time I was. I wanted to be supportive of her, so I went with her to a support group at a local hospital. I found that I benefited greatly from attending those meetings. I highly recommend support groups for a better recovery result. Sharing with others who are going through the same ordeal can be very comforting. Not only do you help yourself, but it makes you feel better when you can help others as well."

Sheila Steinhauser; diagnosed in 1985 at age 41;
office manager; Maryland

"My support group filled in the cracks when I needed it most. We shared everything together and learned from one another. There was a common bond. I met many gals during this period, and we held nothing back."

Alyce Feinstein; diagnosed in 1993 at aged 58;
administrative assistant; Massachusetts

"One of the best pieces of advice I can give is to have someone to talk to—a support group to pick up on the things that you can't do—someone to just hang out with, to lean on."

Michele Marks; diagnosed in 1996 at age 33;
CAD operator; Ohio

"Consider joining a local support group even though it may not be your thing. There, you will always have a place to talk things out, in the company of people who understand."

Mary Raffol; diagnosed in 1998 at age 44;
teacher; Massachusetts

"Get into a support group as soon as you're diagnosed. I got into mine late, which I regret. The place I go has three levels—newly diagnosed and in treatment, after treatment, and a group for people three or more years after treatment."

Sharon Irons Strempski; diagnosed in 1997 at age 52;
registered nurse; Connecticut

"My women's group is a tool all cancer patients need to have."

Nan Comstock; diagnosed in 1988 at age 39;
self-employed; California

"Through my support group, I'm regaining the power that cancer has taken from me. I can now say without reservation, 'God never closes a door without opening a window, and the view from the window he's opened is beautiful.' "

Joy West; diagnosed in 2000 at age 34;
advertising account coordinator; South Carolina

"The breast cancer survivors of the Image Reborn Support Group were my dearest support. My time with them has helped me reach the place in my life where I can say that breast cancer has been a gift. It has changed my life. It took me a while to get to this point, though. In the beginning, when I was in pain, one of the support group facilitators, a breast cancer survivor herself, said that I should feel the pain like a thunderstorm—that it is there and then will pass."

Bonnie Schneider; diagnosed in 1998 at age 45;
audiologist; Connecticut

"I had family members come and help out around the house, and friends bringing meals. At first I felt bad that they were all doing this stuff for me, but by the end of my first four cycles of chemo, I was worn out and knew I needed help. When I got discouraged and fearful, I talked with a nurse. That helped. I also joined a support group. Even though the women were older than me (I was twenty-four), we all had breast cancer in common. They have been a wonderful support for me."

Candice Jaeger; diagnosed in 2000 at age 24;
wife, mother; Illinois

"I contacted Reach to Recovery and found them to be extremely positive and supportive. They put me in touch with others who also had lumpectomies, and I have learned that we do not have to face this alone. Yes, our families are a tremendous support, but it is important to share our feelings with others who know exactly how we feel—and they also know how to help our family members learn how to deal with it too."

Rose Marie Clark; diagnosed in 1996 at age 50;
retired; New York

"I started my own cancer support with women in my area, and I have learned to basically use my cancer as a tool for spiritual awakening. I got my Reiki Master last year, which is a form of energy healing, and I have a nursing background. I have begun a small practice of helping to teach women and men how to use their experience with cancer as their tool for growth by tapping into their inherent wisdom. It is too easy to let the fear and uncertainty that comes with getting cancer take control."

Sandy Rodgers; diagnosed in 1999 at age 44;
homemaker, mom, registered nurse, Reiki Master; Massachusetts

"Four months after my surgery, I looked for a support group. I felt that I needed to be with other women who had been there, so that I could gather some strength and get a better balance in my life. It was a great thing to do. The group was lively and friendly. Newcomers got to meet women who'd had similar surgery. Questions got answered, and fears were understood. No one really knows what you feel unless they have been there too. The truth is, cancer has made my life richer. I never thought I would say that, but it has. I now volunteer in a cancer resource library and help others find information about their disease."

Pauline Hughes; diagnosed in 1997 at age 61;
retired registered nurse; Florida

ONE ON ONE

"The hospital set me up with a 'buddy' who was going through similar treatment and who was around the same age as me. She became one of my best friends during this time. She understood everything about the sickness and anxiety that I didn't want to pile on my friends. It was critical to have someone who really understood what I was going through."

Asha Mevlana; diagnosed in 1999 at age 24;
musician; New York

"I met a wonderful woman while we were both undergoing radiation. She had a great face and hat, so I asked where she got the hat, and we chatted for hours. She has become a very dear friend. She and I feel a kinship that only cancer survivors know. I did find out where she got the hat and have since recommended them to many people."

Susan Clemente; diagnosed in 1990 at age 46;
retired registered nurse; New York

"One of the best things that can happen? Someone answered my e-mail request for information when I couldn't find literature. She became my mentor, giving me questions to ask and explaining what I might have missed."

Anne Jacobs; diagnosed in 1999 at age 62;
managing partner, real estate; Massachusetts

"Six weeks after getting married, I was diagnosed with breast cancer. I was 27. My diagnosis came as a shock to everyone! My former college roommate's mother, a breast cancer survivor herself, called me from two states away. She recommended a book that helped me understand the diagnosis and prepare questions for my doctors."

Beth Compton; diagnosed in 1995 at age 27;
civil engineer; South Carolina

"I believe that developing a positive comradery with a person who has walked in your shoes can be very helpful and encouraging."

Becky Honeycutt; diagnosed in 1995 at age 53;
licensed practical nurse; Indiana

"Get to know some women who are survivors—they are not hard to find! Talking to women who have been survivors for five years, fourteen years, or thirty-nine plus years encourages me. I think of these women's stories when my own fears surface."

Faye Hardiman; diagnosed in 1998 at age 50;
wife, mother, teacher; Georgia

"Find someone who has been down this path to be your mentor! My pastor's wife's cousin, Alma, was sent by God. Although she was less than two years out from diagnosis, she was a tremendous support. We e-mailed and talked on the phone. She told me to ask for tests that would not have been done had I not asked. My husband, Wally, said that it was a big emotional relief for him that I had a 'lay expert' I could turn to at any point."

Monica May; diagnosed in 1997 at age 40;
organizing consultant; New Mexico

"As soon as I was diagnosed, a volunteer from Reach for Recovery came and spent the day with me. She was wonderful! We laughed, cried, and ate junk food. I felt much better by the time she left. She had survived, and I could too."

Mitzi Scarborough; diagnosed in 1999 at age 37;
childcare provider; Arkansas

"Many people, a lot of them strangers, took the time to tell me of their own cancer battle and survival. I didn't even know they'd had cancer. Their stories encouraged me and gave me hope. I try to do the same for others."

Sue Watson; diagnosed in 1996 at age 53;
teacher; Texas

"I am a medical social worker. I might have gotten helpful advice from my colleagues, but I was not comfortable sharing my diagnosis with them for fear of being treated differently by patients and staff. So the most help and excellent advice came from the friend of a friend, whom to this day I have never met. Barbara, who is also a survivor, remained a voice on the telephone who helped me work through treatment choices, and gave wonderful advice as to how to negotiate the next few months of my life. She said that it was okay to not wear a bra if I wasn't comfortable during the weeks of radiation, that it was okay to disagree with my physician (I changed doctors before radiation treatment began), that it was okay to cry and lean on my spouse, and that I do not have to know everything. She said that this time I was allowed to be the patient. I was the one in charge of my life decisions. She helped me to see that I needed to set my coping goals for one minute at a time, one hour at a time, one day at a time—and then to realize, yes, I can do this!"

Nancie Watson; diagnosed in 1995 at age 50;
social worker; Pennsylvania

"I recommend going to your treatments alone. You're bound to meet and talk to your fellow chemo and/or radiation patients. It's almost like a support group. If you have a family member or friend with you, you are less likely to talk to anyone else. Also, going by yourself makes it seem more like just another doctor's appointment, rather than a big ordeal. I got really friendly with a couple of my oncology nurses. They were wonderful . . . and very funny! Sometimes I'd leave there thinking 'How in the world did

I have fun at a chemo treatment?' Not that I wasn't *very* happy when I had my *last* treatment!"

Deborah Lambert; diagnosed in 2000 at age 47;
medical secretary; Massachusetts

"In the paper, I read a letter about a 'must-have' booklet for cancer patients. I called and ordered one. The last question they asked me was, 'Would you like to have a cancer survivor call you?' *No! I would not!* I thought, but instead, the single word, 'Yes,' came out.

"For several weeks, I cried and cried. One particularly bad night, the phone rang. I picked it up. A woman said that her name was Connie, that she was calling from Kansas, and did I have time to chat? 'Yes,' I whispered, and she asked how I was doing. 'Not so good,' I said. 'I can't stop crying. When will I stop crying and feeling sorry for myself?' Connie said, 'One day, it will just stop. You'll be okay. We all need time to mourn, time to be sad, and it's okay to cry.' She went on to tell me about how she cried a lot at first. She gave all her clothes away except a housedress, a skirt, and a blouse. Days, weeks, months went by. She didn't die, but she had no clothes! That was twenty years ago. That night, I began to heal—laughing for the first time in a long, long time. That night, I learned tears are okay. Tears are a part of healing."

Jinny Morrison; diagnosed in 1998 at age 55;
bus aide for mentally retarded adults; Ohio

OFF THE BEATEN PATH

"I found conventional support group meetings difficult, so I formed my own support dinner group. We would dine out every couple of months to discuss having breast cancer. We also shared stories of our spouses, children, and travels."

Deborah J.P. Schur; diagnosed in 1994 at age 43;
sales rep; Massachusetts

"When they found cancer in one breast, I decided on a prophylactic mastectomy of the other. Afterward, I formed what I tenderly call the 'Double or Nothing Club' for all my friends who have had bilateral mastectomies."

Aileen Pandapas; diagnosed in 1989 at age 41;
mom, volunteer, former secretary; Virginia

"The most practical thing I did after diagnosis was to start a support group for breast cancer survivors in their 20s and 30s. We call ourselves the 'Big C Chicks' and now number around fifteen members. Our mission is not only to support and mentor one another, but to educate our peers that no one is too young to have breast cancer."

Joy West; diagnosed in 2000 at age 34;
advertising account coordinator; South Carolina

"We have a large family, and my brother and sister-in-law have a very large circle of friends and business associates. When my sister-in-law was in the hospital, the process of keeping everyone updated was daunting. So my brother set up a website devoted to his wife's health and recovery status. He entered information onto a journal page every day, and visitors to the site were encouraged to sign the guest book, which was a way to send an e-mail to my sister-in-law or brother. It was a fantastic way to keep everyone updated and served as a way for all of us to schedule visits, plus my sister-in-law got to see how many people were out there rooting for her."

Wendy Page;
sister-in-law of Barbra Marcus Kolton; Massachusetts

"I didn't want to go to the minister's fortieth birthday party, but my husband insisted that we stop in for a while. We were met by many familiar faces, helium balloons, food, cake, drinks, and loving hugs. Two friends, each of whom had been free of breast cancer for more than twenty years, shared stories with me. Another friend, who had recently finished chemo, assured me that if I had to have it, the doctors would give me medicine to keep me from getting so terribly sick. My spirits rose. I felt positive again. I could do this thing."

Sandy Williams; diagnosed in 1999 at age 51;

children's public services librarian; Texas

" 'There is no such thing as a problem without a gift for you in its hands.' One of the gifts I received came in the form of a four-day retreat on Madeline Island with the Breast Cancer Recovery Foundation. I was with ten other women who'd had breast cancer. We talked, laughed, and sometimes cried together. We went kayaking on Lake Superior, where I recall seeing trees hanging from cliffs with their roots totally exposed. I commented to the other woman in my kayak, 'Trees aren't supposed to live like that, with their roots all exposed to the elements, hanging from the edge of a cliff. But the will to survive is strong, and we, too, can continue to thrive with less than optimal conditions, just like those trees.' One of the women at this retreat was a petite gray-haired woman, probably in her 60s, who had been blind from birth and had two glass eyes. Our first night, she got up and sang—a rap song no less—about her wahddy dahddy do, which was the name she had come up with for the flap of skin under your armpit after a mastectomy. She had us all just roaring with laughter. She went kayaking for the first time in her life on this retreat."

Gracie Schwingel; diagnosed in 1998 at age 51;

secretary; Wisconsin

"When I was diagnosed with breast cancer, I e-mailed a few friends to let them know. One friend who was not on the list e-mailed me to say, 'We're your friends in the bad times as well as the good!' As a result, I wrote to two lists of friends, whom I dubbed Supergals and Power Pals. I gave them permission to pass on my e-mail to anyone they felt it would help. The list grew over the next six months from fourteen to over two hundred. I sent 'Updates from Deb' periodically to describe what I was going through so they could understand the tests and procedures. Six months later, I'd received over 1300 e-mail messages back. Two of my favorites were 'Because of your updates and courage, my mom went to have a mammogram for the first time in four years!' and 'My mom has breast cancer, too, and is about three weeks behind you in treatment—I've been forwarding your updates and she no longer is afraid, because she knows what to expect.' I've realized that breast cancer was a blessing, not a curse. Discovering that people truly care about me was wonderful. Being able to help others going through something similar was awesome."

Deb Haggerty; diagnosed in 1999 at age 51;

professional speaker; Florida

* * *

"A unique experience I had with breast cancer is that I 'met' a woman online who was diagnosed at the same time I was. She and I found each other at a breast cancer site shortly after our surgeries, and her chemo started the day after mine. We e-mailed each other every day through our treatments—she's in Las Vegas, I'm in the Boston area. We shared our deepest, darkest moments together, but also shared lots of laughter and many tears. In rereading our letters, I realize that I shared feelings with Kym that I didn't verbalize to my husband, children, or closest friends. I think I put on a good front for those around me, because I wanted to protect them. With Kym, I could express all my concerns. Our letters were a safe place for that. Nor were those letters all about breast cancer. We talked about our families and shared day-to-day stories. We refused to allow our disease to define or consume us."

Nancy Lane; diagnosed in 2000 at age 53;

teacher; Massachusetts

"I'm the Las Vegas half of the e-mail penpal duo. Nancy and I literally went through breast cancer treatment together from opposite ends of the country. I initially e-mailed her because I thought I could offer her words of comfort. But Nancy became my comforter, my encouragement. We both had wonderful support systems of family and friends, but we understood everything that was happening to one another in a way that no one else did. I found such comfort in hearing her thoughts, fears, and feelings. We shared day-to-day struggles and triumphs. Nancy's strength, wit, and compassion gave me courage when I couldn't find any of my own. Even though we have never met, I consider Nancy one of my dearest friends."

Kym Dyer; diagnosed in 2000 at age 42;
management; Nevada

RECIPROCITY

"While my extended family and friends all knew about my cancer, I didn't share the information with new friends or associates for many years. Then, around 1990, one of the secretaries in my office developed breast cancer and needed a mastectomy. I came out of the closet for her, and it helped both of us. She was strengthened by seeing my absolutely normal life. And I was strengthened by being able to help someone."

Barbara Jentis; diagnosed in 1983 at age 41;
attorney; New Jersey

"Be a mentor to someone else newly diagnosed in the same manner you chose a survivor to mentor you. You will be surprised how much value your experience has for others."

Kathy Weaver-Stark; diagnosed in 1991 at age 46;
insurance adjuster, instructor; Oregon

"Reach out to others. When my sister wasn't in the hospital herself, she'd go back to visit other breast cancer patients. Focusing on others made her feel better. Giving of herself regenerated her energy."

Barbara Keiler;
daughter of a survivor; Massachusetts

"One of the most rewarding things to come out of my experience with breast cancer is being able to help others. I've had co-workers come to me about people in their lives who had been diagnosed. I'm always glad to be able to help. This is something no one should have to go through alone."

Val Long; diagnosed in 1999 at age 47;
administrative assistant; Massachusetts

"As a professional counselor I felt that my contribution to the cause could be my willingness to be a listener and supporter to others. I tell friends, family, and colleagues that I will talk with anyone they know who is newly diagnosed . . . not for medical help, but with a compassionate ear. Just this past week, I have had two such calls."

Patricia Carr; diagnosed in 1989 at age 51;
community college professor, counselor; New Jersey

"I now call on newly diagnosed women and try to be a resource for them. No question is a dumb question. The unknown is one of our worst enemies."

Judy Peterson; diagnosed in 2000 at age 58;
registered nurse; Colorado

"Over the past eleven years, I have gotten calls from people who know my history, asking me to speak with a friend or loved one of theirs. I always say yes and tell my story. I have been blessed to know that I have helped people get up and move on."

Susan Clemente; diagnosed in 1990 at age 46;
retired registered nurse; New York

"Participate in walks or events that promote breast cancer awareness. Give encouragement to others who are undergoing surgery or treatment. Sending a card or making a call may be as therapeutic for you as it will be helpful for them."

Faye Hardiman; diagnosed in 1998 at age 50;
wife, mother, teacher; Georgia

"I understood that only someone who had been diagnosed with breast cancer could truly know what I was feeling. I became active in the breast cancer movement. I felt that by being verbal and public about what was happening to me, and by helping anyone who asked, I was advocating against the disease. I started a foundation, Art beCAUSE, dedicated to funding research projects which would look at the links between breast cancer and the environment."

Eleanor Anbinder; diagnosed in 1991 at age 50;
sales manager; Massachusetts

"I have embraced my survivor status and have started teaching girls as young as twelve how to do breast self-exams. I have become a Chemo Angel, helping other cancer patients get through the agony of fighting for their lives. And I have become an avid supporter of breast cancer awareness. I am a breast cancer survivor and I am only twenty-seven years old."

Kimberlee Richardson; diagnosed in 2000 at age 26;
mother, Air Force wife, student; Mississippi

"After my diagnosis nine years ago, I decided to do something positive for other women experiencing that scary time in their life. So I've volunteered in the American Cancer Society's Reach to Recovery program. Doing so enabled me to meet many wonderful and courageous women."

Susan Sanford; diagnosed in 1992 at age 48;
retired mortgage insurance underwriter, volunteer; Nevada

"My mother and her mother both had breast cancer, so I was on the lookout for trouble. I found it in 1981 in the form of a tumor on my left breast. A reoccurrence followed two years later, so by age 34, I had bilateral mastectomies. After the surgery, I was visited by an American Cancer Society Reach to Recovery volunteer. She came walking into my house looking fit and healthy, and she was full of energy and wonderful positiveness that gave me hope. She was what I wanted to be—alive and healthy and strong. So I waited the mandatory year after diagnosis and took training in volunteering for Reach to Recovery. It has changed my life, just as I know I have changed the lives of the women I visit each month. I am now that picture of health, that strong woman who has beaten breast cancer not once but twice. I now train volunteers to participate in this wonderful program and urge every woman who is diagnosed with breast cancer to contact her local American Cancer Society office and ask to be visited by a Reach to Recovery volunteer. These are women helping women, sharing their experiences as only women can."

Maribeth Stone; diagnosed in 1982 at age 32;
decorative painting teacher; Massachusetts

"About a year ago, I attended my first breast cancer support group meeting. Paul said I was crying in my sleep that night. It costs me to revisit my experience with breast cancer. But I will always try to be there for any woman I meet who is going through some aspect of breast cancer. I have learned, though, that I cannot routinely 'put myself out there' for meetings and still stay calm enough to live my life and do my work."

Jeanne Sturdevant; diagnosed in 1990 at age 45;
artist; Texas

"I decided not to join a breast cancer awareness group, mainly because I have seen it become a hobby with a few women. All they walk and think is breast cancer. I had it, it's gone, I want to get on with life. However, I am more willing to discuss it and answer questions for someone who might be going through making all the important decisions."

Lorraine J. Pakkala-Lintala; diagnosed in 1992 at age 62; editor, author; Florida, New York

"Less than a year after my diagnosis, my daughter was attacked and almost died. My focus immediately switched from me to her. When she went back to college, I was so grateful for both of our lives that I began doing volunteer work at the hospital where I was treated. I needed to give back. A few years later, I took a part-time job in Cancer Services. Now I can educate other women as they go through the process by letting them know that they have options and that they shouldn't let the fear take over. I am truly blessed."

Marianne Rennie; diagnosed in 1988 at age 39; cancer information specialist; Ohio

"Driving to work one October morning, I noticed lovely pink bows tied around nearly every tree in the business section of town. As I walked around during lunchtime I read many of the inscriptions accompanying the bows. Each was a tribute honoring a woman who had breast cancer, her name put there by a loved one or friend. I was so touched by this beautiful tribute, which I have since seen in other towns, that I have decided to become part of the sponsoring group, the Susan Komen Foundation. Next October, I have names of my own to honor!"

Bobbi Kolton; mother-in-law of Barbra Marcus Kolton; New Jersey

"When I heard the words, 'you have breast cancer,' I knew my life had changed forever. What I didn't expect was the door that opened for me to feel empowered to make a difference. Three days after my diagnosis, I met a new friend at a breast cancer support group. We discovered that we lived a street away and ex-

changed phone numbers. Over the next several months, we
talked and checked in on each other, and a special friendship
began. Together we founded Friends with Hope. Working with
our families and a committee of friends, we organized an annual
5K walk/race and a dinner auction. We have raised over $40,000
for breast cancer research. We now feel that we can do and beat
anything."

Cheryl Cavallo; diagnosed in 1997 at age 35;
homemaker; Massachusetts

"After surviving two bouts of breast cancer, I realized I needed to
give back some of the support and caring that was offered to me.
Fortunately, I live in the town where my treatment was taking
place. Others were not so lucky. I know that in medical emergen-
cies or during long treatment plans, the last thing you want to
think about is a place to stay while treatment is going on. Therefore, I thought, why not build a house so much like home that
everyone who came to stay could relax and concentrate on regaining their health. Thus, the Lewis Rathbun Center, a Hospital
Hospitality House, was born. After much planning, preparation,
and building, my dream to 'give back' came true! The Center
turned seven years old this year and is still going strong!"

Adelaide D. Key; diagnosed in 1978 at age 42;
community volunteer, philanthropist; North Carolina

11 · Humor

You Gotta Laugh . . .

N o way, you're thinking, and it's understandable. The last thing you can imagine when you first learn you have breast cancer and become embroiled in the haze of doctor's appointments, treatment schedules, and family needs is laughter. After a bit, though, the haze clears. You start adjusting to the reality of the diagnosis—finish making decisions, adapt to a new routine—and your mind isn't as cluttered. Nor is your mouth as busy talking with everyone and his brother after that first frenzy. So. That mouth can either turn down, stay flat, or turn up. It's your choice.

Members of the sisterhood opt for the latter. Val Long, who was diagnosed in 1999 at the age of 47, is currently an administrative assistant for the Massachusetts Breast Cancer Coalition. She wrote, "Laughter is a big help. Believe it or not, there are a lot of funny things that happen when you're being treated for cancer. Learn to see the funny side. Everything has one."

Asha Mevlana gives a good example of this. A musician from New York, she was diagnosed in 1999 at the age of 24. "Keeping a sense of humor definitely helped me get through the worst.

Right around the time when my hair started coming out in clumps, my friends and I happened to be out at a restaurant. The food was taking a while, so when the waitress came over, I pretended to get angry. I grabbed my hair with both hands, said I was getting very frustrated that it was taking so long, and pulled huge chunks of hair out in a fit of fake anger. Her mouth dropped. We got our food shortly thereafter."

It isn't just survivors who talk about the importance of humor. Researchers are starting to talk about it, too. While psychologists have long praised humor as a way of decreasing anxiety and stress, more formal studies are showing the actual physiological effects of laughter. Some studies make a connection between laughter and improved circulation and respiration; others suggest that laughter can increase the production of pain-reducing endorphins, or even enhance the immune system. Yet other studies chart a rise in heart rate, circulation, and blood pressure during robust laughter, akin to the most beneficial effects of aerobic exercise.

Floridian Susan Ragland was diagnosed with breast cancer in 1978, well before these studies were done. She has her own thoughts about laughter, as told in a poignant story.

"In November of 1978, at the age of forty-five, I passed the New Jersey State Bar. About two weeks later, I found a lump in my breast. I had a mastectomy, followed by thirty days of radiation therapy, which I tolerated well. By now it was early January. There was snow on the ground, and I was feeling a cumulative fatigue from the treatments. I asked my husband if he could get away to a warm climate, even for a week, just the two of us. He made the arrangements while I called my neighbor, a travel agent. I said, 'Bess, just get me somewhere where there's sun, where it's warm, and where I can just sit and relax. I don't care where it is.' She said that it was a busy time of year, but promised to get right to work on it. In the meantime, my sister, also a veteran of breast cancer, took me for a mastectomy bathing suit. In those days, the makers of such things must have thought a mastectomy meant that somehow your thighs were injured, because the only decent one they had was high on the chest and skirted to the knee. I was very proud of my legs in those days and wanted to flaunt this remaining sexual asset. But I was going away to a warm climate to recuperate and relax. I had a loving, caring, attentive husband, who had literally moved heaven and earth to get away on short notice. So I took the suit.

"My travel agent called me back and said, 'You're in luck. I found a small hotel on the French island of Guadaloupe, where there is guaranteed steady sunshine. I think it's just the ticket.' A few days later, encouraged and optimistic, we arrived in the tropics. What a relief, I thought, to escape the dreary, cold, dismal winter. The only thing I was leery about was my grandma bathing suit. But I said, 'What the hell; who am I here to impress?'

"We went directly to our room. It was lunchtime, and we decided to lunch by the pool and then start our relaxing. Reluctantly, I put on my one-piece swimsuit, which was Kelly green with white piping (I will never forget that suit, although my husband thought I looked very handsome in it), and went off to the pool to have lunch.

"It was then that it hit me between the eyes. Breasts! Everywhere I looked. Breasts, uncovered, everywhere! There were small ones, large ones, perky young ones, and even some droopy old ones. My travel agent had sent us to a topless hotel and beach! Not only was I the only one covered up, but I had this damn skirt down to my knees. All the good feelings about myself, that I'd worked so hard to preserve, suddenly vanished.

"My husband started to laugh, and so did I . . . at first. When we got back to the room, I started to cry a flood. My poor husband didn't know what to do. It was funny, it was a scream, but the thought of five more days of this was untenable. No way could I stay there! We got dressed and went to the hotel manager. He was most sympathetic but informed us that there were only two flights a week in and out of Guadaloupe, and that the next plane out was three days hence. I was trapped. I mustered up my spunk and made the best of it, but on the third day we were up early and on that plane. Much to everyone's surprise, we came home, repacked for a cold climate, and went north to our summer home in the Adirondack Mountains of New York, where we made a fire and sat and relaxed and healed. Only three days there, but I did come home rested—and laughing.

"I am still cancer-free twenty-two-plus years later," she concludes. Me, I like that punch line the best. But there are other punch lines where humor is concerned. For a sampling, read on.

HAIR-HA

"Before cancer, I had bad hair days. After cancer, I had bad hair days, but I could take it off and shake it."

Rosamary Amiet; diagnosed in 2000 at age 48;
program manager; Ohio

"I was standing on the back deck of our duplex home. I had washed my wig and was shaking out the excess water, thinking that I was alone. I wasn't. Our neighbor's three-year-old daughter yelled, 'Jill, what are you doing?' I said, 'Well, I'm drying my hair.' She looked at me and said, 'My mommy keeps her hair on and uses a machine to dry it.' "

Jill Gross; diagnosed in 2000 at 51;
bank head teller; Massachusetts

"When I came home from teaching, I would often take off my wig and set it on a kitchen counter. If I was distracted, then I went off and left it there. When Micah (my son) and his friends would come in, I would hear: 'Jane Barnett Royal-Davidson! Get down here this minute!' Being a good mother, I went downstairs obediently, and there Micah would reprimand me. 'Did my grandmother Royal raise you to leave your hair on the kitchen counter? I think not! Did you raise your children to leave their hair on the kitchen counter? I think not. We take our hair every-

where we go. Now, young lady, I want you to take your hair upstairs to your room and think about what you have done for say,
at least an hour. Then you may come downstairs and we shall
talk.' I would take my hair and go upstairs and lie down for a
much-needed nap. Sometimes a mother has to do as she is told!"

Jane Royal-Davidson; diagnosed in 1996 at age 47;
educator; North Carolina

"I was at a benefit fashion show in my new wig (long, straight
auburn hair) when a slightly tipsy gentleman approached me to
tell me what lovely hair I had. I smiled politely, told him thank
you, and went about my business. Every few minutes, he would
come back over to me to comment on my hair. Each time he was
a little more inebriated, and his comments a little more bold. Finally, barely able to stand upright, he slurred, 'I would just love to
spend the night running my hands through your lovely red hair.'
At this comment, I whipped off my wig, held it out to him, and
replied, 'Knock yourself out. I'm going to get a beer.' After picking his jaw up from the ground, he turned on his heel and I never
saw him again! I'm sure the next morning, he wondered if that
had actually happened or if it was all an alcohol-induced mirage."

Joy West; diagnosed in 2000 at age 34;
advertising account coordinator; South Carolina

"The day after my surgery I got up, drains and all, went to the
sink in the hospital, and washed my hair. The nurse came and,
horrified, said, 'Mrs. Abelmann, what are you doing?' My response was, 'I am washing my hair. I do this every morning!' "

Jeryl Abelmann; diagnosed in 1986 at age 46;
elementary school teacher; California

"One of my best comebacks for someone who complimented me
on my hair was, 'Thanks—want to borrow it?' "

Rosamary Amiet; diagnosed in 2000 at age 48;
program manager; Ohio

BRA-HA

"Shortly after my surgery, my daughter came to check on me. She felt that I couldn't possibly be doing as well as it seemed from our long-distance phone conversations. We were in the kitchen and she had turned, hitting me in my remaining breast. She said, 'Sorry! At least it was the good one!' My reply? 'Honey, it's the only one.' I truly believe that keeping a sense of humor is the single most important piece of advice I can share."

Susan Sanford; diagnosed in 1992 at age 48;
retired mortgage insurance underwriter, volunteer; Nevada

"After my mastectomy, I rescued a German wirehaired pointer. He was in such need of love, and I was in need of being loved, so we were two lost souls together. One morning I showered at 5:30 A.M. and started to get dressed, only to find that my prosthesis was missing from the counter where I'd left it moments before. It took me a few minutes to realize that my dog had it. It smelled like me, so off he'd run with it. I was all over the house chasing this big dog with my prosthesis in his mouth. No matter what I did, he wouldn't let go. I was about to give up and leave him to it, when he dropped it and let me get dressed!"

Jane Royal-Davidson; diagnosed in 1996 at age 47;
educator; North Carolina

"Unfortunately, a prosthesis has no sensation. The husband of a friend of mine inadvertently fondled the wrong woman at a cocktail party, and she didn't even know it!"

Mindy Greenside; diagnosed in 2000 at age 48;
midwife; Maryland

"Humor is most important. I even had to laugh when a large wave crashed against me and took my prosthesis out to the coral reefs of Bermuda. I was never self-conscious of my body. I felt that people cared for me for who I am, not what I look like."

Carol Quinn; diagnosed in 1984 at age 46;
nurse; Massachusetts

"I met my Weight Watcher's goal by going into the dressing room and removing my breast form. I instantly lost 1¼ pounds."

Helaine Hemingway; diagnosed in 1988 at age 41;
teacher; New Hampshire

"Make 'em laugh! That's what I try to do for friends diagnosed with breast cancer. I sent funny cards, even the Hallmark grumpy old lady with the hanging boobs, to two of my friends who'd just had mastectomies. They both said they laughed heartily, and that it felt great!"

Elaine Raco Chase;
friend of many survivors; Virginia

"Before my implant surgery, I wanted to give my plastic surgeon a unique gift. I needed to outmatch his humor for once. The wife of one of my husband's co-workers made me big chocolate breasts, and they were perfect! He loved it! I teased him about using the chocolate breasts for my implant, chocoholic that I was. We took a picture together holding the breasts. He promised to use the picture on those stressful days when he needed to laugh."

Joanne Palmer; diagnosed in 1996 at age 42;
medical receptionist; New York

HAPPY FACE

"Bubble baths were one way I found to be soothing and relaxing. But the best medicine was to laugh as often as possible."

Carol Snyder; diagnosed in 1992 at age 47;
special education teacher; New York

"The best advice I got was from Nanny, my friend Julie's grandmother, who was a forty-five-year survivor of a double mastectomy: 'Just keep on doing the laundry!' "

Betsy Goree; diagnosed in 1998 at age 40;
magazine publisher/editor; North Carolina

"A sense of humor will make the dark days manageable and fun."

Susan Clemente; diagnosed in 1990 at age 46;
retired registered nurse; New York

"The best thing about cancer? I am healthier, funnier, and nicer
than I was before. Now I run, I gave up drinking wine, and I just
started a year off from work to live in style. I really get it now. Life
is short—eat dessert first!"

Sharon Carr; diagnosed in 1997 at age 42;
hospice grief counselor; Rhode Island

"It's a lot better to laugh than to feel sorry for yourself. Go fish-
ing, play cards, do anything to get your mind off yourself."

Billie Loop; diagnosed in 1997 at age 63;
housewife; Missouri

"I got out of the hospital on a Thursday. On Friday, two friends
came and bathed my Newfoundlands, and we were all at the dog
show on Sunday. People kept running up to my friend asking
how I was and whether I was out of the hospital. 'Out of the hospital, hell, she's sitting right over there!' "

Lynne Rutenberg; diagnosed in 1980 at age 35;
retired teacher; New Jersey

"My private joke about tattooing the breast for radiation? I'm single and looking for a boyfriend to play Connect-the-Dots!"

Cindy Ferus; diagnosed in 2000 at age 57;
circuit board technician, former school teacher; Massachusetts

"On the lighter side, when you have cancer, you try to laugh. Three weeks before my mastectomy, my mother and I meet with a plastic surgeon. I pretend I am in Hollywood. I am Cher, who's come in for a facelift. The doctor swivels his chair toward my mother. 'So you're considering reconstruction?' I cut in. 'Wait. It's not her. It's me.' Swiveling in my direction without missing a beat, he starts over again. 'So you're considering reconstruction?' "

Carol Dine; diagnosed in 1980 at age 36;
college professor, writer; Massachusetts

"Humor was most important in helping me survive this ordeal. While my husband was shaving my head and calling me Kojak, I was telling him what a bargain I was, since the family budget for hair care products was just cut in half!"

Renee C. Johannesen; diagnosed in 1993 at age 35;
marketing communications manager; New York

SMILE AND THE WHOLE WORLD SMILES . . .

"I was pregnant with my second child when diagnosed. I had a mastectomy while I was eight months pregnant, and started chemotherapy when my son was one week old. Friends brought our family dinner every night—a lifesaver—and the dozens of cards, notes, and phone calls I received were very uplifting, as was keeping my sense of humor. A close friend, upon hearing of my diagnosis, said in all seriousness, 'Feel free to call if there's anything you need to get off your chest.' I said, 'Actually, I'd rather not!' to which we had a good laugh."

Laurie Bishop; diagnosed in 1998 at age 40;
homemaker, mother; Oregon

"When I told my friend Liesel that I had been diagnosed with breast cancer and was scheduled for a double mastectomy, she asked me if I was planning to have prostheses made. No one else had asked this, so I asked why. With a twinkle in her eye, Liesel sat me down on one of her elegant fur throws and told me about a friend of hers. Apparently, there is a dressmaker in Chicago who had prostheses made out of her pincushions, so that she could conveniently stick her needles and pins into her chest when sewing and making alterations!"

Darlene Jurow; diagnosed in 1995 at age 52;
interior designer; California

* * *

"My son, Wil, was five when I was diagnosed. I explained my mastectomy and reconstructive surgery to him by saying that I had a 'boo-boo' in my chest that my doctor would cut out and that he would put great, big Band-Aids on the cuts. Wil was not bothered by my actual surgery but by the fact that my Band-Aids didn't have Pokemon on them.

"For a long while after surgery, I could only wear sports bras. One day, while I was dressing, Wil came running up carrying my sports bra. He announced, 'Mommy! Here is your booby trap!'

"Before chemo, I explained to Wil that I was going to have to take some medicine that would make my hair fall out. I explained that I would wear a wig, which I described as a hat with hair. A week later, we were in a bookstore ordering children's books on cancer. One of the titles was something like 'My Mommy Has No Hair.' Wil piped up, 'That's okay. My mommy is going to wear a hairy hat!' "

Joy West; diagnosed in 2000 at age 34;
advertising account coordinator; South Carolina

* * *

"I have a rowing friend who is also a gifted jeweler. At my fiftieth birthday party, I opened her gift to me, and it was a gold stud earring mounted with a diamond. The card was sweet and sentimental. It ended with 'P.S. I am so sorry for your loss, but they make them in gold now.' I thanked her graciously. At four A.M. the next day, I sat up in bed, only then realizing that the stud was a gold breast with a diamond nipple! Apparently the other guests at the party had thought I was embarrassed and had let the joke drop. I wear this earring with pride and never think of taking it off."

Diane Cotting; diagnosed in 1999 at age 49;

insurance broker; Massachusetts

"People said some strange things to me during the time I was undergoing treatment and shortly afterward. For example, when my hair first returned, it was jet black instead of the lighter brown it had been before chemo. One asked, 'Is that your hair? I don't believe it. Are you sure that's your hair?' "

Fran DiBiase; diagnosed in 1994 at age 40;

part-time teacher, part-time property management; South Carolina

"My best friend and her family decided to go on vacation during one of her three-week rotations of chemotherapy. She had the first round at home and took the second with her to her destination. When she walked into the hospital where the chemo was to be given, she was met by a young intern. As he was hooking her up he asked, 'Why in heaven's name did you decide to remove your breast?' Janey replied, 'I am a world-class archer, and it just got in the way.' He asked no more questions."

Judy Bayha;

Janey's friend; Indiana

"It's funny. It's almost as though another woman was living inside me and revealed herself just when I needed her. All my life, I had been a prude about undressing in front of other people. But I understood that undressing would be part of the process, and my modesty just seemed to disappear. In fact, I told one of the nurses that I needed to be careful at work, because every time I walked into a small office, I felt the urge to take off my clothes."

Val Long; diagnosed in 1999 at age 47;

administrative assistant; Massachusetts

"To get through radiation, I reached for humor. When I called my mother to tell her the number of radiation treatments had been reduced, I explained that it just takes less time to cook a small pot roast. Friends helped me create humor. For example, there were monitors outside the radiation room. When I mentioned this to my brother, he said that was why there were satellite dishes on the top of the hospital: so the image of me lying there with one breast hanging out could be broadcast everywhere. When I relayed this story to a friend, he carried it further, launching into a conversation between two Martians in a spaceship pointing to the image of me on their radar screen. Whenever I thought of this image, I would laugh—even in the middle of a treatment."

Jeanne Sturdevant; diagnosed in 1990 at age 45; artist; Texas

"My son had planned to marry several weeks before Christmas. Then I was diagnosed with breast cancer. He offered to postpone the wedding, but I told him to proceed. A week before the event, I had my lymph node dissection. On the day of the wedding, I was horrified to find that the drainage tube had fallen out. There was no time for the doctor to put another one in. All I could see was me walking down the aisle of the church with lymph drainage all over my beautiful new dress. So I came up with an idea. I placed a sanitary pad over my surgical site, then put on my bra so it would hold the pad in place. Then I had my husband wrap my body in Saran wrap. I walked down the aisle, with no drainage in sight, and thoroughly enjoyed the reception. That night when I undressed and unwound the Saran wrap, I found there was no drainage at all. The surgical site was stopped up. I laughed, thinking that I now knew what a chicken felt like after being wrapped in Saran."

Voncile Jones; diagnosed in 1994 at age 54; registered nurse; Alabama

"A telemarketer called one afternoon: 'Good afternoon, Jane, and how are you?' So I told him. I said that I was just recently diagnosed with breast cancer. I had a lumpectomy, which was scheduled around my promise to help my juniors review before their exam—and, of course, it had to be scheduled around my summer teaching schedule, and there was Micah's first professional band gig. Then my surgeon decided they needed a cleaner margin, so I had to have a mastectomy, which had to be scheduled around my teaching, too. And there was the decision about what type of chemotherapy to do, and Micah to get off to Israel and Louis to summer school up at VA Tech and Douglas to camp in New York. There were also the flowers that I needed to get into the garden, and then I really needed to get a haircut before all of my hair fell out. So that is how I am, I told the man. How can I help you? He stuttered, and then asked if all of that was true. I asked to be removed from his list, wished him a nice day, and hung up. Louis and Douglas were listening to all this, literally rolling on the floor. Telemarketers stopped calling us for the longest time."

Jane Royal-Davidson; diagnosed in 1996 at age 47;
educator; North Carolina

"When people around you hear the 'C' word, it rocks their world. Once they recover from the shock, odds are they will ask, 'How are you?' followed by the inevitable 'Let me know if there's anything I can do.' After hearing that again and again, I decided to take those who offered at their word. I told them what I needed. And what I needed was to laugh. Instead of crying, or whining, or feeling sorry for myself and asking 'why me?' I needed to laugh. After all, I'd had a sense of humor before I was diagnosed. I wanted it back. So I asked those near and dear to me to send me things to make me laugh. And, lo and behold, they did. My 'laughter therapy' arrived in different shapes and forms. It included a book of Dennis Miller rants, the videotape of a family member at a Comedy Club open mike night, Xerox copies of Doug Adams cartoons, a tee-shirt with the words 'bite me' on it, Woody Allen short stories, shipments of cat beanie babies, rainbow-colored socks with individual toes. Now, cards are sweet and flowers smell good. But in my book, when you are feeling alone and down and somewhat tragic dealing with a health crisis, nothing's better than going to the mailbox and opening a surprise from a dear friend or family member. And if you rip open the package and it makes you smile ear to ear, well, that is what I call healing medicine for the soul."

Alysa Cummings; diagnosed in 1998 at age 45;
educational trainer; New Jersey

12 • Men

By, For, and About

Men play a role in our lives. They may be family members, as in fathers, husbands, or sons. They may be
significant others. They may be simply friends. Or bosses. Any one
of these roles puts them prominently into the breast cancer picture. Members of the sisterhood mention them often—so often, in
fact, that I wanted to know more.

Now, that might surprise you. After all, I have a husband and
three sons, and we're a close family. So I should know how men
feel and what they need during this time, right?

Wrong. Because when you're living it, you don't want to talk
about fears. You have your hands full dealing with a busy daily life
made even busier by breast cancer. Touchy-feely stuff—sensitive
stuff—stuff that shows vulnerabilities and foibles: they're sometimes just too slick to grasp. You satisfy yourself by knowing that
actions speak louder than words.

You finish treatment, regain strength, and life quiets. Time
passes. You move beyond breast cancer. Then something happens—say, *UPLIFT*—and it suddenly occurs to you to wonder

what they were thinking and feeling back then. So you ask. You ask them separately, so they won't feel as though they have to compete with each other for answers. And each of the four, on his own, does pretty much the same thing. He shrugs. He gives a mystified little smile. It wasn't any big deal, he says. You were confident. You promised you'd tell us everything. You never really missed a beat.

Oh, there were other little memories. Tears on the phone. A hug when that was the only thing that brought comfort. Festive holidays. Special Valentines. Lopsided breasts at a law school graduation.

My husband swears that he was never frightened. *Never?* I ask him, wondering if I should be disappointed, worried, *offended.* He shakes his head, as quiet and sure as he's ever been, and it strikes me that we all shared the very same view of my breast cancer. From the start, death was simply not an option.

Those were my men, dealing with our situation in keeping with our own family dynamics. But just as the sisterhood was proving to be a widely diverse group, I knew that their men would be, too. I wanted to hear from those men—wanted to know how they felt when a woman in their life was diagnosed, how they learned about the disease, with whom they talked, who gave them comfort. I wanted to know what advice they would give other men in the same situation—other men who might, just might, pick up *UPLIFT* when they needed a boost.

So I sent an e-mail to each of the women who had already become part of *UPLIFT* and asked if they would try to convince the men in their lives to submit a thought or two. Oh my. Talk about opening floodgates. Based on the immediacy of their replies, these men were *thrilled* to have a chance to speak!

Take Marvin Wilker, who says, "When Helen told me she had breast cancer, I felt like I'd been hit by a fully loaded Mack truck." And Bryan Whittet, who writes, "When my wife was first diagnosed, I was devastated." And George Anbinder, whose first thoughts "were ones of disbelief and denial." And that's only the start. These three and many others have much more to say about breast cancer, not the least inspiring being Dave Schwingel, who wrote about his wife, Gracie, "Cancer has changed her. She is more independent, self-assured, and free. But never alone."

This one's for you, guys. It may validate things you've been feeling. It may give you ideas about where to turn and what to do. It'll certainly tell you that you're not alone.

HE SAYS: WHAT I FELT

"The day of my wife's surgery, I went to the hospital with her. I spent the last part of her surgery crying. I was so afraid she would die. A couple of years later, when she had a biopsy on the other breast, one of our sons sat with me while I cried again. That was almost ten years ago. I have never entirely lost my fear of her dying, but my strength and comfort have always come from my wife. She trusted her doctors and her treatment. We made it through together."

Robert David Vaughan,
Jane's husband; Texas

"When my wife was first diagnosed, I was devastated. We both cried, but I knew I had to calm her down. Our families gave us comfort . . . and, of course, our kids. My advice to other men? Support whatever your wife decides to do, and be patient. Having her breast removed was the easy part; the emotional aftermath may be more of a struggle."

Bryan Whittet,
Debby's husband; Michigan

"I was only seventeen years old, away from home for the first time and in my first semester at college when my mom told me she had breast cancer. I couldn't stop the tears. I thought she was going to die. After my parents left to go back home, I went with some friends and got drunk for the first time! Then I talked with friends. Three guys I lived with all had a story about someone in their lives who'd had breast cancer and beat it, so that helped me a lot. My parents called every day to see how I was. When I told my mom that I was going to come home to help her, she said, 'No. Stay in school and do the best you can do. That will be all the help I need.' I got all A's that semester! I would advise other kids to treat their moms just like they did before. I always made her laugh, and I went back to school thinking she was going to be okay, and she was."

Brandon Whittet,
Debby's son; Michigan

"When Helen told me she had breast cancer, I felt like a Mack truck (fully loaded) had run over me. I remember feeling helpless, feeling that there was nothing I could do to change anything but pray, and pray I did. I wanted to cry but held back the tears. I didn't want her worrying about me; she had enough on her mind. At work, I sometimes broke down, and my colleagues gave me comfort. The person who helped me the most was the surgeon when he said that Helen's chance of full recovery was excellent. I would advise other men in my position to hang in there, think positive thoughts, and look for that light at the end of the tunnel. Who said 'life is fair'? Not I."

Marvin Wilker,
Helen's husband; Massachusetts

" 'Knowing about' becomes 'knowing of.' Learning more about cancer, healing, food, exercise, the spirit, and alternatives were all pivotal to Grace's decisions. I am there when she needs personal support—an ear to listen, an eye to see, lips to smile, a shoulder to lean on, arms to hug her, and a heart to support her always."

Dave Schwingel,
Gracie's husband; Wisconsin

"As the husband of a cancer patient my part has been very limited. I only had to be there on the bad days, and with Kathleen's attitude, those were few and far between. My advice to other men? Don't ever treat the disease with any other thought but total recovery."

Richard Griffith,
Kathleen's husband; Arizona

"My first thoughts were ones of disbelief and denial, but these rapidly changed when we met with the doctors. Ellie's first surgical appointment was with a cold, unfeeling male surgeon. I immediately secured an appointment with a well-known and respected female surgeon. She provided much comfort. I remember most clearly how well Ellie dealt with the entire situation."

George Anbinder,
Eleanor's husband; Massachusetts

"When I first heard my wife's diagnosis, I was frightened for her. Having had combat surgery in Vietnam, I had a sense of what she faced. Christine's doctors gave me all the confidence that I could ever have hoped for. I remember the calm, cool way the surgeon told us how he would approach the surgery, and how he respected Christine's judgment. That first office visit set the tone for everything that followed. All men whose loved ones have breast cancer should meet with the doctors so that they are in on the direction of the treatment, almost as they would be at the birth of a child."

Denis McNamara,
Christine's husband; Florida

"When I first heard that my partner, Dorian, had breast cancer, I felt absolute, complete, utter shock. I'm the type of person who worries and works hard to make sure nothing goes wrong. I double-check that my front door is locked before I go to bed. I always wear a seatbelt. I eat healthy food. To have my partner be diagnosed with breast cancer at age twenty-six was something I couldn't even imagine, a risk I had never prepared for. It still feels almost surreal. The time we spent in a support group for young adults with cancer and their partners was a really trans-formative experience. The facilitator made it clear that if we husbands and partners attended the group with an I'm-just-here-to-support-my-partner attitude, we'd be missing out. Breast cancer impacts the whole family, especially partners. It threw into question some of my unspoken and even unques-tioned beliefs about health and sickness, life and mortality. Being in a group with other people in their twenties and thirties meant a lot to us. As men we're raised to think that it's our job to solve problems. And many of us *are* really good problem solvers. But sometimes with breast cancer there's just nothing we can do. That can be the hardest thing of all: knowing that the woman you so love and care about has breast cancer, and it really, really sucks—and you're utterly powerless to do anything about it. It's not your job to come up with the magical solution and instruct her how to fix it. All you can do is support her and be by her side."

Marshall Miller,
Dorian Solot's partner; Massachusetts

"My first thoughts on learning that my twenty-six-year-old daugh-ter had breast cancer? Disbelief, shock, anger, and denial. There was grief, then acceptance, then the commitment to research and pursue all avenues. Since most research and treatment has been on older women, we felt it was important to consider the long-term effects on a young woman with many years of life ahead of her. I talked about it with everyone, passing what they had to offer on to Dorian. The support was overwhelming. I felt guilty about the outpouring of love for me, which I believed should have been directed exclusively to Dorian. I've come to understand and appreciate that support and how it continues to buoy us. It was wonderful to receive so many calls that it was necessary to allocate whose return call would have to be put off. Ultimately, the greatest comfort came from Dorian herself. I knew that her diligent research, combined with her intelligence and intuition, would lead her to the correct decisions, whether or not they aligned with prevailing practice. Also, knowing that Marshall (her wise and wonderful partner) would be there for her was a tremendous relief. Single moments: Seeing her in the hospital after the first procedure, and feeling the wonder of the fragility/strength balance. Also, having the twisted privilege of being able to take care of her for a few days as she recovered—a treat for me, connecting her childhood to the present—a reminder of our father/daughter/friend relationship and how it continues to evolve. Advice to other men: Place her unique individuality first. Sift through the books and advice with *her* in mind, looking and listening for her needs. Holding hands is good for both of you."

Evan Solot;
Dorian's father; Pennsylvania

"When my twenty-six-year-old granddaughter told us of her diagnosis, I was convinced there was an error. I couldn't associate breast cancer with the child we nurtured and loved. How could we spare her the agony or any pain? How could I sit quietly by to let her make her decisions for her survival? It was difficult for me to discuss this with my male friends, but I was able to discuss this with female friends, who have offered much support. Gradually, Dorian convinced me that hope is there for us, that her remission continues, and that her recovery will be full and complete with the regimen she is following. Her positive approach to her recovery has helped me through this unbelievable event."

Leslie Solot,
Dorian's grandfather; New Jersey

"A woman facing mastectomy, particularly a young woman, might want to videotape herself before surgery. I know this may sound a little ghoulish, but it might be helpful. It is something to share with a current or future lover. I speak as a guy. Sometimes we can't imagine what we can't see. It's often easier to empathize when one knows what has been lost. I don't minimize the value our society places on women's breasts. Even so, there are men who are not breast obsessed. Breast cancer survivors need to know that. A woman's life is so much more than the quantity and positioning of a little bit, or even a lot, of flesh. Breasts don't laugh, smile, share brilliance, or give kindness. Life is the true treasure; otherwise, we'd save the breast and discard the woman. A living woman is beautiful. A dead woman is not nearly so attractive. For the record, I am forty-two, and I really like women."

Alan S. Gardner;
no relation to anyone with breast cancer, just a general good guy; Iowa

"I fell in love with my wife one year after her diagnosis. Part of what attracted me to Cathleen was her strength and her determination to beat the disease after being diagnosed before she was thirty years old. She was so vibrant and full of life that I immediately fell in love with her. About two months after we were married, they discovered a recurrence. This was devastating. Here we had just married, ready to begin our lives together, and the disease reared its ugly head. However, together we attacked this as just a bump in the road. We are forever optimists, insisting that it is better we caught this early. I look at my wife and all she has gone through, and I tell myself that she is one of a kind."

Mark D'Antonio,

Cathleen's husband; Connecticut

"My wife Billie prayed about herself and her breast cancer, and when the doctor had to remove her breast, she couldn't understand why for a while. But we talked about it. I told her I didn't care about her breast. I cared about her. It has been four years now, and everything is going fine. She is still beautiful in my sight. We just celebrated our fiftieth anniversary. We are friends, lovers, and best pals. There is no one in the world I would rather be with. I call her Sug."

Donald Loop,

Billie's husband; Missouri

SHE SAYS: WHAT HE FELT

"My husband's first reaction to my diagnosis was shock. He talks about it with friends and people at work, and all have been extremely supportive. They ask how I'm doing, but also how he's doing, and that makes me feel good. I think it is important to take care of our mates as much as ourselves. His advice to other men? Be there for her. Let her talk, cry, whine, shout—whatever makes her feel better. Go to all her appointments with her, even if it means sitting around being bored. Reassure her that a mastectomy is not the end of the world. Tell her 'I love you—two breasts, one breast, or no breasts.' Most of all, repeatedly tell her that we will get through this, and that she is going to live a long, long time."

Lori Bartz; diagnosed in 2000 at age 41;

customer service representative; Wisconsin

"Whenever my friend Eunice Silverstein went to the gynecologist for her yearly tests, her husband, Stan, worried. Eunice is the youngest of five sisters, three of whom had already had breast cancer. Though all three were survivors, when Eunice was finally diagnosed herself, Stan was very frightened. But he decided he had to put a good face on it, with positive thoughts and comments to Eunice. He felt that fear was contagious, and he didn't want Eunice to catch his fear when she had enough of her own to contend with. So he stayed calm, and discussed his worries only with Eunice's sisters, since they had been through this together. It was a shared family experience. Eunice has been cancer-free now for more than fifteen years."

Rae Shapiro;
friend of Stan and Eunice Silverstein; California

My husband's first reaction was shock. He felt lost, not knowing what to say or do. Then he sat down with me and told me that it didn't matter if I had one or two breasts, because that's not what he married me for. He told me we would get through this together. He took me to get my chemo treatments and made dinner when I couldn't—and he's a good cook! When I came home from the hospital, he didn't want to see my scar. This scared me a little. Then, the next day he did look at it, because he realized what it meant to me for him to see it. Then there was the day he touched it and found it to be just fine. Cancer is tough stuff, but love is stronger."

Mary Ann Budnick; diagnosed in 1991 at age 44;
school bus driver; Michigan

"I asked my son, Tom, who lives in Denver, what he felt when I was first diagnosed. He said, 'I can't remember exactly how I found out about it, but I do remember not being too worried. I know that sounds strange, but I knew that you had a good attitude and good doctors. I just knew you would be okay. Obviously, I was concerned about you having surgery, and it was never a question that I could come to Florida to help, but I looked at this as one of life's lessons and nothing that we would not get over. I remember thinking that we should never be too cocky about all the good things God gives us. I remember thinking that this was His way of keeping us a little humble.' "

Ann Gordon; diagnosed in 1998 at age 73;
retired business executive; Florida

"My oldest male friend, Terry, who has taught with me for twenty-six years, said that his first reaction was fear—fear on many levels. He couldn't imagine the stress and turmoil that I would be in; he imagined himself and his wife in the same situation and tried to figure out what he could say that would support me and give me encouragement. My friend Dickie was scared for me, too, because his mom had succumbed to cancer years ago, when detection and treatment were not at the level that they are now. Once he calmed down, he was totally optimistic. Mike is my chiropractor and a good friend. He was confident that I was getting the best care and that my mental attitude was very positive."

Christine Foutris; diagnosed in 1999 at age 49;
teacher; Illinois

"My husband was as grateful as I for the support of friends and family. His advice to other men: Be patient and understanding during the post-surgery treatment. Chemo and radiation can be physically exhausting and emotionally draining."

Brenda M. Kraft; diagnosed in 1986 at age 60;
retired school teacher; New Hampshire

DIALOGUES

"I felt my lump on Palm Sunday. I thought it ironic that as things grew in the spring, cancer was growing in my breast. I remember putting away the Easter decorations days later, looking out at the daffodils, and saying to my family, 'Next year, as we decorate for Easter and watch the flowers come up, this will all be behind us.' "

Jacki Anthony; diagnosed in 1998 at age 48;
nurse; Massachusetts

"When I first learned about my wife's breast cancer, I felt anger and fear. I was a police officer in a major city, and I was lost at first. Then I went online to cancer sites and read anything I could get my hands on. The information—some good, some bad—was very helpful to me. I went with my wife to every appointment and spoke to the doctors about the procedure, the treatment, and the possibilities. The end results were very good."

Robert Anthony,
Jacki's husband

"My family was very supportive, and in turn I was honest with them about everything that needed to be discussed. My husband and his Pee Wee hockey team were my biggest fans. They dedicated the season and the championship tournament to me, and skated over to me with the biggest trophy I had ever seen. How could I possibly ever forget that moment?"

Jacki Anthony

"When my Pee Wees won the championship, they skated over to my wife and presented her with the game trophy and game puck. This was something we did not expect but will always remember."

Robert Anthony

* * *

"I was at a conference and was with friends when Nina called me to say that she had breast cancer. The friends were a husband and wife. The wife gave me the most assurance that things would be okay, and the husband was supportive, too. The person who gave

me the most strength and comfort through all this, though, was
Nina. She is a very strong lady and had a great positive attitude."

Roger James,
Nina Miller's husband

"My fiancé and I bought a house together in November of 1996. In
December I found a lump. When we learned it was malignant, we
had to decide about the wedding—whether to cancel it, postpone it,
move the date up, or plan it around hair loss and therapy. We decided to wait until treatment was over, but there was no question that
we didn't want to wait for my hair to grow back. I decided to cut back
work to half time during my radiation treatments. I took my afternoons off to plan the wedding. Two weeks after radiation was over,
we had a wonderful, personal ceremony in our church's chapel and
a reception with friends and family in the yard of our new home."

Nina Miller; diagnosed in 1997 at age 40;
manager, oncology social worker; Wisconsin

"We gave each other a lot of strength through those early days
and through the days of treatment. We also had a strong faith in
God that helped us through, and a minister was quite comforting. The thing I remember the most was the early helpless feeling
and the thoughts that Nina was going to die, but the longer she
goes without problems, the less we think about that. The advice
I'd give others is that this diagnosis is not a death sentence and
that one has to be positive and take control of the situation."

Roger James

*   *   *

"When I lost my hair and decided to have it shaved off to avoid
the mess, well, that was hard. But then my husband gave me the
most wonderful gift of love. He had his head shaved also, so I
would not have to go through this alone."

Dee Pobjoy; diagnosed in 1999 at age 41;
sales clerk; Wisconsin

"It was very traumatic for my wife when she lost her hair. I will never forget her surprise when I had my head shaved also. She was speechless, and let me tell you, Dee is never speechless! When she was first diagnosed with breast cancer, I was in shock. Then, all I wanted to do was to hold her and reassure her that she would not be alone in this. My advice to other men? This is not the end of the world, guys. Show your loved one how much you love her, and the rest is easy."

Al Pobjoy, Dee's husband

"When they told me I had cancer, I just shut down. After the surgery, I remembered what a friend told me: 'I have breast cancer, but it doesn't have me.' I kept telling myself that. To me, it was all in the attitude. I am fine now. Yes, I live in fear that it will come back, but if it does, well, I have this experience to give me hope. A positive attitude is just the most important part of dealing with breast cancer."

Dee Pobjoy

"Dee has shown remarkable strength through all of this. She had surgery for breast cancer and was back to work less than a week later. She would have a chemo treatment and would only miss a day of work. Yes, she has cried—so have I—but she has continued to show strength in the most difficult situations. I admire my wife so much."

Al Pobjoy

* * *

"My biggest challenge when my wife went through breast cancer was knowing how to offer support. My instincts in this regard—to be dispassionate and offer advice—weren't always helpful. What worked was to ask Deb what *she* wanted me to do, and to keep this in mind when she needed help. I had a full repertoire of responses, but matching them to Deb's situation was a challenge.

The payoff was the good feeling of doing the right thing during a crisis for someone I loved."

Curt Lamb, Deborah Pierce's husband

"My doctors gave me the option of different treatments. This forced me to do some research. At times the task seemed insurmountable. I was not an expert in the field, and was too involved to see clearly."

Deborah Pierce; diagnosed in 1997 at age 48;
architect; Massachusetts

"One of the things I did which Deb appreciated was to read through some of the very technical reports she received to help her make sense of them."

Curt Lamb

"This helped me to take responsibility for decisions, so that I never felt forced into something that wasn't right for me."

Deborah Pierce

* * *

"I work in a veterans hospital, and while I am in the administrative department, I have learned much about the advances of medicine. Still, it made my stomach drop when we heard the news. A supervisor of mine at the time advised me to give Jeanne all the support I could and to be with her throughout this period, and I was. We had good, supportive friends, and this helped me as much as it did her. I think the hardest part was seeing the frustration, even occasional misery, that she went through. It was hard not being able to do anything to help her."

Paul E. Sturdevant, Jeanne's husband

"My husband has a deep and continuing interest in my physical well-being. Every time I get good reports, he is relieved and satisfied. He almost seems to spin on his heels as he goes on to resume his activities. Even so many years later, I need him to stand there and listen to me talk out my emotions and fears. It may cost him a lot to engage on that visceral level, but that is the level I'm on."

Jeanne Sturdevant; diagnosed in 1990 at age 45;
artist; Texas

* * *

"On the way home from the hospital, still shocked by the diagnosis and the choice I had to make between lumpectomy and mastectomy, I said to my husband, 'If I have the breast cut off, perhaps I could make it an offering, a sacrifice of old things in return for a new life?' That evening, on the back of an old desk calendar, he drew an outline of a lateral view of my breasts. In the center was a black dot—the cancer—with lines that radiated to the edges of the breast. On the side, he wrote, 'All negative energy be gone in the breast of Christine!' Over the next two weeks, I wrote down on this diagrammatic outline all of the negative emotion, the rage, the fear and despair. I finished the night before surgery. It was amazing to see all that stuff out there, outside of me. I was ready to let it go, to let go of the breast that contained the essence of all that pain."

Christine McNamara; diagnosed in 2000 at age 54;
retired physician; Florida

"I told everyone we knew that Christine had cancer. I didn't want it to be a secret just between us. I wanted to use everyone's positive energy to help us face it, just as everyone had helped me after Vietnam. Christine's doctors gave me confidence; I felt they were supermen who could do anything. I remember the calm, cool way the surgeon told us how he would approach the surgery, and how he respected Christine's judgment with regard to her own treatment and destiny. That first office visit set the tone for everything that followed. I think it's important for men in the same position to meet with the doctors, so that they are in on the direction of the treatment. I also advise them to be completely honest about the fear that they have. For me there was no real fear, due to my having had combat surgery, but I think open discussion really helps."

Denis McNamara,
Christine's husband

* * *

"I am a male breast cancer survivor. Nine years ago, I had a modified radical mastectomy and underwent chemotherapy. Because I found the lump early, my prognosis is very good."

David Kingsley; diagnosed in 1991 at age 44;
lawyer; Florida

"When my father was diagnosed with breast cancer, I could not believe it. What he underwent has transformed the way I perceive situations. The meaninglessness of problems comes into perspective when I compare them to what we have overcome. Our family survived a battle that was won by my father's immeasurable courage. We all clutch the hope that life will be fair, yet when it is not, we are awakened. We seek an explanation from somewhere, anywhere. There is none. But I did not become a pessimist. I did not let the disease win. I let it teach me to appreciate everything I once accepted as given. Life is a gift."

Linda Kingsley,
David's daughter

"I am, to my knowledge, the only Reach to Recovery male volunteer in the Southern Florida area, perhaps all of Florida and maybe the U.S. I answer telephone calls from around the country, as well as seeing men in my geographical area. I think it's important for people to know that breast cancer does also strike men and that early detection and treatment is a necessity."

David Kingsley

AND FOR DESSERT—MARS BARS

"My husband is my lifeline. Even when I had no hair and was so sick, he held me and told me I was beautiful."

Kathy Rabassa; diagnosed in 1999 at age 34;
administrative assistant; South Carolina

"My husband's support was priceless. He changed my drain dressing without even making a face—though I can't change a Band-Aid for him without moaning and groaning. Also, he is a very private person, yet he walked in the Making Strides Against Breast Cancer Walk with me. Then, I signed up to be in a trial program to discuss the emotional effect of breast cancer on your family, without realizing that he needed to go with me. He agreed because he knew I wanted to do it. We both got a lot out of it."

Sheila Roper; diagnosed in 1995 at age 57;
homemaker; New Hampshire

"Before I was diagnosed, my husband and I were beginning to drift apart. I often consider that my having had breast cancer was a gift, because the experience brought us closer together. It gave us a true appreciation of life, and we began enjoying each other much more. We came to realize what is important and what isn't. My husband was so happy that I survived that he became attuned to my needs. We were able to enjoy a much richer and deeper relationship."

Sheila Steinhauser; diagnosed in 1985 at age 41;
office manager; Maryland

"What made me feel the most feminine was the fact that my husband wanted to have sex with me."

Frances Gallello; diagnosed in 2000 at age 51;
mental health assistant; New York

"Sex during treatment. That is a good idea. Both of you may cry the first time, but sex will leave you feeling normal. It will make you realize that life goes on, and it's a jumpstart to getting used to your new body image."

Betsy Goree; diagnosed in 1998 at age 40;
magazine publisher/editor; North Carolina

"My whole treatment program lasted a school year—from September through the first of May. On the last day of treatment, my husband took me out for lunch and gave me a rose!"

Fran DiBiase; diagnosed in 1994 at age 40;
part-time teacher, part-time property management; South Carolina

"When my daughter-in-law first told me about *UPLIFT*, I felt that I couldn't contribute. It's been three years since my surgery, and with the exception of the day when I learned that my tumor was indeed malignant, the rest of the time has been only good and positive. What more could I say? Then the letter came asking me about the men in my life, and I knew what to write. The love of my life—my husband of fifty-three years—is the reason my experience with breast cancer was a positive one. When I was given the diagnosis, he held me and told me that he loved me, no matter what happened, and that we would go through this together. Luke and our kids are my personal support group. I thank God every day for their love. My recovery has been so easy!"

Ellen R. Luecke; diagnosed in 1998 at age 71;
retired; California

"The contract with my husband, my partner is very important
Be honest about everything, tell him everything
Get him to go to the doctor and treatments
Tell him how it feels to go for tests and treatments
He will understand

He stands by me and I stand by him
Together, he says, we can go through anything."

Ruth Jones; diagnosed in 1985 at age 51;
housewife, homemaker; Ohio

"My husband tried to balance every trip to the doctor's office or treatment with a fun stop either before or after. Either we stopped at Starbucks for a cup of coffee, or we went into Barnes and Noble to browse, or we went for an ice cream. I almost began to look forward to chemo days!"

Vivian; diagnosed in 1998 at age 36;
professor; New York

"My husband was wonderful. He took over the household chores, was with me for every treatment and every up-and-down swing. We'd make Fridays our Fun Day after each treatment. We went to Chinatown for lunches, Filene's Basement for treats, and day trips to Ogunquit. I found myself looking forward to going to my treatment appointments because of our outings."

Alyce Feinstein; diagnosed in 1993 at age 58;
administrative assistant; Massachusetts

"The most touching, sweet thing happened to me during those trying days when I looked like one of those hairless aliens who stepped off the mother ship in *Close Encounters*. I'd just stepped out of the shower and looked in the mirror to find that the last stringy hair on my head had finally disappeared, when my husband of thirty-five years tapped at the door. He'd never seen me bald; I'd worn a wig during the day and a turban to bed, because I was insecure about my looks. Well, I wrapped my head in a towel and let him inside. I don't know why I finally did it, but suddenly I decided to just take the stupid towel off my head, and I immediately started to cry. Mike held me, smiled right into my lashless eyes, and said, 'So what?' And I thought the best I'd ever hear from him was 'I love you.' "

Lauren Nichols; diagnosed in 2000 at age 53;
writer; Pennsylvania

"I am married to the eternal optimist. When I asked what he thought when I first told him I had breast cancer, he said, 'I knew everything was going to be okay!' My having cancer was a double whammy, since he had been diagnosed with prostate cancer just six months before. We dealt with mine the same way we had with his. He had been such a good patient that I couldn't complain much. By the way, we're both doing great. My last mammogram was negative, the hot flashes are lessening, and his PSAs have all been negative! We have much to be thankful for. And for Christmas, he surprised me with a cruise. We leave next month. We're celebrating thirty-seven years of a wonderful life together!"

Judy Peterson; diagnosed in 2000 at age 58;
registered nurse; Colorado

"On Christmas, after I had finished treatments, my husband gave me a gorgeous ring of rubies and diamonds. He explained that the rubies represented adriamycin (the red devil from chemo) and the diamonds represented cytoxin, which is clear. This ring is a fabulous 'reward' for all I went through, and I strongly suggest that other husbands follow mine's lead. This beautiful ring is less a reminder of my cancer treatment than it is a reminder of how lucky I am to have the love and support of this wonderful man."

Nancy Lane; diagnosed in 2000 at age 53;
teacher; Massachusetts

"The day of my last treatment, my husband's company gave him a surprise retirement party. My daughter and I stood in the back, and as he came in, before acknowledging anyone, he came over and kissed me."

Barbara C. Sumner; diagnosed in 1982 at age 59; homemaker; New Hampshire

"The best thing that ever happened to me happened while I was battling breast cancer. My boyfriend, whom I had been dating for seven years, proposed to me when I looked my absolute worst. I had just finished my fourth of eight cycles of chemo, and had already lost all of my hair. We went to dinner and a play, and as we were leaving the theater, a horse and buggy was waiting for us outside. He said that he wasn't proposing because he thought my time was limited, but rather to give me something to live for. It was the most wonderful thing that could have uplifted my spirits."

Katie Mandra; diagnosed in 1998 at age 22; homemaker; Illinois

"A long-time male friend sent me an e-mail during my treatment that moved me deeply. It still does. He wrote, 'I should really tell you that when times get rough for me, I find the courage and strength I need from the examples set by a handful of people I think of as heroes—one of whom, for a long time, has been you.' As a friend and confidante he was there through two years of breast cancer hell—by phone, by e-mail, or over Kung Pao chicken at the local Chinese restaurant."

Alysa Cummings; diagnosed in 1998 at age 45; educational trainer; New Jersey

"My male friends have been very supportive and are always ready with a compliment to boost my spirits. They're also ready to join me for a spur-of-the-moment dinner out. When my hair started falling out, a very good male friend shaved my head. We didn't intend this, but it was a slightly erotic experience. Later, I ran into an ex-lover whom I hadn't seen in a while. He still wanted to sleep with me, even after hearing that I'd had a mastectomy. He told me flat out that 'it didn't matter.' While I wasn't ready physically or emotionally for a sexual encounter, he made me feel desirable in a way that I hadn't felt in a long time."

Carrie Drake; diagnosed in 1998 at age 42;
administrative assistant; Colorado

"There is life after breast cancer and divorce, because there are many wonderful men out there. I've dated two of them. The first was Jack. After a few weeks, I told him there was something he should know. He said, 'I think I know what you want to tell me. I heard long ago that you had breast cancer. I don't care if you have one breast or no breasts, I love you just the way you are!' The second man, Ted, was tougher because he'd lost his wife to breast cancer. One day, several weeks after we met, he came upstairs thinking I was already dressed. I was in my bra, and when he said, 'Oops,' I said, 'I'm glad you are here, because I have to tell you that I had breast cancer eighteen years ago.' His response was, 'So what? Is that all you had to tell me? So what do you want to do tonight?' When my divorce is final, Ted and I are going to be married. My children adore him and have learned a great deal from this very caring and loving man. He loves my body, and for the first time in my life I feel special and cherished. Most of all, he loves me."

Miriam Cooper; diagnosed in 1982 at age 36;
housewife, mother, volunteer, real estate agent; New Jersey

"When men you don't know look you over and linger at your breasts even after your surgery, that made me feel feminine! Same thing when a neighbor said he'd take me, no matter what. That made me feel good about myself. I found out how much my husband loved me and how much I was loved for being me, no matter what. My husband has since died, and I have a new romantic companion who is fine with the idea that I have only one breast."

Irene Louise; diagnosed in 1995 at age 41;
retired executive secretary; Pennsylvania

"I didn't miss one day of work after my surgery—until the day I retired to get married! I had seen Leonard for the first time in thirty years at the wedding of a mutual friend. He had been widowed for two years. When I realized that he was romantically inclined toward me, I made him look at ONE SIDE of my chest. I watched closely and he didn't wince, just expressed sympathy at what I'd had to undergo. We got married in 1994 and have lived happily ever after."

Lorraine J. Pakkala-Lintala; diagnosed in 1992 at age 62;
editor, author; Florida, New York

"After my divorce, an old friend—male—came back into my life. During my bout with breast cancer, he held me, nurtured me, and made me feel feminine and desirable. It was just what I needed. He didn't care about my scars. So I went on to conquer other problems. I had had a total knee replacement just after my radiation treatments were done, and now I can walk with no pain and know that I am cancer-free at the same time. It's a lot to celebrate, and celebrate I do."

Judy Komitee; diagnosed in 1998 at age 52;
secretary; New Jersey

LAST BUT NOT LEAST

"Consider what it is like to be a man with breast cancer. When I went to a renowned hospital and was directed to the proper department, my daughter, a nurse, and I had a great laugh at the questionnaire I was given to fill out. After the normal name and such, I was asked the following: When did I start my period? How often did I have it? Was it regular? How many times was I pregnant? Have I gone through menopause? Somehow these questions did not fit the patient. The final laugh was when the nurse came out and called for Miss Browne, and my daughter had to point to me as the patient. The good news was that I was told to start thinking years rather than months."

Gerald Browne; diagnosed in 1995;
Massachusetts

13 • Exercise

Making the Body Better

I've always believed in physical exercise. It has been a stress reliever for me since way back when I was a full-time mother with three young, curious, mischievous, conspiratorial, and tirelessly athletic boys at home. I spent years as a swimmer, followed by years as a walker. Then I got breast cancer and, after surgery, found myself with limited mobility in my arms and with chest muscles that were good for nothing. My doctors had given me exercises with the instructions that I should start them immediately, but I had barely recovered from the surgery when I began the saline expansion phase of my reconstruction. Exercise? Are you kidding? I hurt too much for that.

So, ignoring naysayers who warned of permanent disability if I didn't start moving A-S-A-P, I waited until my permanent implants were in and the incision had healed, then began doing exercise videos at home. The videos were basic and didn't take more than thirty minutes on a given day, but they were gentle enough to be fun. Over the next few months I did them four to five times a week—and lo and behold, with barely any pain, I gradually regained the full mobility of my arms. My chest wall settled in and grew stronger, so that I was able to carry supermarket bundles again. But those exercise videos made other things happen, too. My shoulders became broad and my hips narrow. My back grew more flexible and my legs stronger. In short, my post-cancer body became *better* than the body I'd had before!

With this in mind, I knew from the start that I wanted to have a chapter in *UPLIFT* on the merits of physical exercise following breast cancer treatment. Then, last October, I heard about the women who were rowing in the Head of the Charles Regatta wearing pink spandex oufits and sparkly ball caps. All were breast cancer survivors—eight rowers, plus a coxswain—propelling the aptly named One in Nine boat down the Charles River in Boston's premier rowing event of the year.

I was familiar with rowing. Two of my sons had done crew while they were going through school. I knew about the weight watching and body building that preceded a race, and the bloodied hands and extreme exhaustion that followed. I knew how much of a team effort rowing was—and how positively, utterly grueling it was. I also knew that the chest and upper arms were major players in the sport. I couldn't begin to imagine women who'd had breast surgery being able to row. Yet there they were, fully competitive on the Charles.

It took me a while before I was able to get a name and number, but no time at all after that before Diane Cotting, the boat's organizer and a crew member, and Holly Metcalf, the boat's coach, were in my kitchen. While Diane gave me the history of the One in Nine boat, a profile of its members, and a taste of its spirit, Holly explained the mechanics—the theory that after extensive breast surgery, it is necessary to reeducate the muscles, to reconfigure them, so that they work in different ways to achieve the same, if not better, results.

That theory made sense to me. Wasn't I spending my summers kayaking, using my arms and shoulders in ways that would have been remarkable even without my having had breast cancer? Granted, I had no desire to row as these women defined it. But if they inspired me, I knew they would inspire others. With Diane's help, I contacted other members of the team. I wanted to know how and why they rowed.

"I started rowing when I was forty-six," Nancy Oken said. "I was fifty-three and at the top of my form when I got breast cancer. Afterward, I decided that I was not going to reverse the personal strides I had made through my rowing. I rowed in the Masters National in a boat that won a silver metal. I also rowed in a double with another woman who'd had breast cancer. We wanted to prove to ourselves that we were up to the same challenges as the rest of the rowers."

Like Nancy, Diane had rowed before having breast cancer. She had formed strong friendships with her teammates, and those women were her major support group when she was diagnosed. "They called in all their contacts to make sure I was with the best caregivers in the world. But I never stopped thinking of rowing. It was my lifeline to health and personal sanity. I explained this to each of my doctors. They told me they would do everything in their power to get me back on the water."

Beth Meister had never rowed before. She had watched her daughter row, though, and started rowing as a way to control how she looked—"I wanted to be solid and not jiggly"—when her oncologist put her on tamoxifen and predicted she would gain weight. Pat Carr started rowing more as a factor of age than of breast cancer. "I was thinking, 'If not now, when?' Besides, I wanted to find out if I could do it." And Mary Ruddell, who didn't start rowing until two or three years after having breast cancer, said, "No one told me that I couldn't do it—but then, I didn't ask."

These women faced obstacles. But they were determined. "When I first went back to rowing, I felt so weak," said Michele Marks, "but I knew that my strength would come back with hard work." Beth had a problem with numbness in her left arm and hand. "So I chose to row port, which meant that I didn't have to 'feather' (turn the oar blade) with that hand." For Mary, the answer was yoga. "Once I had stretched out the scar tissue with

yoga, I was ready to go!" Diane had had TRAM-flap reconstruction. That meant her stomach muscles were displaced, which
spelled an even greater adjustment. "My plastic surgeon was
afraid that I wouldn't be able to do the sit-up motion necessary to
take a strong stroke. He made me promise that I couldn't do any
abdominal work for six months, and I kept my word. Then, when I
started physical therapy, no one seemed to understand the nature
of my reconstruction. I finally started working with a personal
trainer, who taught me how to strengthen other muscle groups to
replace the muscles I was missing. I learned how to support my
body in new ways, so that I would be able to do the motions necessary to pull hard and row well in a boat."

I asked about setbacks. Other than a passing remark from one
about causing strain by overcompensating, and from another about
once pulling a muscle, none of the women responded. They responded loudly and long, though, when I asked about the rewards.

"Rowing returned my self-confidence," Joyce Abercrombie said.
"Whether physical or psychological or both, the benefits were real.
Continuing to row after having breast cancer helped me to focus
on maintaining a normal life, rather than focusing on the disease." Michele elaborated, "When I'm rowing, all I have to think
about is rowing. Nothing else. It is such a relief and release. Same
with knowing I have the support of the other women, and knowing
I am not alone."

"Rowing gives me a wonderful feeling of strength," said Pat.
Mary added, "In season, I'm on the water three or four days a
week. Rowing allows you to feel alive and one with the earth and
your soul." Beth summed up both thoughts: "Rowing is good for
fitness, strength, and endurance—not to mention an appreciation
of the beauty of the river."

So what, specifically, of the One in Nine boat experience? I
asked.

"The One in Nine boat has given me an opportunity to revisit
my trauma and renew all that is positive," said Beth. "It enables

me to show other women that breast cancer is just another challenge to be won. I'll never forget meeting the other women in the boat for the first time, feeling the positive energy, and seeing the brilliance of their smiles. These things told me that we did indeed share something. We bonded easily. For most of us, it was the first opportunity we had to openly discuss our experiences."

For Pat, rowing in the One in Nine boat meant going public. "Only now, four years later, do people in the club where I regularly row know that I had breast cancer, and that is due to my participation with this boat in the Head of the Charles and the publicity that accompanied it. I never wanted to 'use' breast cancer as an excuse when I was with coaches or fellow rowers."

Not that the women of the One in Nine boat rowed silently. When one wears pink spandex tops and glittery baseball caps, one doesn't have to say a word, and people hear. "The day we got our uniforms for the race was funny," Michele recalled. "We went to try on our tops, and they were all so small that we could see every dent, dimple, and scar. We could also see when one breast was larger than the other. We all commented on that."

Beth had her own thoughts on that uniform. "I like to think of myself as a serious rower. Rowing in the One in Nine boat challenged that image. We were given hot-pink-and-black skintight outfits and pink sequined caps to wear in the race. This was good, because everyone could spot us and cheer. But someone took a picture of me from the top of one of the bridges as we rowed under, and it landed on the cover of US Rowing Magazine. There was no story, just the 'cover girl' picture. To my horror—though I have no idea why I left the house that way that day—I was wearing full jewelry in the race!"

Then she ended with a story that gave me goose bumps. "The One in Nine Boat was rowing up to the start in the Head of the Charles Regatta. We were getting more excited and anxious as we saw the other boats of powerful-looking women who would be our competition. Typically, at the start of a race, crew teams try to scare and demoralize the other crews by looking big and mean. So I was prepared for a cold and threatening reception by these competitors. Instead, as we approached, they began beating the sides of their boats with their palms, unified in a rousing cheer for us— 'One-in-Nine, One-in-Nine, One-in-Nine.' It was an incredible once-in-a-lifetime reception at the start of a regatta!"

Comparing myself with these women, I feel puny. Lest you feel the same, let me bring the rowing experience down to our level by backing up just a bit. Believe it or not, it wasn't so very long ago that Diane was actually afraid to take that first row. "My friends were protective after my surgery, trying to ease me back on the water without putting pressure on me. So one friend told a little fib. She said that her back was sore, and she was too nervous to take a single shell out by herself. She asked me to join her in a double to take the strain off her, in case she ran into trouble. I was paddling away in no time. The feeling was fantastic."

So there. You and I can paddle. Piece o' cake.

IN THE BEGINNING

"Start walking. Put on an oversized button-down shirt, and just do it. You are sure to feel better when you get moving."

Linda Dyer; diagnosed in 1993 at age 40;
magazine editor; New Jersey

"Walk every day—even if it's only a short walk. This is great for everything!"

Debbie MacLean; diagnosed in 1991 at age 47;
volunteer, hospital gift shop and hospice; Massachusetts

"Keep at it. Take it slow, but keep doing it. It will get better, and you will feel better for doing it."

Mary Ruddell; diagnosed in 1992 at age 44;
program manager; California

"The best exercise for mobility: walking my fingers up the shower wall. I felt great excitement each time I climbed another tile!"

Barbara Jentis; diagnosed in 1983 at age 41;
attorney; New Jersey

"Years ago, my daughter gave me a little blue Smurf. When I was doing exercises in bed, I would put him on the headboard. My goal was to touch his nose. I finally did! That arm is stronger today than the other arm!"

Barbara C. Sumner; diagnosed in 1982 at age 59;
homemaker; New Hampshire

"After my surgery, my husband tied ropes around door knobs, set up pulleys, and cut up newspapers for me to scrunch up and throw into a wastebasket."

Irene Louise; diagnosed in 1995 at age 41;
retired executive secretary; Pennsylvania

"I had trouble getting full mobility back in my arm. I actually had pain that came from not using it enough. I was treating it like a useless appendage. My physical therapist said to me, 'It's *your* arm!' Such a simple sentence, but it helped me to remember that."

Judith Ormond; diagnosed in 1996 at age 49;
symphony musician—piccolo; Wisconsin

BECAUSE YOU'RE WORTH IT!

"When I returned to the fitness center, I was treated with special attention. I worked with the fitness instructor, one on one, to make a new program to build myself back up and begin a new healing process."

Sharon Erbe; diagnosed in 1999 at age 54;
nurse educator; New York

"Control of my body became an issue. I exercised a lot, bicycling and running four miles a day, and I learned an incredible amount about nutrition, particularly antioxidants."

Judith Ormond; diagnosed in 1996 at age 49;
symphony musician—piccolo; Wisconsin

"I was diagnosed at forty and am a six-year survivor of breast cancer. One tidbit I would like to offer new patients is to start lifting weights as soon as their doctor allows it. I was not told to do this, and did not realize the benefits as far as building muscle and better use of the arm after a mastectomy."

Fran DiBiase; diagnosed in 1994 at age 40;
part-time teacher, part-time property management; South Carolina

"I like to work out at a health club. Searching for an athletic bra that would utilize my breast form, I discovered 'TurtleShell.com.' "

Helaine Hemingway; diagnosed in 1988 at age 41;
teacher; New Hampshire

"It took me a couple months to feel like exercising after my bilateral mastectomy, but when I did get back to the gym and to a consistent exercise program, it was the best thing I could have done! It made me feel healthy and alive. I started cooking and eating healthy, and I felt, for the first time in my life, that I was taking control and doing something really positive for my body. After being diagnosed with cancer and feeling very out of control, it was wonderful to take charge. A healthy diet and regular exercise—they're good for the body and even better for the mind!"

Julie Crandall; diagnosed in 1998 at age 31;
stay-at-home mom; North Carolina

"Work out in ways you didn't before. My upper body is now stronger than it ever was."

Mindy Greenside; diagnosed in 2000 at age 48;
midwife; Maryland

"After my surgery, I took up walking daily with my neighbor for exercise and also to relieve stress. We still continue this activity. It is the cheapest therapy I know."

Wanda Null; diagnosed in 1986 at age 41;
librarian; Massachusetts

"Try to get out and walk for some exercise, if you find yourself not doing any during treatment. Try indoor mall walking when the weather is bad."

Mary Raffol; diagnosed in 1998 at age 44;
teacher; Massachusetts

"I continued to play tennis between chemo treatments. I had to stop during radiation because my skin was sensitive, but I began it again about three weeks after the radiation ended, when my skin began to heal."

Cornelia Doherty; diagnosed in 1985 at age 45;
mother, widow, speaker; Massachusetts

"I was so excited when I was able to complete a 3.5-mile Walk to Beat Cancer. I was two-thirds of the way through my chemo and couldn't believe how great I felt."

Linda Jones Burns; diagnosed in 2000 at age 40;
high school registrar; New Hampshire

"I am a very active, athletic, and energetic individual. For the past three years, a group of us have participated in the annual Race for the Cure 5K Run/Walk in Helena, Montana. I like to race to win and have won in my division the past two years. One big reason for this . . . is the fact that I enter in the survivor category. I stack the odds, so to speak!"

Kathy Kirkley; diagnosed in 1993 at age 40;
registered nurse, emergency nurse, mother, wife; Montana

"As I recuperated I thought about the things that I wanted to do when I was back on my feet and decided that I wanted to run a marathon. Well, it took me seven years and two attempts to do it, but I did complete the Silicon Valley Marathon in 1999."

Mary Ruddell; diagnosed in 1992 at age 44;
program manager; California

YOU GO, GIRL!

"Nine months after my breast cancer diagnosis, I realized I was going to live. It was time to rebuild my life. I heard another breast cancer survivor speak of her very positive experience doing yoga, and I decided to give it a try. Timidly, I arranged for one private lesson with her very patient and wise instructor. In that first lesson, I learned that I could control my breath, that my worries disappeared while focusing on gentle stretching and the peace of meditation during savasana. I scheduled a few more private lessons, and then tentatively agreed to partner with another breast cancer survivor for further lessons. Together we began to learn how to live in the moment, to breathe into the stiffness for more stretch, to concentrate to hold poses, and the joy and healing of deep relaxation. I realized that I did have some control over my body. My arm mobility improved. A friendship developed. Months later, a third breast cancer survivor joined our group. A fourth has now been invited. Yoga on Friday evenings is one of the highlights of my week. I am more at peace with my post-surgical body. Despite the fact that breast cancer is what brought our group together, breast cancer does not exist during that weekly hour."

Sandy Gabriel; diagnosed in 1999 at age 45;
medical physicist; New Jersey

"About a year after my surgery, I started taking yoga lessons. The classes were great, as I was able to stretch various muscles and move in gentle ways that I had not been able to before. It was very freeing to be able to move in ways I had not moved in over a year."

Mary Ruddell; diagnosed in 1992 at age 44;
program manager; California

"I was having trouble getting my mobility back in my arm after the mastectomy. I began yoga and swimming. At first I could barely make it across the pool. Now I swim a mile easily and it feels wonderful."

Diane Wilkinson-Codon; diagnosed in 1999 at age 53;
massage therapist, nurse; Nevada

"Only a few short weeks after surgery, I was back in the pool swimming. The mastectomy bathing suit that a friend told me about is not necessary. My chest looks normal in a regular swimsuit with a shoulder pad sewn in one side."

Marcia Gibbons; diagnosed in 1991 at age 52;
artist; Maine

"Where I live in upstate New York, we have forty-six high peaks that hikers climb. My friend did this while undergoing her treatment for breast cancer. It gave her a challenge and the hope that she could beat this disease, and she has!"

Stephanie King; friend of two survivors;
New York

"I like to hike. During the time when I wasn't strong enough to do that, I tried to take little walks, extending the length of the walk a bit each trip. It was good just to be outdoors, enjoying the sights, sounds, and smells of my surroundings, which just happen to be pretty darned awesome."

Carrie Drake; diagnosed in 1998 at age 42;
administrative assistant; Colorado

"Before I was diagnosed with the cancer, I had been losing strength, in my legs especially. I was unable to get out of the bathtub or to get up off the floor, and I had extreme difficulty getting out of a chair or a car. The doctors were puzzled, and I had many tests, but all were normal. After my cancer surgery, I started to gain strength back. I saw a neurologist, and he confirmed that I was regaining my strength. The weakness could have been from my body fighting the cancer. I have since heard of others who have also experienced weakness before cancer was diagnosed. We still don't know for sure, but I do know that I am feeling fine now and am quite active. I am a square dancer and have my old stamina back now, so I am able to do a whole weekend of dancing at a festival."

Diana Vise; diagnosed in 2000;
civil service, retired; Texas

"I had just achieved my black belt in karate, after three years of hard work, when I was diagnosed with breast cancer. I feel that being in good physical shape definitely helped me get through the treatment. I continued to exercise and walk daily, which helped me bounce back faster after each treatment. Exercise also helped me have some kind of control of my life again. I felt alive and healthy when I worked out. I also play piano, and I continued to work my forty hours a week during the whole thing. It's a way to heal yourself mentally."

Kathy Rabassa; diagnosed in 1999 at age 34;
administrative assistant; South Carolina

"Two things helped me a lot, and these had to do with mental attitude and how I felt about myself. First, I continued to work out on my treadmill even when I didn't want to, and my reward was feeling proud of myself and giving myself pats on the back. Second, I had someone around who made me smile. During the worst of it, my youngest son brought me little black-and-white cows to put on the handlebars of my treadmill to keep me company, and he came home every night and made me giggle over new stories of where he worked. He also prodded me to eat and take my medicine, but it was all done with a grin. If attitude is important, then feeling good about yourself and learning to look for the smiles should be at the top of everyone's list of survival tools."

Barbara Hutchinson; diagnosed in 1995 at age 62;
retired; New Hampshire

"I'm getting around to exercise this year as I battle with the aftermath of breast cancer—menopause! Who knew that estrogen could be so helpful with so many little things? Ah, well, hot flashes too will end."

Christine Foutris; diagnosed in 1999 at age 49;
teacher; Illinois

14 • Recurrence

Come Again?

I wanted no part of this chapter. I don't like seeing, hearing, or even *thinking* the word "recurrence." There's a part of me that is just superstitious enough to fear that mere mention of the word will bring on the real thing. And I'm not alone. I warrant that if breast cancer survivors were to cite the single most terrifying word in the world, "recurrence" would be it. Besides, I reasoned, this book was supposed to be about positive stuff, and recurrence is a downer.

So I didn't address the issue in the original version of *UPLIFT*. I would have been perfectly happy never to do so. Then several readers caught me short. They loved the book, they said, only they *have* had experience with recurrence and would like to hear from other survivors who have, too.

Then publication of the paperback version of *UPLIFT* appeared on the horizon, and my editor asked if I wanted to include new material. Did I? I certainly did! I had plenty of new material. It had been coming in from a bevy of gracious and generous contributors to the guestbook at the *UPLIFT* site at www.barbaradelinsky.com. I could easily add new material to any number of chapters.

Well, I could. But then there was recurrence. I still didn't want to see it, hear it, or think it. But it was real. And readers had asked for it. And as much of a downer as recurrence was, I was willing to bet that some who've had experience with it had encouraging words to say to others, and that was the purpose of *UPLIFT*.

So I sent out a mailing asking for submissions, figuring that if none came in, I would be spared having to see, hear, or think recurrence. No such luck. Submissions streamed in—and something really interesting happened to me. P.J. Wamble, a magazine editor from Tennessee, who was diagnosed in 2000 at age forty-five, put it well: "The fear of a second round might be diminished by reading what others have to say." Indeed, as I read what others had to say, my fear *was* diminished. I began to see that recurrence was do-able.

Mind you, the element of my superstition was still a problem. I had no sooner begun to organize these new submissions when I woke up one morning and saw something on my reconstructed breast. It was right on the surface, just as my oncologist had warned that a recurrence for me might be, and it did look like the mosquito bite she had alerted me to. I tried calamine lotion, but the red spot remained. I tried cortisone cream, but it didn't fade a whit. I tried, alternately, witch hazel, Vaseline, and Visine. Visine? Yes, Visine. Models use it to take the red out of zits, and praying that this was only a zit, I tried it.

Nothing.

After looking at that red spot for two days, I was convinced that this was *it*, that I'd better clear my schedule to allow for surgery and chemo, that I did *not* want to tell the boys but that I'd have to, that perhaps this was payback for my hubris in daring to publish *UPLIFT*. I mean, my mind went on and on.

When I finally came to my senses, I called my doctor, who saw me the very next day. She took one look. That was all she needed. Dermatitis, she proclaimed. Cortisone cream, she suggested, but not just for a day. May take up to a month, she predicted. Radiated tissue doesn't have the circulation of virgin skin, she explained, and is therefore both more susceptible to irritation and slower to heal.

Heal it did, though it took the full month. And the moral of this story? As so many of the submitters to this chapter will say, at the first sign of a problem, check it out. Check it out, ask questions, nip potential problems in the bud. The diagnosis may be recurrence or not, but if there's one advantage we now have by virtue of being breast cancer survivors, it is the privilege of having even the tiniest things taken seriously.

One last word. Recurrence takes different forms. There's the kind that results from a spreading of the initial cancer. And there's the kind that is separate and new, a second occurrence independent of the first. For the purposes of this book, I am clumping these together, so that recurrence is defined, most simply, as a second diagnosis of breast cancer.

Have I had a recurrence? Yes. I had breast cancer in my left breast one year, treated by re-excision and radiation. The following year, I had breast cancer in my right breast, treated by (bilateral) mastectomy.   Funny, though, I didn't think of the word "recurrence" at that time. Breast cancer is breast cancer. It came, and I dealt, which is what I'll certainly do if it dares come again.

OH NO! NOT AGAIN!

"We were all devastated. My kids, now eleven and eight, took it harder this time, because they are old enough to really understand what is happening with their mommy. But after a good family cry, we knew we would face this new turn of events with the same, if not more, tenacity than we did before."

Kimberlee Richardson; diagnosed in 2000 at age 26;
mother, Air Force wife, student; Washington

"Two weeks prior to my daughter's wedding, one week prior to her college graduation, and six years in remission to the day, I found out I had breast cancer again. At first I was devastated, much more than the first time. I was sure it could not happen again. I had done everything the doctors had told me to do, but there it was again. After all that, I decided that with everything else going on, wedding and graduation, I just really did not have time for this.

"It has been four years since that recurrence. I don't have the view that I will never have it again. In fact, I probably am even more determined to live for the moment, having experienced the recurrence."

A survivor

"When I was first diagnosed with a recurrence of cancer, it came as a total shock to my husband and me. We spent countless hours looking for answers. How could this happen? Why did the cancer recur?

"The first decision I made was to have a bilateral mastectomy. The cancer was in my right breast. There was no evidence of cancer in my left breast, but I wanted it removed anyway. I know this is not a decision that everyone would make, but it was right for me.

"As for my prognosis, it's great as far as I am concerned. My doctors agree that I should live a long life after my treatments are over, but they don't know for sure, and neither do I. I will live with the uncertainty forever, but I will live well."

Helen Zibuda; diagnosed in 2001 at age 42;
wife, mother; Massachusetts

"I was originally diagnosed in 1997 and had a local recurrence in 1998. It really wasn't half as scary as everyone makes it out to be. I had survived eight rounds of chemo and ten hours of reconstruction, so what was a little local recurrence?"

Monica May; diagnosed in 1997 at age 40;
organizing consultant; New Mexico

"Being told I had a recurrence was worse than first being diagnosed. The second time around was more difficult to come to terms with. This is when I finally learned to take one day at a time. I learned to stay in the moment and try not to worry about tomorrow. Every day that I am here to complain means I'm still alive, and that is a good thing!"

Helene Deutsch; diagnosed in 1997 at age 40; school assistant; New York

"God never promised us that life would be fair. Just the opposite. In this life, we will have trials and tribulations. God did, however, promise that He would cause good to come out of bad, and I cling to that."

Nancy Ellis; diagnosed in 2000 at age 53; quality technician; New York

"People sometimes say to me, 'Why you? This isn't fair!' I hope they wouldn't say that if I won the lottery. Although I appreciate their indignation on my behalf, this isn't about fair. This is just something that happened. My friend Mary says, 'There's only one fair, and they hold it in Del Mar in June.'"

Lynnette Moore; diagnosed in 1997 at age 45; education; California

A NEW ATTITUDE

"I feel that I am a different person since my second bout with cancer. The first one left me kind of numb and in shock. The second came so quickly that it made my head spin, but it has also focused me. I no longer worry that someone might think I'm odd when I carry my breast cancer care bear to doctors' appointments. And do you know? No one even blinks an eye."

Dianne Bouford; diagnosed in 2001 at age 54; homemaker; Maine

"Round One with breast cancer, I was scared, humbled, but determined to be brave.

"Round Two with breast cancer, I was furious, raging, and ready to charge into battle. My feelings and approach were completely different this time.

"I love the saying, 'I am not a survivor—I am an overcomer.'"

Sue Braun; diagnosed in 1988 at age 41; homemaker; Ohio

"I've had breast cancer two times, the first in 1992 and the last in 2000. The last one was much easier because it was found so very early, and because I knew what was ahead for me. It is still very frightening to be told the word 'cancer,' no matter how many times it recurs. But at least you have some idea of what will happen in the months ahead."

Caroline C. Hudnall; diagnosed in 1992 at age 55; retired legal tech in the Supreme Court of Alaska; Montana

"The good thing about losing your hair a second time is that you KNOW it will grow back."

Lynnette Moore; diagnosed in 1997 at age 45; education; California

"With a recurrence and taking chemo again, you know what to expect, because you've been there before. Every chemo has different side effects, but you learn to live with it. You learn to live with treating the disease, and try to chase it out of your body."

Paula Porter; diagnosed in 2000 at age 47; telephone operator; New York

"Perhaps the most difficult challenge of all is managing my mind. I suffer thinking of the past (shoulda woulda coulda) and of the future (do I have one?). Learning to be here now and live moment by moment works. It's simple, but not easy. One gift of this recurrence has been the beginning of a spiritual exploration. It is in this domain, which is new to me, that I find peace."

Susan Zimmerman; diagnosed in 1978 at age 38;
collagist; California

"When you have another diagnosis delivered to you, don't panic. Just regroup and think carefully. It is not the end of the world; it really isn't. Remember to trust your instincts and request tests that you may want. Me? After the mastectomies, reconstruction, and recovery period, I am ecstatic! I feel and look better than before, and more than anything, the peace of mind is priceless. I know that there is always the chance of recurrence, but I also know that with diligent follow-up care and basic common sense, I am able to deal with the situation."

Cathy Hanlon; diagnosed in 2000 at age 42;
school researcher; New York

"It has been two years since my first surgery and one year since my second. These were two different primaries. I feel very grateful that both cancers were found at early stages. I found I had many more friends than I thought, and they were great spirit-lifters."

Wendy Golab; diagnosed in 2000 at age 63;
nurse; Connecticut

"I have come to the conclusion that God gave me cancer the first time to get my attention and to tell me I was not living up to my potential. He gave it to me the second time because I didn't listen. Believe me, I listen now!"

Adelaide D. Key; diagnosed in 1978 at age 42;
community volunteer, philanthropist; North Carolina

"My way of dealing with this reality is to view the cancer as part of who I am now, rather than as some monster that is threatening to destroy me. The cancer cannot ruin today for me—only I can do that to myself by succumbing to hopelessness and fear.

"I have always been frightened of flying. Within just a few weeks of my recurrence, I flew across the country to visit my brother and sister-in-law. I realized how silly it was of me to be afraid of flying when I am living with cancer every day. I am planning another trip in the spring. My recurrence has made me braver in many ways."

Christine Bohnet; diagnosed in 2001 at age 53;
data processing coordinator; Michigan

"These days I spend in gratitude. I try to make each day count. My family is everything. I try not to get so angry or emotional over things anymore. Cancer? Heck. I'm not afraid of it so much anymore. Chemo? Baldness? Wigs? Meds? Been there, done that. It's time to move on. There's a life to be lived, and I'm living it. And if I do just one thing each day, however small, to make the world a better place, everything I have gone through will have been worth it. Life is beautiful. And it's a gift."

Barbara Hartman; diagnosed in 1999 at age 53;
homemaker, proud grandma; New Jersey

"I know that each recurrence is seen as a setback. It's hard to get past the latest test results for a little while, but we have to keep thinking positive thoughts and planning for our futures. For me, it helps to have fun things planned, like scrapbooking time to work on my photo albums with friends up in the mountains, or a road trip to northern California."

Gwen Loverink; diagnosed in 1994 at age 34;
police dispatcher; California

"I have learned to laugh along with my tears and have come to appreciate every minute of every day. I am determined to fight this 'beast.' Breast cancer isn't like others. It is a chronic illness for which we need to find a cure."

Lynne Andrus; diagnosed in 1998 at age 47;
teacher; New Hampshire

NEW JUICE

"The eight years between my two BCs, as I call them, have found so many new techniques. My wise surgeon told me that looking at my 1992 case was looking back into the 'dark ages.'"

Caroline C. Hudnall; diagnosed in 1992 at age 55;

retired legal tech in the Supreme Court of Alaska; Montana

"I've had two recurrences since my original diagnosis in 1995. I am so thankful for the new drugs that are coming out. I have been on Herceptin off and on for the last three years. I am cancer free at this time and praising the Lord!"

Helen Kim; diagnosed in 1995 at age 55;

retired medical receptionist; Michigan

"I have had a recurrence of breast cancer after almost six years in remission. I have an exceptional oncologist who is very much into the mind, body, spirit approach to cancer. I buy into that philosophy also."

JoAnn Cámara; diagnosed in 1996 at age 53;

early intervention specialist; Ohio

"When my cancer returned, I felt this was really it for me, that it was only a matter of time. But my doctor assured me that we could fight it. This time I went through chemo, a stem cell transplant, and radiation. The whole process took a year. It is now five years since I finished it, and I am still cancer free. I really want to let cancer patients know that there is always hope. The scientists are always coming up with something new. If you can hang on, the next treatment may be just around the corner!"

Regina Vaughn; diagnosed in 1993 at age 45;

drapery shop owner; Ohio

"I thank God every day for the newly developed breast cancer medications I am being given. After only a few treatments, my liver enzymes have returned to normal and the pain in my hip has significantly improved. My doctors are ecstatic, and I am feeling strong and hopeful."

Christine Bohnet; diagnosed in 2001 at age 53;
data processing coordinator; Michigan

"If I should have yet another recurrence, I know that the longer I'm able to keep fighting, the better the chances of finding a cure, and having it apply to me!"

Cathleen D'Antonio; diagnosed in 1994 at age 28;
benefits analyst; Connecticut

WHAT HELPED ME . . .

"My first recurrence 'struck' a month after my husband and I were married. I was devastated, not only that IT was back, but that it had nestled in my skull. This time around, though, I had an even larger support system—my husband's family as well as my own. Believe me, going through three stem cell transplants was not easy, but their optimism and faith, along with my positive resolve, kept me going. We got through that ordeal, along with three other 'recurrences' in the bone. I am living proof that, YES, you can survive multiple recurrences!"

Cathleen D'Antonio; diagnosed in 1994 at age 28;
benefits analyst; Connecticut

"After I finished my first set of radiation treatments, I contacted a support group. I had only attended two of the monthly meetings when I had the second cancer diagnosis. I barely knew these women, yet many of them sent cards and called me during my treatment. It meant so much to me to find a card in the mail. Some names I couldn't put a face to, but they all cared. I have found that a good support group is especially helpful when cancer comes back."

Dianne Bouford; diagnosed in 2001 at age 54;
homemaker; Maine

"First, listen to your body. If you feel deep down inside that something is wrong, then you need to push the issue. Ask for a blood test, a CT scan, PET scan—whatever. Don't take 'no' for an answer. Second, try not to completely lose it if the words 'persistent' or 'residual' come up. If that happens, remember that you beat this once before, so you know you have the strength to do it again. Third, make sure you do research and ask a lot of questions before deciding on your new course of action. Ask to be paired up with someone who has been in a similar situation. It is such a comfort to talk with someone who has been there."

Kimberlee Richardson; diagnosed in 2000 at age 26;
mother, Air Force wife, student; Washington

"It is a year ago this month that I was originally diagnosed with breast cancer. I had only been finished with my chemo for four months when tests indicated some spots on my liver and my hip bone. I was devastated. My team of doctors quickly rallied around me. I was amazed when they told me they were not giving up on me! I was even more amazed when they shared stories with me of other breast cancer patients with similar metastases, who have been receiving treatment for years and are still living meaningful lives. They explained that I must now view my illness as chronic, and learn to live with it and with the treatments needed to extend my life for many years."

Christine Bohnet; diagnosed in 2001 at age 53;
data processing coordinator; Michigan

"One of the things I did this time around was to let my family and friends know I needed continuing support. I told everyone to do whatever felt right to them, that I would take all the help that was offered. I received such an outpouring of love and support that it nearly overwhelmed me."

Dianne Bouford; diagnosed in 2001 at age 54;
homemaker; Maine

"I have been bald twice and have purchased three different color wigs. I feel my attitude is a good one, and that this is what helped me get through not one but two bouts with breast cancer. I feel that we are all put on this earth to help one another, and since I am a two-time winner in this game, I have been able to help other women diagnosed with cancer understand and walk through the fear."

Mary Stewart; diagnosed in 1998 at age 44;
claims adjuster; California

HERE'S MY STORY

"My first diagnosis in 1995 was a small tumor. My second tumor was large and aggressive, which really surprised me, since I was so diligent in monitoring. I was diagnosed right before my son's wedding. That's what kept me going initially. I knew I had to remain upbeat for him. I finished chemo three weeks before the wedding, and let me tell you how I danced and celebrated at the wedding. What a wonderful day!"

Rozanne Perlman; diagnosed in 1995 at age 48;
travel agent; California

"My recurrence was found through a simple tumor marker test done by my oncologist every year. I realized that if not for this test, the tumor might have been found when it was too late, and I could have died. My tumors are both gone now. I am praying that no new ones appear. But I have learned to live with cancer. One of my goals in life is to see a preventive vaccine or a cure for this disease."

Marcella Malamut; diagnosed in 1983 at age 50;
homemaker; New Jersey

"I was thirty-five years old when I discovered the lump in my breast. Six months after my treatment ended, I discovered another lump under my arm. How do you deal with this? How do you remain positive when ill-informed friends have you on your deathbed?

"What did I do? I laced up my boxing gloves once again, I smiled, and I stepped into the ring. My opponent has seemed to score more than I have, but I'm certainly not down for the count. I keep getting back up, taunting the enemy. I've humbly learned to place myself in God's capable hands, and we have this agreement that we'll take this thing one day at a time. He's certainly more experienced than I, and He even possesses miraculous healing capabilities.

"Recurrence, even metastatic recurrence, is not the end of the world. In fact, there's usually plenty of time to figure out who you really are, and who you want to be. Always remember, you have a choice."

Julie Jarzynski; diagnosed in 1999 at age 36;
hairdresser; Illinois

"I was working on my computer when it hit me. I sat back to watch a program download and absentmindedly put my hand to my neck—and felt a lump the size of a marble. I panicked. I was sure I was going to die. I thought, 'This is it. It comes back a second time, and you're dead meat.'

"Tests proved that it was indeed a malignancy. I had it again. But here's the thing. Weird. It was totally contained in that little lump. It didn't spread. It didn't go anywhere."

Barbara Hartman; diagnosed in 1999 at age 53;
homemaker, proud grandma; New Jersey

"I was originally diagnosed with breast cancer in March of 2001 at age forty-one after feeling a lump in my right breast. My treatment ended in October of 2001. I had a mammogram and physical exam in February of 2002 and was given a clean bill of health. Less than two months later, I felt another lump in the area of my lumpectomy scar. This resulted in a diagnosis of recurrence in May of 2002.

"My second tumor was even smaller than my first one. I feel very fortunate that my cancer was caught early on two separate occasions."

Helen Zibuda; diagnosed in 2001 at age 42;
wife, mother; Massachusetts

"I was diagnosed just three years after my twin had breast cancer. The treatment I chose was lumpectomy with radiation. My recurrence came one year later, with additional DCIS found in the same breast. I chose re-excision. My next recurrence came one year later, with more DCIS found in the same breast in new sites. I had mastectomy with immediate reconstruction. I felt changed, finally free, yet fully natural. It was the best decision I could have made.

"Then, with recovery, I found NIA (neuro muscular non-impact aerobics). Twice each week, I move, exercise, and dance with other breast cancer survivors. The instructors are also breast cancer survivors. There is tremendous hope in the framework of dance. I would recommend breast cancer support based on movement to all survivors."

Debra DeSocio; diagnosed in 1997 at age 41;
special education teacher; New York

"I had recurrence in the same site two years after my original lumpectomy and radiation. The first time, I declined chemo; the second time, I had a mastectomy and chemo. The recurrence put me into a serious depression. I had recovered very quickly after the original diagnosis, but now I was really sick. The hair loss was much harder to bear than the breast loss.

"I think the recurrence put me in close touch with the meaning of friendship. I moved out of the depression slowly and into a most positive place. It was the kick-start allowing me to continue to play and enjoy my life even more. It was after the recurrence that I took up rowing.

"I had another scare three months ago, but life goes on. In two weeks, I will celebrate my sixty-fifth birthday with lots of friends, songs, live Irish music, and plenty of Irish whiskey and wines. Life is just fine, thank you."

Patricia Carr; diagnosed in 1989 at age 51;
community college professor, counselor; New Jersey

"I was first diagnosed in June of 2001. Five months later, I went to my surgeon for a follow-up visit. I had one rather large lump in my right breast. It had already been through two mammograms, and my surgeon had been sure it was cystic in nature. Now, because of my new history of breast cancer, he took a closer look. It turned out to be a very slow growing cancer.

"When friends react with pity or horror to the news that I had a second cancer so soon after the first, I tell them that if the mammogram hadn't found the first one, who knew how long it would have been before my doctor and I realized something was seriously wrong with the second one. My second cancer needed to get our attention. For that reason, I am grateful for the first one.

"The third lump got everyone's attention in a hurry. It turned out to be a cyst. So take heart, girls. Every lump you find after breast cancer isn't necessarily a new cancer. Get it checked out promptly, but don't feel doomed."

Dianne Bouford; diagnosed in 2001 at age 54;
homemaker; Maine

"I was first diagnosed with breast cancer in 1994. In 1999, I had a recurrence in my lung. Fortunately, it was operable, and I have been cancer free since then. I had scans every three months for about a year and a half, and now have them every six months.

"The first few weeks after part of my lung was removed, I was a basket case. I have three young daughters, and I decided that if I was going to die, they were going to remember me as a fighter, not a cry baby. I prayed and asked God to give me the peace that passes all understanding. It was as if a burden was lifted off my shoulders.

"While dying is in the back of my mind, I have decided to live life to the fullest for as long as I can. No one is guaranteed a to-morrow. It's 11:08 PM right now, and my five-year-old daughter is calling me to do the Electric Slide. Life is GOOD! Gotta go."

A survivor

"It was at my five-year check up for my first cancer when my doc-tor questioned a lump in my other breast. My reaction was differ-ent this time. Even with my husband's gentle support, I doubted my future. I was angry and scared.

"I did get through it. My treatment was more aggressive than the first time. Donning a new plaid turban, I picked up my beau-tiful, angel-faced child at school. Upon seeing my head wrapped, he looked up with the most compassionate face and asked, 'Your hair came out today?' My reply was, 'Yes, honey, it did.' Then, as only a child can do, he said complimentarily, 'You look like a swami!' He touched me deeply with his simple, sweet acceptance.

"Six years have passed since I've been called a swami."

Diane Loughran; diagnosed in 1991 at age 44;
teacher; Massachusetts

"My daughter was living in New York City and rode her bike to work every day. One day, while she was visiting someone, her bike was stolen. She was very upset and went looking for a cop. When she finally found one and told him her story, his response was, 'So what? This is New York City. What are the odds of finding your bike?' She said very proudly, 'My mother has had breast cancer three times, and she is still alive. What are the odds?' He put her in his car and they actually found the bike and the guy who stole it.

"What are the odds? Apparently, they have never been better!"

Lyn Rosenthal; diagnosed in 1989 at age 36; medical center manager of volunteer services; Florida

SEEING THE LARGER PICTURE

"Things happen in our lives over which we have no control. The events of September 11 changed thousands of lives in an instant. Breast cancer changed me and my focus in life. Yes, there is life after breast cancer. Since I have been blessed to have that life, I'm not going to waste it."

Rozanne Perlman; diagnosed in 1995 at age 48; travel agent; California

"During my second round of chemo, the world collapsed. My daughter called me on the morning of September 11. I watched as much TV as I could. One tower had already collapsed. You can see New York City from the top of the hill on my block. I walked up the hill and looked. In the distance, the remaining tower stood, looking bluish-grey in color, smoke billowing from the roof.

"And here I thought cancer was the worst thing that could happen to you. I was in the middle of cancer treatment for the second time, and I had a chance. Those people never did.

"I know that cancer is hardly the worst thing in the world that can ever happen to a person. What's worse? Hate, anger, prejudice. They are far more deadly."

Barbara Hartman; diagnosed in 1999 at age 53; homemaker, proud grandma; New Jersey

"Recurrence of breast cancer is a scary place to be, because there is no cure. But the tragedy of 9/11 showed me that I was not really so bad off. I am alive. I can fight this disease. I know who my enemy is. "Even though this is a frightening thing to live with, I do live. I live every day with a basic attitude of no regrets. I make sure that there is no wasted time or feelings. When the flowers smell fragrant, I know it, because I take the time to stop and smell them."

Lynne Andrus; diagnosed in 1998 at age 47;
teacher; New Hampshire

"Having this disease has left me free from personal fear of things like terrorist attacks and flying. I realize I can dwell on the uncertainty of the future and go crazy and feel sorry for myself (which does happen from time to time), or I can dwell in the blessings of the present, which are too numerous to count."

Diane Phillips; diagnosed in 2001 at age 58;
UCC minister, nurse; California

"September 11 should have taught all of us how unpredictable life can be. None of us has a guarantee that we will live until tomorrow, but we are here today, so we need to make today worthwhile."

Christine Bohnet; diagnosed in 2001 at age 53;
data processing coordinator; Michigan

LONG-RANGE

"I am a recurrence survivor. I was initially diagnosed with breast cancer in 1982 at the age of forty. Five years after my initial diagnosis, I was diagnosed again. Things were different this time. I had six months of chemo, followed by radiation. I had many positive happenings during this trying time. With the help of my breast cancer support group, family, co-workers, and friends, I knew I was not alone in this battle.

"Cancer definitely changes your life. It is a word we all fear.

But if I learned one thing, it is that cancer does not always mean a death sentence. I know. I am a twelve-year recurrence survivor!"

Adelaide Carrara; diagnosed in 1982 at age 40;
retired school secretary; Massachusetts

"We are monitored so closely by our doctors that recurrences are usually found quickly and can be acted upon immediately, thus improving our chances of long-term survival."

Christine Bohnet; diagnosed in 2001 at age 53;
data processing coordinator; Michigan

"Breast cancer is a chronic condition—it is never truly 'gone.' And one can live WITH it for years, as I have. You accept that YOU are 100% responsible for your own health and well-being. Your body is designed to heal itself, given conditions and an environment in which it can do so. It is up to you to provide them."

Susan Zimmerman; diagnosed in 1978 at age 38;
collagist; California

"I am a long-term survivor—twelve years, to be exact. Having survived this disease more than once, I am much more aware of 'time' and how quickly it passes. My journey has been a tough and daunting one, but a rewarding one as well. I am a survivor who is still standing, laughing, and living each day."

Susan Clemente; diagnosed in 1990 at age 46;
retired registered nurse; New York

"It has been almost twenty-five years since my first diagnosis and seventeen since the second, yet I am busier and happier than I have ever been. I won't tell you that cancer won't come back, but it is going to have to run like hell to catch me!"

Adelaide D. Key; diagnosed in 1978 at age 42;
community volunteer, philanthropist; North Carolina

15 · Religion

Bringing In the Big Gun

When I initially conceived of *UPLIFT*, I had no plans for a chapter on religion. It wasn't that I didn't think religion was a major factor in many people's lives, especially those who were ill—because I knew that it was. But I felt that there were already plenty of other "inspirational" books on the shelves. I wanted *UPLIFT* to contain the kind of practical info and upbeat stories that hadn't yet been published.

So I didn't mention religion in the guidelines. Nor, though, did I discount submissions that mentioned it from inclusion in the book when they did indeed arrive. How could I? The religion-health link has been documented. Studies have found that when anxious people turn to God, their anxiety is reduced, and when their anxiety is reduced, both their immune systems and their cardiovascular systems get a boost. Moreover, members of the *UPLIFT* sisterhood repeatedly name their church and its members as a very special kind of support group.

The premise of *UPLIFT* is to tell the good stuff. If faith helps a woman make it through breast cancer with a smile on her face and makes her palm's lifeline longer than ever, those submissions fit the guidelines to a T.

Here they are, short and sweet. Enjoy.

HAVING FAITH

"The most settling thing I did after hearing my diagnosis was to take a walk along the path by the shore of Lake Mendota. At one point, I stopped, leaned on a railing overlooking the lake, and looked back at the land. After a while, I simply said, 'God, I don't want to deal with this. I'd like you to handle this one for me. Okay?' That was it, but amazingly then, I was able to let go. Not that I didn't do my part in taking very good care of myself, but I never fretted about my diagnosis after that. I just did the next right thing that came along."

> Gracie Schwingel; diagnosed in 1998 at age 51;
> secretary; Wisconsin

"My daughter left a framed saying next to my bed. It said, 'God is watching you. I know because I asked him to.' "

> Corda M. Gilliland; diagnosed in 2000 at age 72;
> retired, widow; Pennsylvania

"We have a deep faith, and this is what sustained us as a family. We prayed frequently together. I attended daily mass with my husband as often as I could."

> Cornelia Doherty; diagnosed in 1985 at age 45;
> mother, widow, speaker; Massachusetts

"The most constructive thing I did after hearing my diagnosis was to have a heart-to-heart talk with God. The most *helpful* thing I did was to learn that one of the members of my church was a ten-year survivor."

> Debby Whittet; diagnosed in 1996 at age 43;
> household technician, part-time library worker; Michigan

"A phone call soon after my diagnosis prompted my involvement in my local religious organization. The people there were so welcoming that it opened up a whole new world for me with a renewed spirituality in my faith. This has given me a new and ongoing support system of wonderful people who care about me."

Linda Perkins; diagnosed in 1999 at age 35;
project manager; New Jersey

"When my mother was diagnosed, I was only twenty and had no idea of the ramifications of it. Through two years of her surgery and treatments, I encouraged her and celebrated with her when it was finished, and she still survives. Then, I was expecting my fourth child when my own diagnosis came. It was overwhelming and humbling. What helped me to endure the treatments with four small children? My friends and my church. Being headstrong and independent, I had to learn to receive their kindness. The outpouring of food was so incredible that we had to set up a schedule because the refrigerator was overflowing. I was grateful for their generosity, as I certainly didn't feel like cooking. It turned out to be a double blessing. Those who shared their gifts were also enriched. I learned that sometimes I am able to do Christ's work by helping others, and at other times I was to be helped so that my neighbor could be Christ for me. My faith grew in leaps and bounds! Less than two years later, my sister was diagnosed with cancer. Somehow I couldn't be sad, though I knew how hard her next few months would be. God was working through her as well. I knew that we are survivors. How lucky our family is—and my cancer experience continues to be a blessing. As I work in the pharmacy, many of my patients receive the same diagnosis. When I tell them that I have had cancer and am a survivor, it gives them hope."

Jane Zinda; diagnosed in 1987 at age 33;
mother, pharmacist; Ohio

"It's not that I ever laughed at people involved in prayer chains, but I was sincerely grateful when they included me."

Kathi Ward; diagnosed in 1994 at age 47;
merchandiser; South Carolina

"Jeremiah 29:11 has been such a help when I begin to doubt. 'For I know the thoughts that I think toward you, saith the Lord, thoughts of peace, and not of evil, to give you a future and a hope.' "

Judy Peterson; diagnosed in 2000 at age 58;
registered nurse; Colorado

"Among my cancer blessings were the 'signs' of love I received from God. For example, for weeks I saw a heart outline on a tarnishing sink drain. I'd never seen it before and have never seen it since."

Diane Bongiorno; diagnosed in 1998 at age 43;
instructional aide; New Jersey

* * *

"When I told a dear friend of mine about my diagnosis, she told me about a dove that had been hanging around her house in Texas. This dove should have been long gone, since winter was near. But this dove served a purpose. It brought peace somehow to people who saw it. One day my friend mailed me a feather from this dove with a note saying, 'Remember, sometimes God's word rests on the wings of a dove.' It was a sweet reminder of trust in God, and He would give me peace.

"The morning of my mastectomy I was in the shower when I heard my son yelling about a bird in the house. Since we have several caged birds, I assumed one of them got out. When I got out of the shower, I asked him what all the commotion was about, and he said, 'A bird flew in the house, made one lap around the living room and flew back out.' When I asked him what kind of bird it was, he said it was a white dove. My sister had seen the bird and agreed with that. I knew that God had sent that dove to give me peace and remind me that He is in control. During my recovery and chemotherapy I remembered the dove, God's promise, and my favorite verse, from Proverbs 3:5 and 6, 'Trust in the Lord with all your heart and lean not on your own understanding; in all your ways acknowledge Him and He will make your paths straight.' "

Tammy Delin; diagnosed in 1997 at age 33;
teacher's aide; California

* * *

"My friend Alice hated going in for her radiation treatments. The lying still really got to her. She finally discovered that if she said the 23rd Psalm, she knew exactly how many times to say it and where she would be when it was over. When I passed this hint on to another good friend, June came out after her treatment one morning with a smile on her face. 'It works,' she said. If you don't know the 23rd Psalm, sing your favorite song to yourself. That works, too!"

Donna Palmer;
friend of a survivor; Michigan

"To strengthen my belief in God, in myself, and in life during the chemo, I read an uplifting perpetual calendar verse and psalm daily—and still do."

Sue Braun; diagnosed in 1988 at age 41;
homemaker; Ohio

"I was given a prayer that I said before each treatment, and it comforted me then and still comforts me now. 'The light of God surrounds me. The love of God enfolds me. The power of God protects me. The presence of God watches over me. Whatever I am, God is, and all is well.' "

Christine Foutris; diagnosed in 1999 at age 49;
teacher; Illinois

"I awoke one morning realizing that I had entered into another part of my grieving process. I was sad to be losing a part of my body, but I visualized our Lord on the cross, and I thought of the pain that he must have suffered. He did so much for me. I could do this."

Sandy Williams; diagnosed in 1999 at age 51; children's public services librarian; Texas

"Life is a series of choices. My friend Sheryl sent me a story about a carrot, an egg, and a coffee bean. The story went like this: 'When life throws you in hot water, you can choose to be a carrot, an egg, or a coffee bean. A carrot becomes soft and pliable, giving in to the adversity, giving up. The egg hardens and refuses to conform. The coffee bean, however, turns the water into a steaming, flavorful drink.' 'You,' Sheryl wrote to me, 'chose to make coffee.' In the past, when my husband or children or close friends have been ill, I had actually prayed to God to give me the illness, to let me carry it. When I knew that I might be facing cancer, I felt God telling me, 'Now's your chance to make coffee.' "

Rosamary Amiet; diagnosed in 2000 at age 48; program manager; Ohio

"I owe my survival to the Lord Jesus Christ. Every time I go for radiation treatment, I surround myself with prayer. I pray right through the radiation."

Jennie Isbell; diagnosed in 1999 at age 76; retired, housewife; New York

"The thing that helped me get through this the most was my faith in God. I have never prayed so hard in all my life. I put everything in God's hands, and asked Him to help me."

Paula Porter; diagnosed in 2000 at age 47; telephone operator; New York

"How to deal with the worry? That was a hard one, because two years after my diagnosis, there was another lump. So I turned to God. I had been floating. He grounded me once more. I got the news that it was nothing, but I want to stay grounded. I can face anything laid before me . . . with God."

Pam Waddell; diagnosed in 1998 at age 38;
writer, teacher's aide; Texas

"This Buddhist prayer helps me to begin each day: 'May all be loved. May all be healed. May all be sheltered. May all be free from fear. May I be loved. May I be healed. May I be sheltered. May I be free from fear.' "

Deb Haney; diagnosed in 1996 at age 48;
administrative assistant, artist; Massachusetts

"Cancer, for me, was an agenda, giving me permission to live the way I had been living for years, by faith. God has blessed me with twelve years of survivorship and many wonderful friends, fellow cancer survivors, and their families!"

Aileen Pandapas; diagnosed in 1989 at age 41;
mom, volunteer, former secretary; Virginia

"Looking back, I realize that I have a greater appreciation for the joys of life, a calmness I never had before, and a deeper faith in God. What more could I ask?"

E. Mary Lou Clauss; diagnosed in 1991 at age 55;
homemaker, retired registered nurse; Pennsylvania

"Today is June 8, 2000. You ask what is so special about this day? Well, let me tell you, God has blessed me with nineteen cancer-free years! I thought of many ways to celebrate this day, and finally decided to do a walk called "Making Strides Against Breast Cancer." My goal was to raise $1,900 for breast cancer research, $100 for each of the years I have been cancer free. Well, I did the

walk and raised even more than that. Thank you, Lord, for one
more time blessing my steps. I can't wait for next year!"

Debbie Roberts; diagnosed in 1981 at age 22;
housewife, mother; Kentucky

* * *

"Someone wrote, 'Having cancer was the best thing that ever
happened to me.' Originally, I thought this was a stupid statement. I could not comprehend how anyone could say this. But,
after the past year, I agree. My wife having cancer was the best
thing that ever happened to us. In looking back, I was a religious
snob. I felt that going to church weekly, saying my daily prayers,
and occasionally volunteering for our parish kept me in touch
with God and my salvation. But I stopped going through the motions when Joanne was diagnosed with breast cancer. I started to
pray with my heart. I found prayer an answer to life's problems.
Had it not been for my wife's cancer, I would have never reached
this level of understanding."

Gene Palmer;
Joanne's husband

"We named my cancer Jack. During the weekly trips to the hospital with my husband, 'Hit the Road, Jack' and 'You Are My Sunshine' became our theme songs. Jack did indeed hit the road.
Prayer was powerful."

Joanne Palmer; diagnosed in 1996 at age 42;
medical receptionist; New York

16 • Pure Uplift

Wrapping It Up with a Bow

So we've discussed specifics, like hair, food, and clothes. We've talked about what we want, how we feel, and what others can do to help. We've gone through tactics for regaining control. We've done the positive attitude thing. What's left? Nothing but wrapping it up. This chapter is a catchall for miscellaneous thoughts of the sisterhood that might just as easily have fit several other chapters but didn't instantly slip into any one.

We're talking some wonderful bits of philosophy here, like that from Rosamary Amiet, who wrote, "My single most important piece of advice for a friend is, don't spend time worrying how to live with breast cancer. Spend your time learning how to live life." And that from Sallie Burdine, who wanted to pass on something she'd read: "Attitude is the mind's paintbrush. It can color any situation." And from Betsy Ellis Bowles, who wrote, "We do have *some* control over the length of our lives, but the real kick comes from knowing that we have *much* control over its width and depth. If we're not doing what makes our hearts sing, we're wasting precious time."

And then, there are a few special anecdotes, like this one sent in by Darlene Jurow: "My breast reconstruction involved using stomach tissue to form two new breasts. Due to the incision from hip to hip, I had trouble standing up straight for several months. Upon seeing my distress, my husband ran out and bought me three antique canes. One had a built-in flask . . . a wee nip for the time when the pain was gripping. One had a concealed dagger to poke those who jokingly called me an old crone (I was only fifty-two). The last had a compass in the handle to always direct me back to family. These three treasures have been my 'support.' They represent comfort, self-esteem, and love. Internal strength comes in strange packages!"

Not so strange a package, by now, is *UPLIFT*. You may already be well versed in the attitude, but a little more never hurts. Read and reread. As so many members of the sisterhood say, "If it feels good, do it!"

SO MUCH TO APPRECIATE

"Breast cancer has helped me not to take anything for granted. I'm content with even the smallest of things, like working on cross-stitch, having time to read, talking and visiting with my family and friends, or watching my cats play and sleep. These are all special moments."

Gwen Loverink; diagnosed in 1994 at age 34;
police dispatcher; California

"I was thirty-six years old and six months pregnant when I was diagnosed, and had a mastectomy and chemo treatments during my pregnancy. I certainly never expected this at a time that should have been so happy, but we are certainly happy now. My child and I are both survivors!"

Tammi Keller; diagnosed in 2000 at age 30;
mom; Pennsylvania

"My sister and several of my friends have had breast cancer, and all are doing well. When I was diagnosed, I told myself that if they got through it, so would I. Now, after thirty-three radiation sessions, I am a survivor, too. The key to success, I think, is a positive attitude and a good outlook."

Ellie Meyers; diagnosed in 2000 at age 70;
retired federal employee; Maryland

"I will never forget the feeling of warmth and caring I received when a total stranger approached me in a department store at the time when my 'chemo hair' was just starting to grow. She had the courage to ask me if I had undergone chemotherapy and was it for breast cancer. When I answered yes, she gave me the longest, hardest hug of encouragement, and I nearly cried. She had a daughter who was a recent survivor, and she wanted to pass on the feeling that 'you can do it, too.' This unknown woman has made me want to be just as courageous and pass on the needed hugs, so my eyes and ears are always open. I am very proud to be recognized as a survivor and never want to lose that image, so I am keeping my hair short and wispy as a sign to everyone."

Sarah Stuart; diagnosed in 1999 at age 52;
banking human resources assistant; Vermont

"A positive attitude makes such a difference. It is a fact that it affects survivor rates in cancer patients. Quality of life is also improved by a positive attitude. How to stay positive? Take one day at a time, and deal with each problem as it comes. Don't let your mind anticipate new ones. They might never occur."

Judy Peterson; diagnosed in 2000 at age 58;
registered nurse; Colorado

"How is my post-cancer body better? Physically, I'm a bit leaner, so I feel better about my shape and weight. Mentally—more importantly—I appreciate so much more, each and every moment that makes up the day. *And* I no longer tolerate rude or narrow-minded people!"

Carrie Drake; diagnosed in 1998 at age 42;
administrative assistant; Colorado

"I've always felt thankful for the wonderful people and things in my life, and I continue to do so. Whether my appreciation of these things is part of growing older, or getting cancer, or what, I don't know. I sincerely hope that my compassion, volunteering, fundraising, or whatever small part I can play will help someone else with breast cancer."

Sheila Roper; diagnosed in 1995 at age 57;
homemaker; New Hampshire

"Now, at the dinner table, each member of our family says what we are thankful for. It doesn't have to be a serious thing—it may be soccer—just as long as we are all appreciating the abundance in our lives. We are all so blessed. Let us pay attention to what is right instead of what is wrong."

Sandy Rodgers; diagnosed in 1999 at age 44;
homemaker, mom, registered nurse, Reiki master; Massachusetts

"I ate well during chemo in order to keep my blood counts as high as possible. I cried when I had to and smiled the rest of the time. I counted the days when chemo was over and then breezed through radiation. I kept saying over and over, 'This too shall pass.' Now, when bothersome little things happen, I compare them to that time in my life, and it puts everything in perspective. This Christmas was wonderful. I enjoyed every moment and never complained. I plan to enjoy many more!"

Frances Gallello; diagnosed in 2000 at age 51;
mental health assistant; New York

"You know that saying about taking time to smell the roses? Nothing could be truer, especially for those of us who've had breast cancer. I just went to Paris with three girlfriends, and I don't work Saturdays now or allow for the stress I used to feel. I just bought an older MBZ 450SL hardtop convertible. I had always said that one day I'd have one, and even though I couldn't afford a newer one, this one is gorgeous and I love love love driving it!"

Patti R. Martinez; diagnosed in 1999 at age 54;
realtor; California

"I was diagnosed a year and a half ago and had a lumpectomy and radiation therapy. Having been an oncology nurse for several years, I must say that it was both frightening and enlightening to have the shoe on *my* foot! My breast cancer was discovered from a routine mammogram, as so many are, and my experience was a positive one."

Donna Barnett; diagnosed in 1999 at age 40;
registered nurse; California

"My mother is grateful for the benefits and blessings she has received regarding her bout with breast cancer. She believes that breast cancer survivors, those currently undergoing treatment for breast cancer, and those whose lives have most recently been turned upside down because of a mysterious lump are truly a sisterhood and family whose collective motto includes strength, determination, optimism, love, and prayer."

John E. Schlimm II;
son of survivor Barbara Schlimm; Pennsylvania

"Never ask yourself 'Why me?' It's not only a waste of time and energy; it's a misconception. Look around you at those less fortunate. The world is full of victims—wonderful people who have had bad things happen to them, too. Be faithful, thankful, grateful, and keep an open mind. You never know what tomorrow will bring, and it just might be a cure."

Kathy Weaver-Stark; diagnosed in 1991 at age 46;
insurance adjuster, instructor; Oregon

EVERY DAY IS A GIFT

"I am a seven-and-a-half year breast cancer survivor whose disease was diagnosed during my eighth month of pregnancy. Now, as I walk in the New York Race for the Cure every September with my beautiful daughter Eve (Hebrew for Life), who has a sign on her back that says, 'In celebration of my mama,' I realize that God had presented me with a challenge, but he also gave me a great gift."

Renee C. Johannesen; diagnosed in 1993 at age 35; marketing communications manager; New York

"It has been seven years since my diagnosis, and I live life as fully as I can. When I hesitate to take that trip to do something I'm too tired to do, I push myself. I thank God every day for this strength and for giving me another day."

Alyce Feinstein; diagnosed in 1993 at age 58; administrative assistant; Massachusetts

"I am a very lucky forty-two-year-old married woman with three sons aged sixteen, thirteen, and nine. I believe that we are given this 'gift' of illness to see how special and fragile life is. The gift may not be wanted, but it can teach a most valuable lesson: to love and live fully in our day-to-day lives."

Cathy Hanlon; diagnosed in 2000 at age 42; school researcher; New York

"Say to yourself daily, 'I can beat this.' A positive attitude will give you the courage to go on when things get rough. Most important, remember that you are not alone!"

Cheryl Cavallo; diagnosed in 1997 at age 35; homemaker; Massachusetts

"My treatment began in the fall, right in the middle of football season. In Oklahoma, football is taken very seriously, and both of my children were actively involved. Our son, Jay, was a member of the varsity football team, and our daughter, Kelly, was a varsity cheerleader. It was our son's senior year, and we had tried not to miss any of their activities. As the weather got colder, though, my doctor warned me about staying well and told me—absolutely—not to attend the football game the following Friday night. I explained to our son that I wouldn't be able to attend, but that I would listen to the radio and cheer for him from home. He left the house at about five o'clock, saying that he understood and that he just wanted me to be well. At about six o'clock, I got a call from the football coach asking if there was anything wrong. I told him about my precarious health and explained that I shouldn't be out in the rain and cold. The coach had seen that Jay and his friends were down, and was worried that if I wasn't there, they might not be able to concentrate on the game. Then he asked to speak to my husband.

"My husband hung up the phone, bundled me up in my coat, boots, hat, and gloves, and off we went to the football field. When we arrived at the visitors' gate, we were waved through and were met by the school athletic director, holding a huge umbrella, who walked us up to the stadium section reserved for the media and coaches. In this booth, they had a cozy chair, an electric heater at my feet, and a nice stadium blanket, just in case I needed it. The head coach came in and asked about my comfort, and then asked me to do him a favor. He asked me to watch him on the field during warm-ups, and when he waved to me, for me to stand up. He left and went to the field and called the players together. He then waved to me, and I responded by standing and gave a wave of my own. The boys saw me in the booth, pointed up to our position, and began clapping Jay on the back. It seems that our son had told his friends that I wouldn't be able to attend the game. I believe he did understand but was still worried about his mom, which in turn worried the other boys. Two of his good friends had gone to the coach to have him check on me, and he decided that they wouldn't believe I was truly well unless they saw me. I can't tell you who won that football game, but I can tell you how uplifted I was by the show of love and kindness on the part of those big burly boys and the coaches, not only for me, but for our son as well."

Brenda Carr; diagnosed in 1988 at age 40;
wife, mother, retired school counselor; Texas

"When I see my tattoo marks from radiation or my lack of a breast and begin to feel sorry for myself, I stop short and remember that since my diagnosis, I have seen my son marry and my daughter graduate from high school and go off to college. Every day is a gift."

Joanne Tutschek; diagnosed in 1988 at age 55;
research communications director; New Jersey

WHEN I GROW UP

"I don't recommend getting breast cancer as a way of helping you decide what you want to be when you grow up, but for me, the diagnosis and subsequent mastectomy and chemotherapy were the wake-up call that helped convince me to abandon a grueling one-hour-each-way commute to a windowless office in Washington, D.C., for a job closer to home. I had always wanted to be a novelist, and as I faced my own mortality I thought, *if not now, when?* Eighteen years later, I am the author of three published novels (whose heroine is a breast cancer survivor), one collaborative novel (with twelve other women), and a slew of short stories."

Marcia Talley; diagnosed in 1983 at age 39;
mystery novelist; Maryland

"Getting my diagnosis in 1992 gave me the courage to pursue my lifelong dream of becoming a nurse. I felt that if I could beat cancer, I could do this. Going back to school at the age of thirty-nine was great for my self-esteem. I found that I was able to talk to the younger women about the importance of self-exam. I calmed their fears. They told me that I was an inspiration to them and their mothers, because I had a zest for life. Well, I'd been able to get rid of all the negative things in my life. For me, life truly began after breast cancer."

Deborah Parker; diagnosed in 1991 at age 34;
registered nurse; Tennessee

"After I was diagnosed with breast cancer, my realization that I was not, after all, immortal led me to focus on what I have long believed is the one thing that I have a responsibility for improving: public education. That was more than eight years ago, and I am still doing everything in my power to see that public education in general, and the teaching of reading and writing in particular, improves."

Annelle Houk; diagnosed in 1988 at age 59;
writer, editor; North Carolina

"I took a course offered by the hospital that pointed out the importance of a positive outlook. This was not an easy course, because it talked about giving yourself time for things like meditation and paying attention to your own needs. It didn't tell you how to start doing this after spending forty-seven years without. Around this same time, I was told of a woman psychotherapist who specialized in treating cancer patients. I went on to have many sessions with her, concentrating on cleaning out my psyche of old hurts and grievances. Then I radically changed my life. Among other things, I moved to New York for an academic year, going back to the art I enjoyed when I was younger. During this time, I learned to see myself separately from my family, and, as a result, could cope much better with everything. The best part is that I am now an emerging artist."

Carol Pasternak; diagnosed in 1986 at age 47;
artist; Ontario, Canada

"What have I done in between chemo and radiation? I started oil painting again after fifteen years. And I started an afghan. I hadn't made one in years. The one thing I'm really proud of is that I'm going to open my own business in two months. I saw a great need for a wig store in this area. Having had cancer, I understand the importance of looking good as you go through treatment. Everything has fallen into place for the store, which tells me this was meant to be. The landlord of the space is supporting me all the way. We have lots of renovating to do, but my boyfriend is a jack-of-all-trades, and the few people who know of my plan have volunteered to help! Who could ask for more?"

Sharon Daniels; diagnosed in 2000 at age 49;
hairstylist, wig store owner; Massachusetts

LONGEVITY

"At age thirty-four, I thought I was too young for cancer. But I wasn't. I had an eight-year-old daughter and a budding career and no time for something like this. The hardest part was the seven months of chemo. I figured that if I could survive the cure, I'd be fine. I'm proud to be approaching my twentieth anniversary, and am a huge proponent of self-exams and regular checkups. Women owe it to themselves to do this!"

Marti Devich; diagnosed in 1980 at age 34;
sales, business owner, writer; Minnesota

"When my radiation ended, I bought a five-year-calendar. I am proud to report that the pages of that calendar are now only a month shy of being full of five wonderful years. I just bought another one!"

Suzanne Pollock; diagnosed in 1995 at age 50;
stationer; North Carolina

"Seven years cancer-free is marvelous!"

Alyce Feinstein; diagnosed in 1993 at age 58;
administrative assistant; Massachusetts

"My husband was quite ill when I was diagnosed with breast cancer. I was only home from the hospital for a few days when he
died, and I had to face the anguish of that. After my incision
healed, I had thirty-eight days of radiation, and every day I would
take off alone to go eight miles away for the treatment. It helped
that after each one I would go to lunch, shopping, or to a movie.
I will be eighty-six on my next birthday and have just moved into
a beautiful retirement home. They take wonderful care of me
here. What a life. God has been good to me."

Dorothy A. Wilson; diagnosed in 1995 at age 80;
retired; Florida

"My mother was a long-time survivor who lived to see her *grandchildren* graduate from school, get married, and have children of
their own."

Betty Pollom;
daughter of Frances Davis; California

"It's okay to be afraid. Watch your own body and mind, and react
with your doctors if you don't feel that something is right. Don't
be afraid to advocate for yourself—but don't worry. After a few
years, you won't think every headache is a brain tumor, and
breast cancer will *not* be the first thing you think of when you
wake up in the morning."

Eleanor Anbinder; diagnosed in 1991 at age 50;
sales manager; Massachusetts

"I was given the best piece of advice by my oncologist when I
raced in, terrified because I'd found a tiny lump on my leg. 'Yep,
it's a lump,' he said. 'You're going to get lots of lumps and

bumps, and you're entitled.' I think every cancer survivor feels a panic over every ache, pain, lump, or bump for quite a while. Don't be foolish; get them checked if they hang around. But these are no more likely to be cancer than they were before you had your mastectomy."

Lynne Rutenberg; diagnosed in 1980 at age 35;
retired teacher; New Jersey

"Aches and pains are a problem. So is growing older. I mean, I'm only fifty-five, but my body doesn't recover from bruises and sprains as quickly as it did when I was twenty. Add to that the fact that I'm now into working out and 'power' walks, and you have muscle sprains and aches that last a while. When to worry? I asked my doctor about this. She said she would be glad to check out anything that gave me pause, if it would put my mind at ease. She also said that as each year passed, I would become more comfortable with those aches and pains. She's been right on both counts."

Barbara Delinsky; diagnosed in 1994 at age 49;
writer; Massachusetts

"When I returned home from the hospital, it was July. The flowers were blooming profusely, the grass was pretty and green, the sun was shining bright, and I marveled at the beauty of God's earth, which I had not appreciated like this before. That was forty-six years ago. I have lived to see my grandchildren and great-grandchildren. Some of the happiest days of my life have been since then."

Willie Mae Ashley; diagnosed in 1954 at age 37;
writer, retired saleslady; Tennessee

"My mother had a radical mastectomy during the 1930s. She also had to go the radiation route. Her body was scarred, but she had no recurrence. She lived to be ninety-one!"

Alice Bruneau;
daughter of a survivor; Florida

"It has been more than eight years since my mastectomy. In that time, my cancer has been transformed from a 'C' to a 'c.' After thinking I'd been given a death sentence, my stubbornness and determination took over. What had been fear and rage now became 'get out of my way; I have work to do.' I was determined to continue teaching, finish my master's degree in special education, and get back on the tennis courts as soon as possible. But if we want to talk of fearless survivors, I have to talk about the special kids with whom I've worked over the past thirteen years. These are kids unable to attend school because of physical and/or emotional problems. My job is to go to their homes every day for one to two hours of instruction. There have been kids with broken legs and some who suffer emotionally. Some are stricken with AIDS, sickle cell anemia, or cancer. As I struggled to keep working through my treatments, these kids kept me going, telling me to eat well, to get lots of rest, and do all the things that make me smile. They would call my home on treatment days to tell my partner what side effects might occur and how to deal with them. As the years have passed, my concerns have slowly but surely disappeared. With each year, my level of physical and emotional well-being has become stronger and stronger. It's okay that my body is shaped like a pear. I am comfortable with myself. After all, I am here. I am a survivor."

Carol Snyder; diagnosed in 1992 at age 47;
special education teacher; New York

"My friend Ruth and her husband Marshall were part of our poker group for nearly forty years. When Marshall was diagnosed with lymphoma, Ruthie spent that entire time with him, sharing a semiprivate room. She went home only to bathe, feed the cat, and check the mail. Then, one month after Marshall died, after being his bulwark for nearly five years, Ruthie was diagnosed with breast cancer. Who would be her support? We always teased the Pollacks about the number of children they had—three girls and two boys—a 'full house.' Ruthie tells us that her great 'hand' and

their spouses saw her through her mastectomy and reconstruction. Fifteen years have passed since then. Ruthie has travelled to
all the states that she missed with Marshall, plus many foreign
countries. Beyond her travels, she is particularly proud of completing the fifty-five mile walk from Santa Barbara to Malibu in
1999—the Avon Breast Cancer Awareness Walk—during which
she turned sixty-five. What a way to celebrate a birthday, and what
a woman! She is a role model for us all!"

Rae Shapiro;
friend of Ruth Pollack; California

"The mantra I was given to repeat daily: 'Anything less than growing old is simply not acceptable.' "

Betsy Ellis Bowles; diagnosed in 2000 at age 57;
private mortgage banker; Massachusetts

THE BEST THING ABOUT HAVING BREAST CANCER

"Breast cancer, like any other illness, is one of life's teachers.
What do we take away from it? That depends on each of us. We
can't change our situation, but we can make the most of it. We
can take time to slow down and really care for ourselves, something that is often hard for women to do. We can also become
more compassionate about the suffering of others, and there are
plenty with worse problems and challenges than ours. We can become more spiritual, more physically healthy, more focused on
what is really important in our lives. We can be more thankful for
the love that surrounds us."

Deb Haney; diagnosed in 1996 at age 48;
administrative assistant, artist; Massachusetts

"For me, breast cancer was a wake-up call. I worry less about things
I have no control over, and focus on what is important to me."

Debby Whittet; diagnosed in 1996 at age 43;
household technician, part-time library worker; Michigan

"Breast cancer has changed my life in a way that is almost hard to describe. There is no room for negativity in my life now. Everything and everyone are more special to me than ever. I try every day to recognize my wealth of good family, good friends, and good attitude."

Jennifer Wersal; diagnosed in 2000 at age 30;
marketing; Texas

"I wouldn't wish breast cancer on my worst enemy, but for me, it was one of the best experiences of my life. It gently moved me along on my spiritual journey and made me stop and rethink priorities."

Sandy Williams; diagnosed in 1999 at age 51;
children's public services librarian; Texas

"I have heard some women say that they were glad for their cancer diagnoses. I wouldn't go that far, but it did make me take stock of my life and decide what was important and what was not. Although I have always been a Christian, I am more spiritual now and, I think, a much better person. My husband, Jay, and I always talked about buying a big truck and hitting the road when our kids were old enough. We did that the year after my diagnosis. It has been a great experience. We have been in almost all of the states and have enjoyed every minute of it."

Rebecca Clarkson; diagnosed in 1997 at age 45;
trucking; Utah

"In less than two years, I experienced breast cancer through my two best friends. It changed all of our lives, because we realized that the silly things in life that we took so seriously before weren't so important after all. The words of the old expression 'When you have your health, you have everything' are the truest words ever written."

Grace Trocco;
friend of two survivors; New York

"My best friend was diagnosed nearly two years ago, and what a frightening thing it was! She had two young children who really needed her, along with her family and friends. We fought together, laughed together, and cried together—and she is wonderful today! No more wigs, no more chemotherapy; she is clean! What a joy! It makes all of us appreciate life and love so very much!"

Pat West;
friend of a survivor; Indiana

"I see the world differently now. I don't take life so seriously. Since being diagnosed, I have traveled to all the places I wanted to see. I'm more spontaneous. I lost my beautiful blonde curly hair and every single hair on my body, but that meant I didn't have to shave or shampoo my hair. It meant that I had a low-maintenance body and could be ready to go anywhere in seconds, instead of hours. I was proud to be bald, because I was alive. I'm not afraid or embarrassed to tell people I love them. I am living with a vengeance."

Cindy Bird; diagnosed in 1998 at age 39;
human resources generalist; Colorado

"This has been a tough battle, but it's also been one of the most wonderful journeys I've ever taken. I've met the most remarkable people. I've learned that the human spirit is truly alive and well. I can honestly say that I do not regret having breast cancer."

Val Long; diagnosed in 1999 at age 47;
administrative assistant; Massachusetts

"Since having breast cancer, I am less afraid in some ways and more in others. I now ride on roller coasters and helicopters, and take physical risks more often, and I feel great about having done them. I am, however, much more neurotic about every little bump, lump, or pain."

Suzanne Pollock; diagnosed in 1995 at age 50;
stationer; North Carolina

"Going through breast cancer is no piece of cake, but the benefits are endless. I believe that fear is the single most deadly emotion I had to deal with."

Alyce Feinstein; diagnosed in 1993 at age 58;
administrative assistant; Massachusetts

"Only positive things have come out of my having breast cancer. I have learned to enjoy the smallest of life's pleasures. I have learned that nothing is a crisis unless it is fatal. I have learned not to complain about getting up in the morning. My circle of friends has become larger than life—all kinds of friends, all very important to me. I've learned to take time each day to be thankful for what I have, not what I want. I remember that God only gives me what I can handle."

Jacki Anthony; diagnosed in 1998 at age 48;
nurse; Massachusetts

"I learned to let family and friends take care of me. My husband went with me to the first chemo treatment, but after that a different friend accompanied me each time. Friends cleaned my house, brought food, took me shopping, and sent me books. My children 'created' a tee-shirt with all their names on it—including a two-year-old handprint and a grand-dog pawprint. Another thing I learned? To let people pray with me and for me. These gestures of love, friendship, and faith generate a wonderful sense of well-being."

Faye Hardiman; diagnosed in 1998 at age 50;
wife, mother, teacher; Georgia

"Perhaps the most significant outcome of my battle with breast cancer is that I have changed my outlook on life. I now regard life as precious and try not to focus on negative things. Eliminating stress and resentment from my life and concentrating on the positive things has become my goal. I am now more at peace with myself."

Sandy Mark; diagnosed in 1998 at age 55;

administrative assistant; Connecticut

"Breast cancer has taught me to accept what I cannot change, to listen with an open heart, and to love myself. It has taught me to look at small wonders; to appreciate sunshine, rain, and wind; and to value the love of family and friends. I have a wonderful sister, and our time together is precious to me. At a special time of day, we each light a candle and think of each other."

Nan Comstock; diagnosed in 1988 at age 39;

self-employed; California

"Cancer has changed me more than it has changed my life. I have always laughed a lot, and I continue to do so. But my soul is deeper and wiser, and I can see the small stuff from the rest. I don't save my china for a special day. Every day is special!"

Dot Heimer; diagnosed in 1999 at age 56;

certified dental assistant; Missouri

"It seems weird to say that breast cancer could in any way improve my life, but it has. I am halfway through chemo, and it is rough. But I have found that I am the one who has taken my marriage, family, and life for granted. My husband is two hundred percent there for me, and I have found so many wonderful qualities in him that I never would have known if it were not for this disease. It's too bad that it took something like this to make me realize what a good life I have."

Lori Bartz; diagnosed in 2000 at age 41;

customer service representative; Wisconsin

"The best thing about breast cancer? I am truly happier now than I was before the diagnosis. Slight fear of recurrence is my friendly reminder to live fully. After every doctor's visit, I celebrate. We have a special dinner, and I dance around, knowing that I'm healthy. It more than makes up for the nervousness I feel before each visit. More than most people, who have check-ups less often, we get the 'good news' of good health every few months. I feel a lightness of being incomparable to anything I felt before cancer."

Sharon Carr; diagnosed in 1997 at age 42; hospice grief counselor; Rhode Island

"I was diagnosed in March and operated on in April. Chemo began in June and ended in August. They were six months that totally changed my life and that of my family, but given the option, we would do it all again! Why? I found out that my husband loves me for who I am, not for my breasts. My family was drawn closer together and even closer to God. We do not take any day for granted. And best of all, we've had the opportunity to encourage others in the same situation."

Patti Dempster; diagnosed in 1998 at age 45; homemaker, wife, mother; California

"Looking back over my experience, I realize how much I have gained. Having breast cancer was an opportunity to live my life to the fullest. This is not to say that I was dancing with joy when I heard the diagnosis. But you can learn that you are stronger than you thought. You just face it and let it flow over you. It does not define who you are. It is something that comes along just like anything else, and you decide how to live through it. We don't get to choose when we are born or when we die, but we can choose to be happy and fully present in the time between the two."

Adelaide D. Key; diagnosed in 1978 at age 42; community volunteer, philanthropist; North Carolina

"I learned that I am my own best friend, and that the inner me is stronger and braver than I'd ever thought possible. I learned to feel comfortable saying 'yes' when someone offered to run an errand or cook dinner. I learned to take naps in the middle of the day—first by setting the kitchen timer for ten minutes and making myself close my eyes until it buzzed. I learned that my two dearest friends know what to say and when to say it. I learned how important it could be to receive a telephone call or greeting card. I learned that it's really okay to cry, even in public. I learned how to leave a little present for myself on the seat of the car so it would be waiting for me after each chemotherapy session. I learned how to leave my spirit outside the door of the treatment room so that the chemo would hurt only the ghost I took in with me. Now I'm the one devoting herself to the Race for the Cure. Now I'm the one sharing my belief that a person who *used* to have cancer was wheeled out of the operating room and that the person in the recovery room is already a survivor. Now I'm the one offering to 'show,' to lend an ear and give encouragement."

Kathi Ward; diagnosed in 1994 at age 47;

merchandiser; South Carolina

"How can cancer make life better? The answers are still coming, four years after my diagnosis. You learn to see that each person who enters your life is a potential gift, and that you are buoyed by a web of beautiful souls. You learn to discard old acquaintances and unsupportive friendships, to weed out those relationships that 'don't work.' You learn to make space in a busy workday for moments of appreciation, beauty, and love. You learn to make choices that feed rather than drain you. You learn to take care of yourself, to take naps, eat good food, drink water, go to bed early. You learn to pamper yourself—to read only books you like, take walks, go out in nature more often, get massages and healing treatments. You take time for art, for tea with friends, for crafts, reading, or whatever it is that nurtures you and heals."

Deborah Pierce; diagnosed in 1997 at age 48;

architect; Massachusetts

"I'm tremendously grateful for all I learned from breast cancer. Yet, the journey for me is not best expressed by the term 'survivor.' I'd rather call myself a 'breast cancer emerger,' because I emerged from it a different person. I didn't just survive. I became someone new and better. I became a person who believes in the power of hope, and who understands the importance of opening her heart and inviting love to come in."

Holly Marion; diagnosed in 1996 at age 49;
fundraiser; North Carolina

17 • Fast Forward

Five Years Later

'll spare you the banalities about time flying when you're having fun, and simply say that I was stunned to realize, in the fall of 2005, that it had been five years since I first sought out the advice of breast cancer survivors for this book. Where were those *UP-LIFT*ers now? What were they doing with their lives? I really wanted to know, and I figured that if I wanted to know, you all would want to know, too.

So I asked, and it was a delight reading the material that poured in. My only problem was cutting it down to the thirty pages that my publisher allotted me. Rather than the snippets of advice that comprise so much of the rest of *UPLIFT*, here we have little stories. There are stories of fears that never materialized, careers changed for the better, new adventures dared—and they are written with such heart that it broke *mine* not to be able to include every word. I've done my best to capture the feeling, and sincerely apologize for paragraphs that had to be left on the cutting-room floor.

And what about me? What have I done in the last five years? I've written five more novels, for one thing. For another, I've had a second nonfiction collection published, this one a Q&A about lobsters and lobstering called *Does a Lobsterman Wear Pants?* With the entirety of my proceeds from *Lobsterpants* (as my publisher and I fondly call it), like those from *UPLIFT,* going to research, we come to a third thing I've done since *UPLIFT* was first published. I've funded a fellowship at Massachusetts General Hospital. In its third year now, the fellowship gives a surgical oncologist an additional year of training focused on innovative breast cancer treatments and research. The fellowship is a springboard for now three doctors to spend the next thirty years doing research. I'd call that money well spent.

Oh, and one more thing. Last December, I marked the tenth anniversary of my mastectomy. Actually, I hadn't been keeping track. When my doctor pointed it out, I was stunned!

Ten years is an amazing milestone. But then, so is five years—and twelve and a half—and fourteen—and twenty-four—all of which are marked by various women in this chapter. Moreover, keep in mind that by the time this book hits the stands, another year will have passed since these newest *UPLIFT*ers wrote to me. So add a year. And smile. We're all alive. World, watch out!

HOW LUCKY WE ARE

"Thirteen is supposed to be an unlucky number, but I consider it a lucky one for me. It's been over thirteen years since my diagnosis of Stage III breast cancer. I thought my number was up then. My only child had just turned three, and I remember thinking, 'Who is going to raise her if I'm gone?' My mother had died of breast cancer in 1983, and my husband, well, I just couldn't see him parenting a small toddler by himself. As I began my battle with breast cancer, I started thinking, 'Hey, I'm going to be the one to raise my daughter. I'm going to take her to her first day of school. I'm going to help her choose her first prom dress.' And guess what? I have.

"I am also lucky enough to be working with one of the largest breast cancer studies in the nation, the Sister Study. I am helping recruit fifty thousand women from all over the country to be in the study. These women have not been diagnosed with breast cancer but have a sister who has. The study is looking at environmental factors along with genetic factors."

Cat Andrews; diagnosed in 1992 at age 42; recruitment coordinator for Sister Study breast cancer research; North Carolina

"Who would have thought I would be here writing to you after being a cancer survivor all these years? My diagnosis wasn't 'hearts and flowers'—not at all. It was bittersweet. After hitting rock bottom, I slowly began to climb up the ladder and fight this deadly disease. And guess what? I'm still here. It's been twelve and a half years now, and in that time my husband and I have celebrated two weddings and three grandchildren!

"Life has been very good to me. I'm feeling well and have a wonderful life. My husband and I retired two years ago, and our days are filled with exercise, fun, and relaxation with wonderful people we've met. However, I never forget the 'old days' and try to help as many as I can who are going through that difficult time in their lives."

Alyce Feinstein; diagnosed in 1993 at age 58; retired real estate administrative assistant; Florida

"Here I am celebrating fifty-eight years of age and a proud fourteen years as a survivor of breast cancer. It's been a long haul, but I have made it and loved every minute. I have met so many beautiful people and done things that I might not have done if I hadn't had cancer. In 1998, I got my picture taken with Olivia Newton-John at the Race for the Cure in Michigan, and another one with Lynda Carter—Wonder Woman! Then came the book *UPLIFT*, and now I'm in print. Life is good!"

Mary Ann Budnick; diagnosed in 1991 at age 44;
retired school bus driver; Florida

"It was September of 1995, and I should have had my mammogram seven months earlier, but kept putting it off. Well, thank goodness for that mammogram. It saved my life! I am a nine-year survivor now and every year I walk the 3K in the Race for the Cure. It just makes me feel good to do that. Having breast cancer was the most frightening thing I have ever experienced in my life. But I feel great now. It's amazing how surviving this changes your life. You look at life differently—you don't let the petty things bother you. I am just so happy and grateful that I am a *survivor*!"

Carol Contrino; diagnosed in 1995 at age 44;
circulation assistant at public library; Texas

"After trying on bathing suits in the spring of 1992, I decided to have a breast reduction. I was forty-four, married for twenty-three years to a wonderful man, with a daughter in ninth grade and a son in second grade. Not quite two weeks after the surgery, my doctor told me that cancer had been found in the tissue he had removed. I will never forget that moment—the reduction mammoplasty saved my life! There was no history of breast cancer in my family.

"After my diagnosis, I did what I do best. I educated my family, my friends, my colleagues and students at Plainfield High School, where I have taught for thirty-six years. I presented a program about breast cancer at local service organizations, and hosted an information table at my church. I have also coordinated an annual Rally for a Cure. This year, we raised a total of $90,191. My illness thirteen years ago changed me profoundly. It made me think about who and what is really important."

Tiffany Corbett; diagnosed in 1992 at age 44;
high school teacher; New Jersey

"I have been cancer-free for ten years. I feel very lucky. My grand-daughter was five months old when I was diagnosed, and is now a beauty at eleven.

"I received *UPLIFT* on my sixty-fifth birthday, and realize that many of the ladies had a much more difficult time than I had. I chose not to have reconstruction and have never been sorry. I am grateful that we have a choice."

Virginia Danczak; diagnosed in 1995 at age 59;
communications; Nebraska

"I am happy to say that I am a five-year survivor. I look at my life a lot differently now. I am more outgoing and much happier, and am now helping other women who have breast cancer. I am so glad that I have been given a second chance in life."

Maryann Eberhard; diagnosed in 2000 at age 43;
school monitor; New York

"I found the lump in my right breast in January 2001, and decided to have a double mastectomy. I told my family, friends, and even my customers what was going on, and the emotional support I received was phenomenal. In March 2001, the surgery was done. I decided against reconstruction, because that wouldn't be me. I kid around about my flat chest and my zippers—my badge of courage!"

Bonnie Fergerson; diagnosed in 2001 at age 54;
sales/customer service representative; New Jersey

"I was devastated when I was told I had breast cancer. However, I now feel that it was a gift. I learned so much about myself and reprioritized my life to focus on what really mattered to me. I had been a workaholic and felt I had to be in control of everything around me. While in chemo and radiation, I didn't have the energy to be in control, and I just 'let go.' It was wonderful how my husband stepped up and did housework. I now enjoy my life much more, spending quality time with my kids and grandkids. I'm grateful for my doctors and all the women I've met who have inspired me and made me proud."

Donna Garrison; diagnosed in 1998 at age 56; notary public and package store associate; California

"I am so grateful to Barbara for writing *UPLIFT*. The stories touched my heart. It's seven years now since I had the shock of hearing the dreaded words 'breast cancer,' the discomfort after surgery, and the tough decisions to be made regarding treatment. I am now free of cancer and will continue to be."

Pat Mohr; diagnosed in 1998 at age 59; retired accounting technician; Manitoba, Canada

"I had problems with pain, and my left breast had started to become larger than the right one. I went to the doctor and was told that I was fine, that I didn't need a mammogram, that I was too young to have cancer, and that I should lose weight and come back in two years. When I continued to have problems, I went to another doctor. He sent me to a surgeon, and I did lose the breast.

"This was back in the '80s. I have lived twenty-four years more and have been able not only to see my children grow and get married, but to enjoy my three granddaughters. My advice to all is never to let a doctor pass up your feelings. If something has changed, and one doctor tells you nothing is wrong, get a second opinion."

Vicky Pakso; diagnosed in 1981 at age 37; housewife; New Jersey

"I am a cancer survivor. I was diagnosed in 1992, had a lumpectomy and radiation. I wake up each morning and thank God that I have been able to live and enjoy retirement with my husband, Jim. We were fortunate to celebrate our fiftieth anniversary last

December and took a wonderful cruise to Hawaii. I used to have mammograms every six months, but now have them only once a year. Each year I feel fortunate again."

Barbara Phelps; diagnosed in 1992 at age 58;
registered nurse; Illinois

"On September 20, 2005, I had my five-year check-up with the surgeon who performed my lumpectomies. His words to me were, 'I told you that you weren't going to die from this!' It's difficult to describe the many emotions I felt when he shook my hand and told me that I was released from his care. I was elated, but I also got choked up. He was an excellent surgeon and during the five years I saw him, I valued his opinion and trusted his judgment. This may sound crazy, but I will miss him and his staff."

Janet Whitaker; diagnosed in 1999 at age 41;
insurance agent; North Carolina

OPPORTUNITY KNOCKS

"Wow, I cannot believe it has been seven years. I could not be in better shape. I have lost twenty pounds, go to Curves three times a week, and work full time. I look and feel good. I have a wonderful life with a very supportive husband and daughter, and four super grandchildren. What more could I ask?"

Jacki Anthony; diagnosed in 1998 at age 48;
purchasing agent; Massachusetts

"Thirteen years cancer-free! When I was diagnosed with aggressive Stage II cancer, everything in my life seem to stop, including my running. I went through a year of chemotherapy, three months of radiation, three surgeries, and premature menopause. I put my running on the back burner for a while, secretly wondering if I would ever go back to it.

"Here I am, almost fifty-two years old, and my running has never been better. I am healthy and happy, and I know what is important in life. I am able to be more caring, compassionate, and understanding. I can love deeper and stronger because I know how precious life is."

Jacqueline Hickey; diagnosed in 1992 at age 39; special education administrative assistant; Massachusetts

"While I was at home recuperating from surgery, I wrote and received a grant to conduct a reading project for kindergarteners in my hometown. When people questioned my energy level, I responded that breast cancer was a condition of my breast, not my brain. I never say I had breast cancer. I say that I *encountered* breast cancer and beat the living daylights out of it.

"I was particularly proud of the tummy tuck that I received during reconstruction in 2002. I purchased a bathing suit that showed my flat stomach, and wore it while visiting Mexico that year. Two of my daughters got married in 2004, so that year was indeed hectic but joyful. I am now expecting my first grandchild."

Elise Bourne-Busby; diagnosed in 1999 at age 57; elementary school principal; New Jersey

"One beautiful bright sunny Mother's Day I was sitting in my daughter Lisa's yard when a butterfly flew onto my arm. It was the same side where my breast cancer was. I was in awe! I couldn't stop staring at its magnificent colors, its beauty, its gracefulness. I believed that this butterfly was a sign from God, telling me that I was going to get better. I was still going through my treatment at that time. The butterfly sat there for quite a while. Before it flew away, it went behind me, then flew back to the same arm, and then took off in flight.

"I now have a permanent picture of a butterfly on my leg, a tattoo created by my son Jason, who is a tattoo artist. I've just turned sixty, and this Mother's Day marks five years since that butterfly visited me. I'm very blessed. God has sent our family another grandson and two great-granddaughters. That makes me a grandmother of five boys and two girls."

Joann Connor; diagnosed in 2000 at age 55;
medical librarian; New Jersey

"Happy Anniversary to all of us! Proudly, this is my third *UPLIFT* entry. I was in the first two books, and those were two of my proudest accomplishments. I was initially diagnosed in August 2000. The following year it came back in the same breast, and I opted for a double mastectomy. I had immediate reconstruction, which was awesome. I wake up each day with gratitude and a sense of hope. I am determined to focus on the here and now, not the when and if. I've learned to take something good out of every situation."

Cathy Hanlon; diagnosed in 2000 at age 42;
volunteer; New York

"I have been in remission for over eighteen years. In that time, I have changed my profession from a quality control inspector for a company that did not care about the individual, to a certified nursing assistant, home health aid, and a Reiki master teacher. If it wasn't for breast cancer, I would not be where I am. I am now living in Florida, helping others, working as I need to and enjoying my life, family, and especially my year-old grandson."

Ellen Hurteau; diagnosed in 1987 at age 34;
certified nursing assistant, home health aid, Reiki master; Florida

"What a shock it was to hear that I had breast cancer! Of course, that first day, I felt that I would soon die and the tears were streaming down my cheeks on the way home from the surgeon's office. I thought of my two little grandsons who were in kindergarten, and wondered if I would see them grow up. My husband

had retired just three weeks before, and the plan was that I would
continue working at home as a medical transcriptionist, but I
wondered what would happen now. There were so many un-
knowns, so many fears. Little did I know how my life would
change, and for the *better*.

"Shortly after my surgery, I joined a breast cancer support
group called Friends in Touch Care Team. Not only did I find
support, but I met other survivors who were newly diagnosed. A
year later, I was asked to be a member of the management team
and am doing that to this day. I absolutely love it! I celebrate with
joy my fifth year of survivorship on Valentine's Day 2006."

Karen Lange; diagnosed in 2001 at age 56;
medical transcriptionist; Michigan

"It's been five years, nine months for me, but who's counting! I
still think about my cancer, but less and less. I dwell on the positive and live each day knowing I've conquered it. I recently read a
sign that said 'A positive attitude may not solve all your problems,
but it will annoy enough people to make it worth your effort.' I
loved it. Keep smiling, and that too makes people wonder what
you've been up to!

"I'm exercising more now. I really found out how good it was
after my surgery and got into a program for cancer survivors. I
only wished I had started earlier in life. Now, I faithfully visit the
Y to start off my day."

Judy Peterson; diagnosed in 2000 at age 58;
nurse; Colorado

"When I was diagnosed, I didn't really think, 'Why me?' because
so many women are diagnosed. But I did wonder, 'What for?' I
thought there must be a reason, and while feverishly working
through the whole process, including radiation, as if each day
was just like any other, I realized somehow I had to find time to
better care for myself.

"I started a diet—no fads, no organizations, just sensible eating, which I always knew was appropriate. I began to exercise, finally colored the gray from my hair, and began a transformation. Today, I am a size 8 (from a hefty size 18), work with a personal trainer, eat healthy every day, and look better than ever. I hope everyone can find the 'what for?' for them."

Arlene Petty; diagnosed in 1999 at age 49;
president of insurance brokerage; New Jersey

"Wow, six years out. I have a party every spring to celebrate another year of being cancer-free. I invite a lot of friends, and we just have a blast. Friends are so important to me now.

"I make it a point now to relax more. I tend to let the housework go at times and just appreciate kicking back. We finally bought our dream home two years ago, and I just love coming home. I tend to spend a lot of time just sitting on the porch swing listening to nature. Don't get me wrong—I am still anal about having a clean, organized house. But I have come to realize that tomorrow is another day, and cleaning can wait if I want it to."

Kathy Rabassa; diagnosed in 1999 at age 34;
administrative assistant; South Carolina

"I am writing about my very dear friend Bev, who has been a survivor for five years. She was so brave going through every stage of her treatment. It was like she had the flu or something. She would always be the one to laugh and uplift her friends. She is so healthy today, and someone you always want to be like. She is still working with us and always comes into work smiling and ready to do whatever needs to be done. I have learned so much from her."

Valerie Swett; friend of woman diagnosed in 2001 at age 65;
retail; Maine

FAMILY JOY

"Every day is a gift, isn't it? I have had the joy of attending my son's wedding and seeing the miracle of my new granddaughter, born to my daughter. I have been able to help my mother, a survivor for even more years than me, through the loss of my dad and into her aging. Much as I cringe at how high the number is getting when I have a birthday, I'm just celebrating the fact that I *am* having another birthday. I'm amazed at how many I know who've gone through this as well. There's hope, gratitude, and joy at having come this far."

Janice Austad; diagnosed in 1998 at age 50;

IT manager; Minnesota

"After my mastectomy, breast reconstruction, and chemo, I decided that the worst was over. I looked normal with my wig, and shortly thereafter my hair grew in. I never looked back, and my life went on as though there had been no interruption. For this, I thank my husband, my three sons, and my wonderful friends."

Ruth Berler; diagnosed in 1996 at age 76;

retired teacher; Connecticut

"At the time of my diagnosis, my daughter was nine years old. My hope was to be able to live and raise her. Today my daughter is twenty-six; I have been privileged to see her marry and give me three wonderful grandchildren. I feel very fortunate to be a survivor of seventeen years."

Debra Gainey; diagnosed in 1988 at age 36;

office manager for large manufacturing corporation; Missouri

"I had a choice of just losing one breast, but I chose to lose both. I knew I didn't need either to define who I was. I was a mom, friend, lover, aunt, grandma and great-grandma, and the man I loved, loved me just as I was. What is really funny is I have eight great-granddaughters and one great-grandson, and guess who can always put them to sleep when no one else can? Mamaw (that's me). So, ladies, there is so much more to you than your breasts. So much more of love to give and receive. You can change someone's life, bring laughter and happiness to them."

Nancy Brown; diagnosed in 1995 at age 57;

computer operator; Ohio

"My experience with breast cancer was not a negative one. I came through it with a new perspective on life. I realized what is most important to me—the unconditional love of my family. I have lived to see my son graduate from college, start his own company, and get his pilot's license. I have seen my daughter get married. She has given me two beautiful grandsons, now ages eight and six. They are the loves of my life. They laugh at so many things, and have taught me to do the same.

"My significant other and I have a terrific relationship. When I was going through chemo, all he wanted to do was feed me. As most of you know, that was the last thing I wanted. But his thought was so generous and kind."

Carol Fischer; diagnosed in 1993 at age 48;

retired; Maryland

"I hit my five-year mark on April 2, 2006 and now have thirty-month-old twin grandsons, who are the joy of my life."

Bruni Levine; diagnosed in 2001 at age 49;

customer service; Connecticut

"It was May when I was diagnosed, and I was pregnant with my daughter Eve. Every year, Mother's Day has special significance for me—another year of health and happiness.

"I have turned my experience into positive energy. Never one to sit back and dwell on the negative, I am active in the American Cancer Society's Relay for Life and Making Strides walks, and the Komen Foundation. Words cannot express the emotion I feel when I see so many women come together, united for a cause. Even more rewarding—and significant—is that as I walk the three miles, my daughter is by my side."

Renee C. Johannesen; diagnosed in 1993 at age 35; manager, marketing communications; New York

"It has been twelve years since I was given the news that would change my life forever. A mastectomy, chemotherapy, and lots of support from my friends later, I am here to tell you, each day is sweet. I have seen grandchildren added to our family, have been able to support my parents and in-laws in their old age, and also helped my husband start his own business. I thought my life was over, and just look at what I have experienced!"

Suzanne Mann; diagnosed in 1993 at age 49; retired registered nurse; South Carolina

"I have been cancer-free for five years. After first being diagnosed I found out that I would be a grandma. Now I have a four-year-old granddaughter, a two-year-old grandson, and a one-year-old granddaughter. Nothing could be sweeter than having these precious babies around to laugh and fill my home with joy and love."

Midge Mohler; diagnosed in 2001 at age 54; seamstress; Minnesota

"It has been five years since I was diagnosed, and I often wonder how I got through those eight months of treatment without falling apart. Somehow I did, with the love and support of my husband, son, and many friends. I know that this will sound funny, but I am sure you have heard it before. Breast cancer changed my outlook on life. It provided me with a greater appreciation of what is important and what is not worth getting stressed about.

"When I was diagnosed, my son was sixteen. All I could think about was whether I would be there when he graduated high school. Well, I saw him graduate in 2002. He has attended Emerson College since then, and I am looking forward to his graduation in May."

Roz Rowley; diagnosed in 2000 at age 54;
teacher of the visually impaired; Massachusetts

"I was diagnosed in February 1996, at the age of thirty-six. I was married and the mother of a fourteen-year-old son and twelve-year-old daughter, and had no family history of the disease. My first emotion was complete fear that I would not see my children grow up, graduate from high school, go away to college, get married, or have children of their own.

"My son graduated from college in 2003 and got married in 2004. My daughter is a senior in college. A cancer diagnosis is not a death sentence. You can survive!"

Cindy Sloan; diagnosed in 1996 at age 36;
claims analyst; South Carolina

"There isn't a day that goes by that I don't think about having had breast cancer. It was just eight years ago that I had my mastectomy.

"I have been teaching preschool for seven years now and love it. I feel great. I think it's because I have a wonderful husband and children who truly love me. My kids are getting older; Josh is finishing college, and Traci is sixteen. They were so young when I was diagnosed and really didn't understand what was happening. Traci now joins my husband and me on breast cancer walks and seems to be learning what the fight is all about."

Tobi Stelzer; diagnosed in 1997 at age 40;
preschool teacher; New Jersey

EVEN BETTER TO GIVE

"I am a twenty-four-year breast cancer survivor and share my experience with many through my volunteer work with the American Cancer Society. I take part in two annual walks each year and, next month, I will participate in a twenty-four-hour Relay for Life. I am very lucky to have my adult children take part in these events also. This past summer I attended my forty-fifth class reunion. How very proud and happy I was to be there!"

Rosemary Bentley; diagnosed in 1981 at age 39;
accountant; California

"As a fifteen-year breast cancer survivor, I encourage newly diagnosed women to seek support from other survivors. A couple of days after my bilateral mastectomy, I was visited by a Reach to Recovery volunteer from the American Cancer Society. Her visit had such a positive impact on me that a year later I also became a Reach to Recovery volunteer. I visited newly diagnosed breast cancer patients in their homes and the most common remark from them was, "You don't look sick." I told them that I was never sick and neither are they, that they have just experienced a temporary setback and that they would bounce back. One of the older women that I had visited through Reach to Recovery told me that I gave her such hope that she called me every Christmas for the next ten years. She has since passed away—from heart problems, not breast cancer—and I miss her calls."

Billie Bules; diagnosed in 1990 at age 54;
homemaker, retired sales manager; Arizona

"Breast cancer was a blessing in disguise. I have learned so much about myself, my beliefs, and my faith. I became a Reach to Recovery volunteer. All the people I have met have given me strength in so many different areas.

"My children are now grown, and I have a beautiful granddaughter who is almost one year old. I hope and pray for a cure for cancer, so that my baby and now her baby can continue to shine in this world."

Linda Jones Burns; diagnosed in 2000 at age 40;
secretary; New Hampshire

"I find it hard to believe that five years have passed since *UPLIFT* debuted. Life goes on. I would not have survived without the help and support of my wonderful husband and some really great friends who sat with him while I underwent surgery. He always says he is not nervous, but I know the truth. He has shown enormous courage. It is very hard on caregivers to worry and wait.

"I have been blessed with terrific doctors who call me a role model and an inspiration. I love that label because I work hard at getting up and out to help others newly diagnosed through an organization called Cancer Hope Network. Cancer does keep us strong."

Susan Clemente; diagnosed in 1990 at age 46;
retired registered nurse; New York

"Six years and counting. . . . Wanting to give something back, I heard about an 'Angel Network' of men, women, and kids jumping in to help an individual or family in crisis. I started the 'Sudbury Angel Network' just five months ago, and we have fifty-six volunteers. Angels do live among us!"

Susan Grayson-Johnson; diagnosed in 1998 at age 50;
retired; Massachusetts

"I was diagnosed with DCIS in my left breast when I was fifty-three. I decided on a mastectomy with immediate breast reconstruction. I recovered and returned to my job as an administrative assistant, and soon realized it was time to make a change. My co-workers' priorities were not mine. They were

working for selfish reasons. My husband came out of his early retirement and found a supplemental job, so that I could quit
mine.

"Early the next year, breast cancer was found in my right
breast. I decided to have the same surgery with the same doctors.
I recovered quickly and, grateful for my now-good health, I
reached out to other survivors through Reach to Recovery, Susan
Komen Breast Cancer Foundation, and Carol Baldwin's Breast
Cancer Research Foundation. Yes, I am very thankful for five
years of good health. Breast cancer has made my life richer. I
have met many wonderful people and am proud to have made a
difference in their lives. I keep busy working on fund-raisers and
collecting donations for various breast cancer walks. I have a
seven-year-old granddaughter and until there is a cure for breast
cancer, I can't do enough."

Judy Hooper; diagnosed in 2000 at age 53;

administrative assistant; New York

"I am Marie, and I live in Reston, VA. In 1999, I had a surgical
biopsy which showed cancer that had not shown up on X-rays
and mammograms. Prior to my mastectomy, I went online to a
good breast cancer chat room—BCANS, out of Nova Scotia—
and learned much there. Post-surgery, I was able to help many
women and their men and families, also, through this chat room,
and that was very satisfying.

"With breast cancer, especially, women have two choices: either
to tell others about their situation or to tough it out privately. I
chose to tell and give out information as I learned it along the
way. I had to get used to everyone looking at my chest when they
first spoke to me post-surgery, which was a hoot! As time went by
they treated me normally again. I am fine now, six and a half
years after surgery."

Marie Johnson; diagnosed in 1999 at age 56;

retired—now a quilter; Virginia

"When I was diagnosed with breast cancer, I was serving as the President of the Pennsylvania Business and Professional Women's Organization, with more than three thousand members. During this time I had to provide articles for our mailings and magazine. I always included something about what was happening with my treatment, and these articles proved to be my forum and therapy. The support I received from the members of the organization helped me more than you can imagine!

"I am pleased to tell you that I will be serving as the chair of the 2006 Komen NEPA Race for the Cure. By doing this, I hope to make a difference and pray that my nieces (and nephews) will not have to worry about this disease when they get older."

Annmarie Kiehart; diagnosed in 2000 at age 43;
production coordinator; Pennsylvania

"After a routine mammogram, I had a follow-up biopsy that confirmed I had breast cancer. Everything went well after the lumpectomy. I was able to return to my teaching position, though I was still receiving radiation treatments. At a friend's insistence, I became a member of R.I.S.E. (Reaching and Inspiring Survivors Everywhere), a newly formed support group in my community. I am enjoying each day to the fullest!"

Barbara Mulvey; diagnosed in 2000 at age 50;
retired teacher; New York

"Cancer is a scary diagnosis. Back when I was diagnosed with breast cancer, I wished there had been more people giving me the thumbs-up and reassuring me that cancer is not a death sentence. As a fourteen-year survivor now, I advise others to have a positive attitude, a bit of faith, and the determination to help others. This gives you a reason to hope and persevere.

"Just a few years ago, I found the website called ChemoAngels. Here, they assign you a patient, and it is up to you to send cheery cards and/or small gifts to your assignee. The astounding thing is that complete strangers are helping sick people at a most vulnerable stage in their lives. I thank God for having found a way I can give back something to others facing cancer. Through adversity, I think I have found my purpose in life."

Dorothy Padilla; diagnosed in 1991 at age 39;
homemaker/mother; Connecticut

"I am a thirteen-year survivor! Probably what I have appreciated most are all the wonderful friendships that developed because of my diagnosis. It's amazing how many people have been touched by breast cancer in one way or another.

"Over the years, the fear diminishes. I have found helping others to be therapeutic. As a twelve-year Reach to Recovery volunteer, I now have my own breast cancer resource center at a local medical center, and I have served on the local affiliate board for Komen.

"My advice to those newly diagnosed? Try to make this very unpleasant period of your life as positive as you can. The unpleasantness will pass!"

Susan Sanford; diagnosed in 1992 at age 48;
mortgage insurance underwriter/retired; Nevada

WHO'D'VE THOUGHT . . .

"In December of 1996, I had a routine mammogram that looked suspicious. My doctor said there was nothing to worry about and suggested I have a follow-up mammogram in three months. Having two young children, and being a full-time high school guidance counselor, I put it off for four months. The suspicious area proved to be a malignant tumor. I started radiation, but I was determined to fight this, get well, and move on with my life.

"I took a promotion to Head Guidance Counselor that August, a position I had wanted for several years. But in the spring of

2000, my world was again turned upside down when my mammogram showed calcification in the other breast. I decided to have a bilateral mastectomy with TRAM-flap reconstructive surgery at the same time. My family and my dearest friends were all there. They cared for me, cooked, baked, cleaned my house, and encouraged me every step of the way.

"Three years later, when the mayor of my hometown asked me to spearhead a program for local women affected by breast cancer, I jumped at the opportunity. We created the Nutley Thriving Survivors Program, which I still chair today. Through the Nutley Thriving Survivors, I have met some of the most beautiful people I know."

Michele Fleitell; diagnosed in 1996 at age 48;
educator; New Jersey

"If anything good can come from having breast cancer, then it happened to me. After being diagnosed, my creative energies started to flow and I began painting. I painted pink ribbons on everything that didn't move! I am pleased to say that I had two of my breast cancer designs published in magazines, and I'm looking forward to having more in the future. Until there is a cure, I'll paint pink ribbons!"

Janice Ferrari; diagnosed in 1998 at age 47;
housewife; Pennsylvania

"I am five years out. I've reached the time doctors told me that I should 'throw a big party' to celebrate 'having made it.' It sounded so far away when they talked about it during those early discussions when I was first diagnosed.

"During treatment, I often thought about how I hadn't made time to meet the man of my dreams, get married, and have children. Well, the man of my dreams found me, and I did marry him in 2004. I am now the proud stepmom of two smart, interesting girls, and we're planning to adopt, as well. My husband wasn't with me during the cancer year, but when he hugs me tightly and tells me how sorry he is that I had to do it but how grateful he is that I got through treatment and am healthy, I feel he, too, understands the significance of my being here."

Kym (Dyer) Hills; diagnosed in 2000 at age 42;
management consultant; California

"I was diagnosed eleven years ago! What have I done since? Well, I finally finished my degree, an achievement that I had been delaying for a long time. I have been enjoying life without tamoxifen and hot flashes. I have resumed the normal routine of living without fear (except at mammography time). And most important, I have regained control over many of the things that I lost when fighting breast cancer.

"For instance, for years I allowed my doctors to dictate when I would have my mammograms, which was always right before Thanksgiving. Several years they found 'something' that required further testing, and I had a miserable holiday season until the final diagnosis came in late January. Now, I insist that my mammograms not be done until January, so that I can enjoy the holidays.

"I have also learned to slow down and smell the roses. My husband and I bought a cabin near the Canadian border. We spend as much time there as possible, snowmobiling in the winter and kayaking in the summer. I feel normal again—even when the lumpectomy scar gets sore after kayaking for eight or ten miles. I consider those little tweaks a minor inconvenience and a reminder of how lucky I am!"

Pam Lord; diagnosed in 1994 at age 41;
human resources benefit coordinator; New Hampshire

"My treatment for breast cancer took about a year, and it was a difficult year physically. I was sooo tired! But as I was going through this, I could hardly believe how wonderful my life was spiritually and emotionally. I never knew that I had so many good friends, neighbors, co-workers, acquaintances, and especially family! It seemed that I was surrounded with love, joy, prayers, kindness, and just plain good positive energy. It was the best year of my life."

Sharon Matsumoto; diagnosed in 1999 at age 49;
bookkeeper; California

"I can't believe that on December 5, 2005, I marked my five-year anniversary of being cancer-free! Life has been so good. Sure there have been ups and downs, but what would life be if there weren't? Aside from my full-time job, I work as an ACS Reach to Recovery coordinator. I have met wonderful women who have shared their experiences with me. We all make it through this, coming out stronger than before.

"I've decided to finally do something for myself that I haven't done in years. I'm going back to school in a nursing career. I've thought about it now for a few years but have just started the courses recently. I think having been diagnosed with breast cancer has pushed me into pursuing my lifelong dream. I'm very excited and scared about doing this at the age of forty-eight, but if I can fight cancer, then I can fight to become a nurse!"

Liz Nippert; diagnosed in 2000 at age 42;
unit coordinator; Massachusetts

"Greetings Dear Sisters! Two years after my diagnosis, I decided to live life my way. John and I bought a home in a Florida retirement community, where I have served on the board of directors of our homeowners association, started a monthly program on healthcare topics, and served on numerous committees. My husband and I walk in the sunshine together, ride our bikes, invite friends over to play cards, help our neighbors through good times and bad. We were blessed with two precious grandsons and, after forty years of marriage, we learned to ballroom dance! Now we have a date every Friday night to waltz, rumba, foxtrot and cha-cha the night away! I am alive—and well! Please celebrate with me in spirit—hear the music inside you—feel the blessing of being alive!"

Louise Norville; diagnosed in 1998 at age 54;
registered nurse; Florida

"My, my, my. Five years. I prayed so very hard I would live to see that day on my calendar. April 12, 2005. Yes. I made it. In the past five years, I have gone in for a dozen or so CT scans, and every time I sit on the exam table waiting for my doctor to come in, I break into a cold sweat. What a roller-coaster ride it is! But all of my labs, exams, and scans have come out well.

"These past five years, I have seen my husband finish his degree and become a commissioned officer—his lifelong dream. I have seen my son grow from a boy to a handsome young man, seen him enter high school and get his first crush. I have seen my daughter blossom into a beautiful, caring person, with a bigger heart than I ever thought a child could have. We have been transferred to three different states. That means three different medical facilities, three different schools for my kids, and three different squadrons for my husband. But, I love it. I love our life. It makes us who we are and who I am. I am a survivor."

Kimberlee Richardson; diagnosed in 2000 at age 26;
fitness technician; Nebraska

"I can't believe it's been five years since my diagnosis. What I thought was the end is only the beginning of a new life!

"I opened my wig store five years ago, when my own treatment was done, and I have learned so much from my cancer customers. I tell them I am a survivor, and we are instantly connected! We share our fears, treatments, and hopes of a better future. Most women are horrified to lose their hair. I make light of how easy it is—no more time-consuming styling, costly hair products or salon expenses for a while. We all agree that Chinese food is the only thing that tastes good when having chemotherapy.

"I have two adorable new grandsons and another on the way, for a total of five grandchildren so far. And in April, I married a wonderful man who has supported me in everything I've gone through in the past ten years. So you see, there is life after cancer!"

Sharon (Daniels) Schmitt; diagnosed in 2000 at age 49; hairstylist/wig store owner; Massachusetts

"It's hard to believe it's been five years since *UPLIFT* first came out. I am blessed to say I am thirteen years post-cancer. I've had a scare or two in the last five years, but all is *well*. The best news is that my daughters, ages thirty-two and thirty-six, were married within six months of each other, and I was there! How blessed I was to be strong and healthy enough to dance the night away!

"Needless to say, I am still working overtime. Yoga, tennis, aerobics, photography, cooking, and teaching occupy most all of my time and energy. More news—my photographs of former synagogues, architecture, names, and faces of the Bronx have been put on display. The other wonderful news is that my partner of sixteen years and I are getting married. Both of our families will be there.

"Recently a doctor considered me 'cured.' What could be better!"

Carol Snyder; diagnosed in 1992 at age 47; special education teacher; New York

"More than five years have passed since my breast cancer surgery. Where have the years gone? After my treatments were complete, my husband and I decided it was time to smell the roses. He wanted me to make a list of things I wanted to do, and so I did. Five months after completing my treatment, I rejoined my Sweet

Adeline's Chorus and prepared to go onstage at the International Convention. We also went to Florida to visit my sister, and then to California, so that I could wade in the ocean. Before I knew it, I realized that, hey, I wasn't getting ready to die—I was going strong!"

Florence Wade; diagnosed in 1999 at age 63;

manager of retirement apartment community; Arizona

"I have been busy! I am nearly five and a half years beyond diagnosis and only go to annual check-ups now. They're a little scary, but such a relief when they are done. I'm just glad to have good follow-up from my doctors.

"My husband and I had been married for six years. Our original plan for Y2K was to start a family. With my diagnosis, our plans changed, and we fought breast cancer instead! Once treatment ended and I got the okay from my doctors, we resumed the Y2K plan and had a healthy baby boy in April of 2002. Carson is the light of our lives. He's our miracle, and we couldn't imagine life without him now! I am fortunate enough to have been able to stay home with him for most of his first months and then gradually took on marketing contract work that I could do from home. I began to volunteer for the local Komen Foundation, and then was offered a part-time job as Events Coordinator. I now work two days a week in the office and at home when Carson is napping. I am *so* lucky to be here, to have my family, and to be able to work at a job that I love.

"I have given *UPLIFT* to so many people—not because I'm 'in it,' but because of its helpful and inspiring messages. It's good to know that there is a light at the end of the breast cancer tunnel."

Jennifer Wersal; diagnosed in 2000 at age 30;

marketing; Texas

"Breast cancer is a gift, an opportunity to learn that life is sweeter because we taste every moment, savor every encounter, and never take for granted the special people who love us and whom we love dearly.

"My journey with breast cancer took me from working on Wall Street to taking a detour and being a yoga instructor. I decided to take a break from the stress of New York City after two recurrences of cancer, and to focus on caring for my body. A series of coincidences led me to a yoga teacher training course, and I found my new passion! I am able to care for my body, mind and spirit, and inspire others to do the same. My life has new meaning. I live with compassion and an open heart, loving every moment!"

Penny Williams; diagnosed in 1998 at age 41;
yoga instructor; New Jersey

FEAR-LESS

"Five years ago, I thought my world had come to an end. I had breast cancer. Me! Then I got angry. Why do so many women still get breast cancer? Why is the treatment so debilitating and disfiguring? That anger mellowed to determination—determination to survive, to learn as much as I could about breast cancer, to take control of my own health care, and to encourage women with breast cancer to take charge of their lives and their care."

Deb Haggerty; diagnosed in 1999 at age 51;
author, consultant, speaker; Florida

"I have a lot to be thankful for, and a lot has happened. On October 19th, I will be celebrating my five-year anniversary as a survivor. I was diagnosed at the age of thirty-two.

"I moved back to New York from Jacksonville, Florida, after living there for seven years. I am glad to be back home! I have learned to live life to the fullest. I enjoy every day and spend as much time as I can with my family. I have learned to conquer fear and live with hope by trusting God and appreciating life."

Charron Walker; diagnosed in 2000 at age 32;
client account specialist; New York

"I always knew at some point in my life that I would be diagnosed with breast cancer. I just did not plan on being diagnosed six weeks after the birth of my son, Sam! During my six week check-up, my doctor asked about a lump that he felt. Having worked with him in surgery for so many years, I could tell by the look on his face that he knew what he had felt was not good.

"The day before surgery, I was having breakfast with my daughter, Caitlin, who was five at the time. Out of the blue, she looked at me and said, 'Fear not for I am with thee.' She had learned this verse at daycare. It became my mantra during the rough times with chemo and trying to have a normal life. I now celebrate twelve years of being a member of the Sisterhood of Breast Cancer Survivors!"

Sallie Barron; diagnosed in 1994 at age 35;
surgical nurse; Arizona

"I completed five years cancer-free this year. When I was diagnosed with breast cancer, it was an emotional shock, as I had been a caregiver to a dear friend with cancer, and now I was on the other side. I was the patient. My friend had been so positive with his therapy, even knowing he was terminal. The only way I could face my cancer was to be positive; anything less would have been an insult to his memory.

"My positive attitude allowed me to face radiation with no fears or anxiety. Halfway through these five years, they found a lump in my liver, but it turned out to be a blood clot and dissolved on its own. My oncologist introduced me to an organization called Healing Odyssey, which has weekend retreats several times a year. This is a great group of women—*just like us.*"

Lois Brender; diagnosed in 2000 at age 68;
retired secretary; California

"Six years have flown by, and I have pushed the idea of having cancer to the back of my mind. I have traveled much—to Tahiti,

New Zealand, France, Greece, and, of course, to the mainland of the U.S. to see relatives and friends.

"Water aerobics has helped me a lot. It's a great outlet for telling friends how you feel that day, and knowing that no one will judge you. This is one more way in which you can put cancer out of your mind, and get on with living and appreciating your family and friends."

Ellinore Eckel; diagnosed in 1999 at age 61;
retired; Hawaii

"Wow, it's been five years since my diagnosis of breast cancer. This past July I learned from my eldest son and his wife that I was going to be a grandmother. Life was looking pretty good. Then I had my yearly mammogram and was told that there was a significant change in the area of my previous surgery. Of course, I thought the worst. I especially thought of the irony that I was finally going to have a grandchild but would not live to see it grow up. But the news was good. The change in breast tissue was a result of the radiation. The doctor explained to me that even after five years, the radiation can still alter the scar tissue and surrounding area.

"I feel so blessed to have my good health and my loving family. The best present of all will come next spring when I help to welcome my new grandchild into the world."

Fran Hegarty; diagnosed in 2000 at age 47;
librarian; Massachusetts

"I was twenty-four when I was diagnosed. The cancer had invaded my lymph system and my brain. In one year, I had three brain surgeries, radiation, and four rounds of chemotherapy. That was six years ago. At one time we were hoping that I would turn twenty-five! Today I am married, have a house, and an adorable little doggie. I am alive and kicking!"

Kim Lang; diagnosed in 1999 at age 24;
executive assistant; Illinois

"I was diagnosed with breast cancer in 1995. In 1996, I had a double mastectomy followed by chemo. In late 1996, a lump was found in the incision site, so it was removed. In three weeks, I returned to my job part-time with the help of my boss and co-worker. They would pick me up and then return me home when I got too tired.

"My sister is a beautician. When I lost my hair, I surprised her by going to her beauty shop. I walked in with my scarf and hat, walked over to her and said, 'Bonnie, I need to talk to you about my last perm!' I then took off my hat and scarf. Her face was a picture of shock. The lady who was getting a perm softly said, 'What kind of perm did you give her?' We all laughed, as I confessed why I had really lost my hair. My sister still tells people what I did to her."

Barb Seyl; diagnosed in 1995 at age 55;
retired; Montana

"Nine years ago I went into the operating room telling my surgeon to do whatever was necessary to keep me alive. Eight years ago, after completing chemo and radiation, I knew I was cancer-free. Since then, my two daughters have graduated from college and have begun their own careers. I went back to teaching my wonderful high school students who keep me young and teach me the phrases I need to understand them."

Penny Trosterman; diagnosed in 1996 at age 45;
teacher; New York

I DO BELIEVE

"My sister gave me a copy of *UPLIFT* for Christmas. It was a very moving book to read, and it rekindled many past memories. I immediately went searching for the journal that I wrote during my breast cancer time. As I read it, I could see how frightened and scared I was, then as I continued, I could see how my inner strength gradually built. My faith in God played a big part in this. Without prayer and blessings, I do not think I could have had the strength I did.

"A wonderful lady came out to see me from Reach to Recovery. She remarked on how positive I was and said I should think about volunteering. A year later, that is exactly what I did. Knowing that I could give one person hope and peace was the greatest feeling in the world."

Lorraine Colavito; diagnosed in 1989 at age 48;
homemaker; New York

"My story is very simple. I was thirty years old, a young Navy wife with four children under the age of twelve, and there was no history of cancer in my family. I found the lumps myself while showering at the gym. My husband made me call the doctor immediately.

"I refer to the early '70s as the 'dark ages' of breast cancer surgery. But I was in the right place at the right time, a small military hospital to which my surgeon had recently been transferred after his surgical internship at a teaching hospital in Texas. He told me that both lumps were not only malignant but of a type of malignancy not normally occurring in the breast. My course of treatment was daily radiation.

"Never did I fear I would die. Although I had not considered myself a deeply religious person, I did believe in God and consider myself somewhat spiritual. I was certain I'd live a long, healthy life and raise my children, and I have!"

Beatrice Flannagan; diagnosed in 1972 at age 30;
mortgage and real estate broker; California

"I went to the doctor because I felt a pain in my right breast. After the mammogram, I was sent for a biopsy, and I did have cancer! I was shocked and scared. My doctor suggested a lumpectomy and radiation.

"The head of the radiation unit was just one of the people who gave me the hope and strength I needed. I had an incredible group of nurses who treated me like I was special. Also, my dear sister had wrapped up thirty-three presents, so I had one to open on each day of my treatments.

"When the treatment was over, I went into a down spiral, feeling that nothing more was being done. So I read everything I could, talked to my friends, who gave me tremendous support and love, and put my life in God. I also had therapy, which helped. I now no longer live each year waiting for follow-up mammograms, but just go day by day. I watch what I eat, stay active, and listen to my own body, but the best thing I do for myself is to love life."

Karen L. Graves; diagnosed in 1997 at age 53;
retired bookkeeper; Minnesota

"My diagnosis came just before Christmas. The news blindsided me. My faith in God as the ultimate healer carried my emotions.

"I was home alone after the biopsy when the surgeon called to say I had breast cancer. I called my husband who was at work, and could barely get out the words. He came right home, and we held each other tight. 'Everything is going to be all right,' he said. 'We will take one day at a time.' I am now in my seventh year as a survivor of the most dreaded news any of us go through, and I am feeling great."

Ruth Hill; diagnosed in 1998 at age 60;
retired teacher; Michigan

"I'm doing fine—just this year finished my five years on tamoxifen. Now I'm taking Femara, which is supposed to be very effective. I thank God daily for good health and energy."

Phyllis Jezequel; diagnosed in 1999 at age 66;
missionary; Florida

"Since I was initially diagnosed, I have learned that hope is real. I have made it day by day, month by month, year by year, so I know it's possible. I think my primary lesson learned is that all the garbage in life no longer merits my tears and nerves and depression. 'Don't sweat the small stuff' is so true.

"I have been blessed with an outstanding husband, my family, my inspiring grandson Trent, and friends, but first and foremost I 'praise God from Whom all blessings flow.'"

Dixie Stoller; diagnosed in 2000 at age 47;

executive secretary; Texas

"From the first time I heard 'breast cancer,' I was calm, and just wanted to take care of it. My calmness came from Jesus. Through my prayers, and the prayers that were said for me, my whole ordeal was not upsetting. The best thing I can offer anyone in the way of advice is to trust in the Lord. He will give you peace and walk through this with you."

Cheryl Wagner; diagnosed in 2000 at age 52;

administrative assistant; Illinois

"I celebrate twenty years of surviving breast cancer. It is truly a celebration. I knew what my chances were, since the cancer was also in my lymph nodes. But from the start, I felt positive that I would beat the odds, and I have. I had wonderful support from family and friends during this time. That, along with a strong spiritual belief, got me through. I never dwelled on the fact that I had breast cancer. I think the most important thing is to have a positive attitude."

Mary Wise; diagnosed in 1985 at age 40;

administrative assistant; South Carolina

"Being diagnosed with breast cancer was the most devastating occurrence in my life. Although I discovered the lump in my breast,

I never considered the possibility it was cancer. After the call from my doctor, I was shaken beyond belief.

"Despite the numerous doctor visits, treatments, medications and very ill days, I grew stronger. I now have a renewed perspective on life. I have changed my diet and established a fitness plan to help me get and stay in shape. Breast cancer was not a death sentence for me, but the path to a healthy and spirit-filled closer relationship with God."

Oglatha Williams; diagnosed in 1998 at age 41;
Texas

18 • Fast Fast Forward

Ten Years Later

I'm not one to keep track of how long it's been since *UPLIFT* was born. Honestly, I'm too busy living to be constantly counting the years. But the original version came out three days before the World Trade Center fell, and with the tenth anniversary of that date approaching, there have been one too many reminders.

Ten years since the original publication of *UPLIFT*? Hard to believe! But then, I have to pinch myself to believe that it's been nearly seventeen years since my own diagnosis of breast cancer. I had been waiting for breast cancer all my life, so my diagnosis was in many regards a relief. It identified something I had feared, and treated it. For the very first time, I realized I would die of something else.

Well, here I am, alive and well—and bolder than ever, my husband would say. Initially, he blamed my new speak-my-mind mode on menopause. Hah! It had nothing to *do* with menopause and *everything* to do with beating a certain disease and feeling empowered.

Empowered? Actually, that's pretty funny. I now have six grandchildren, and if there's one thing I've learned, it's to keep the old

mouth shut when it comes to child rearing. No criticism. No unso-
licited advice. I had my turn as a parent; now it's my kids' turn.
The upside of that, of course, is that being free of responsibility, I
can simply have fun with these little ones.

But being a grandmother is only part of what I've done in the
five years since the last edition of UPLIFT was published. I've also
written five more books, each one different from the last and more
finely tuned, both in content and style. I've learned that one really
good adjective is better than three lukewarm ones, and that in this
fast-paced life of ours, my stories have to move. I've learned to
blog. I've learned to do live chats. I've learned that Facebook is my
BFF when it comes to communicating with readers.

Between economy woes and the advent of ebooks, the field of
publishing has experienced a tsunami. Does this depress me? Absolutely not. I beat breast cancer, didn't I?

In gathering material for this tenth anniversary chapter, I heard
from many women who were in earlier editions of UPLIFT.
Though I have met only a few in person, I think of them all as old
friends. I've loved reconnecting and hearing what they're doing. In
that vein, if you see discrepancies between their earlier credits and
their current ones, it's because they have changed occupations or
moved. Indeed, as I write this, eleven-year-survivor Flo Wade has
e-mailed to say that she and her husband have just been hired to
work this summer season at the Old Faithful General Store in Yel-
lowstone National Park. "Yes, I'm excited!" she writes. "Each day
is a new adventure."

Each day is a new adventure. I like to look at it that way, too. Do
I ever think about cancer? Of course, I do. With each little pain
that lasts longer than a day, I briefly wonder at its cause—and the
older I get, the more little aches and pains I feel. But I've come to
realize that there's always another explanation. If it isn't fasciitis in
my heel, it's tendonitis in my wrist or arthritis in my knee. Does this
depress me? Absolutely not. It's the price of living—now—into my
sixties. Yikes!

Life is about growth. It's about moving forward. That's what my characters do in every book I write, and it's what I try to do myself. And I'm not alone in this. Among old and new UPLIFTers, those who've passed the ten-year-mark exude enthusiasm.

Read on, dear friend, and smile.

LEAVING TREATMENT BEHIND

"It's hard to believe it's been over ten years since I was diagnosed. Chemo was by far the worst thing I went through, and I still credit my wonderful husband for helping me through. I fear recurrence, but I don't let it hold me back. I thank God for the last ten years and am hoping for thirty or forty more!

"I now make time for things, rather than putting them off. I don't take life for granted, but I am thankful for every breath. I enjoy volunteering as a way of showing my thanks for all the kindness I was shown.

"My life is good. I still have the most awesome husband, and we are fortunate to have healthy children. We even became dog people and now can't imagine life without our little mutt."

Lori Bartz; diagnosed in 2000 at age 41;
legal secretary; Wisconsin

"I am a breast cancer survivor—twice. The first time was twelve years ago. Then, when a tiny bump was found again in April 2010, I had a second mastectomy and elected to have radiation. It was one of the most rewarding experiences of my life. Radiation showed me a strength in myself that I didn't know I had. It gave me the courage to speak my mind, to not settle, to know that I have been through a battle and that I am a survivor."

Michele Darby; diagnosed in 1998 at age 52;
retired administrative manager; New York

"Ten years ago, I was in the middle of radiation for breast cancer. Five years ago, I was holding my daughter's hands as she had chemotherapy for the same disease. And today we are both alive and well and celebrating each day as the gift that it is!"

Gwen Angstrom; diagnosed in 2000 at age 59;
retired; Washington

"As far as I know, I am doing fine without any breasts. It's really quite wonderful not to have to wear a bra. I am supposed to be wearing my prosthesis daily, but I find they are heavy, so I don't wear them. Naughty! It's liberating not to have to carry round those poor, dear breasts that I had before the double mastectomy. Life has never been better. I am enjoying every minute!"

Hilary Prince; diagnosed in 2009 at age 73;
retired; Prince Edward Island, Canada

"I'm headed into eighteen years of remission!"

B.C.; diagnosed in 1995 at age 32;
event coordinator; California

"I was first diagnosed with breast cancer in 2000. When I had a recurrence in 2008, I decided to have double mastectomies and chemo. I don't regret that one bit, as I found out later that there was a precancerous lesion in the other breast. Now we're still enjoying life to its fullest, and I know that the best is yet to come. I'm more daring and try new things that I've always wanted to do. We're spending our kids' inheritance, too! Last year, we went to Italy and then to Greece. This year we're heading for Scandinavia. We're having a party for our seventieth birthdays in the mountains in September. And my hair is finally returning!"

Judy Peterson; diagnosed in 2000 at age 58;
retired RN; Colorado

"I was diagnosed with breast cancer in 2001, and had chemo and radiation. I was teaching preschool and handicapped preschool at the time, and never missed a day of teaching."

Angela Moore; diagnosed in 2001 at age 64;
retired teacher; New Jersey

"Breast cancer seems to touch the lives of more and more each year. When I meet someone shocked to find herself in this situation, I tell her that in retrospect, the diagnosis is probably the worst part of the whole process. After that, we pick ourselves up and get busy *doing* whatever we have to do to get through, survive, and thrive. I am happy to report that I am doing great and enjoying life!"

Deb Haney; diagnosed in 1996 at age 48;
artist; Massachusetts

"Anniversaries of being cancer free? I celebrate each day. I had my left breast removed in December 1990 and my right breast removed in March 1998. Having cancer twice keeps me in the reality and blessings of each day.

"I was in a relationship when I had both surgeries. That relationship ended, but I moved forward with my life, knowing I would find my way. I retired in 2005 and have traveled my home state on part-time work assignments, enjoying each one and all the new people. I have never felt my breasts defined me as a woman. I am in a sexual relationship today and am open about my surgeries."

Sandra Haymart; diagnosed in 1990 at age 47;
retired chief deputy circuit court clerk; Missouri

"I am a survivor of twelve years come March 3rd of this year. I had bilateral mastectomies with tissue flap reconstruction on that day in 1999, one day before my thirty-eighth wedding anniversary. I could have had a lumpectomy but chose to rid myself of the problem entirely. I had no problem making that decision. For me, it was the smart thing to do. By doing the tissue flap reconstruction, I used my own body's parts to reconstruct. I wear normal clothes, normal bathing suits, and need no extra anything. I was able to do lots of normal things after just six weeks. Ladies, just do it!"

Marie Johnson; diagnosed in 1999 at age 56; retired; Virginia

"Participating in the original *UPLIFT* was life changing for me as I completed chemo and reconstructions and looked to life after breast cancer. Now, more than ten years from my diagnosis, I have five grandchildren, am retired and living life to its fullest."

Rosamary Amlet; diagnosed in 2000 at age 48; retired, part-time consultant; Ohio

"I have been cancer-free for sixteen years. Time goes so fast!"

Virginia Danczak; diagnosed in 1995 at age 58; retired; Nebraska

SCHOOL DAYS

"In the years following my breast cancer diagnosis, I earned a master's degree and then a PhD. I supported my children by teaching school. Later I worked in aerospace, and eventually started my own business. Breast cancer was my wake-up call. It sparked me to take charge of my life and make dreams come true."

Mimi Mills; diagnosed at age 28; author, educator; Colorado

"I've had so many things happen to me since I was diagnosed with breast cancer. I'm sixty-one and in law school, and sometimes I wonder what I was thinking! What keeps me going are my grandchildren, the trips I take, and volunteering."

Donna Danzis; diagnosed in 2002 at age 54;
child abuse case worker; Florida

"I was diagnosed in 1993 while pregnant with my daughter. On Mother's Day 2011, I will be celebrating my eighteenth birthday. I consider it my birthday as opposed to an anniversary, because my diagnosis was part of a new chapter in my life, the birth of a fresh start. My daughter is beautiful, healthy, and heading off to college in September. She serves as a constant reminder that when diagnosed early, breast cancer is not the end of your life. I continue working with the organizations that supported me during my recovery. I also started another chapter of my life by going back to school and fulfilling a long-ago dream by getting my master's degree in education."

Renee C. Johannesen; diagnosed in 1993 at age 35;
teacher; New York

"I was diagnosed in 1997. Since then, I have completed my master's degree in nursing and now work part-time as a clinical instructor. We are cruise fans and have traveled the Caribbean, the inside passage in Alaska, and the Mexican Riviera. I have had one cancer-related surgery since my initial diagnosis, but otherwise my health has been great. There is life after diagnosis."

Alexandra Koffman; diagnosed in 1997 at age 40;
RN; Massachusetts

"I am a thirteen-year breast cancer survivor and feel wonderful. I've been teaching preschool for the past twelve years and am loving it."

Tobi Stelzer; diagnosed in 1997 at age 40;
preschool teacher; New Jersey

"For the past three and a half years, I have been a special needs preschool para-educator. Five months ago, I started a new venture. I am now back in school getting a degree in speech-language pathology assisting, and I'll finish at the same time my daughter graduates high school. I am very blessed. Life is good."

Kimberlee Richardson; diagnosed in 2000 at age 26; special education para-educator, student; Washington

WE'RE IN BUSINESS

"Update from one of the original *UPLIFT* sisterhood members! In the fourteen years since my diagnosis for breast cancer, I have continued to focus on my creative side with growth in my jewelry and artisan creations. I convinced my husband to rent our home to our son and move to the ocean, which was a lifelong dream. I have continued to work in several of the shops where my jewelry is sold and enjoy the friendship of the many creative friends who inspire and color my world."

Deb Haney; diagnosed in 1996 at age 48; artist; Massachusetts

"When I was diagnosed in December 1999, my world turned upside down. But it has changed my life for the better. Six months after I finished treatment, I changed jobs, something I had been reluctant to do in the past. When I was laid off from that job in 2009, I started a home-based business, a very risky move at a time when the economy was in the basement. But having survived breast cancer, I knew I could do anything! Yes, breast cancer was the worst thing that ever happened, yet it was the best thing, too! It changed my life in the most positive ways."

Joan Merritt; diagnosed in 1999 at age 53; retired; California

"I can't believe that another five years has passed. That makes me an eleven-year breast cancer survivor, and ten years since I opened the wig store. It's humbling to know I've helped hundreds of women feel good about themselves despite losing their hair. It's a woman's thing—we need our hair! I really can relate. When I let them know I'm a survivor, you can just see their shoulders relax.

"I now have a total of five grandchildren. I graduated and don't have to see my oncologist anymore. I started oil painting again after twenty years. And I have a *big* birthday coming up and feel blessed that I am here to celebrate it!"

Sharon (Daniels) Schmitt; diagnosed in 2000 at age 49;
hairstylist, wig store owner; Massachusetts

"I was a waitress at the time I was diagnosed, and after chemo and radiation, continued raising two beautiful boys. They are now ages twenty-two and nineteen. Four years ago, I opened a restaurant (so much for stress free), and I am married to the same wonderful man, who was always there for me through it all."

Donna Troiani; diagnosed in 2000 at age 42;
restaurant owner; New York

"It's been over sixteen years since I was diagnosed with Stage II breast cancer—sixteen years in which to evaluate the priorities in my life. I have concluded one thing—never overlook an opportunity for pleasure. If you've always wanted to learn to play the piano, then find an instructor and begin. Want to throw a pizza party for your grandchildren, then do so!

"Set goals, even if they're small ones. There's nothing like the satisfaction I feel when I have attained a goal. I am especially proud of one: I published recently a novel that takes place in my beloved New Hampshire. It is such a thrill to meet my readers and see the wonderful reviews they post.

"It's so easy to get caught up in our day-to-day lives that we tend to lose touch with those we care about. Skip the e-mail and pick

up the phone. Make a date to have coffee. Give of yourself. You
may like your 'return on investment.' I know I do."

Pamela Lord; diagnosed in 1994 at age 41;
human resources manager; New Hampshire

VOLUNTEERING

"When I was first told I had breast cancer in January of 2000, I became angry—angry that so many of us get breast cancer, angry
that the treatment is still so disfiguring and debilitating. In the
eleven years since my diagnosis, I have worked to end breast cancer. I serve as chair of the board of directors of the Florida Breast
Cancer Foundation, and I have a website designed to encourage
woman with breast cancer to control their own health care. Most
of all, I talk with anyone and everyone about breast cancer and
what they can do to end this war. I am very fortunate to be one of
the 'thrivers' with no signs of a recurrence and the ability to help
others in return for the help I was given."

Deb Haggerty; diagnosed in 1999 at age 51;
author, speaker, breast cancer advocate; Florida

"I am eleven years cancer-free. I was diagnosed at the age of thirty-
two in October 2000. In 2006, I started Young Survivors Network,
a program for young women survivors of breast cancer. Our mission is to educate, support, and advocate for young women who
have been diagnosed with this disease. I have learned that everything I go through is to help someone else. A quote I live by: 'God
spared me for a reason, and this is my purpose in life.'"

Charron Walker; diagnosed in 2000 at age 32;
founder, director of Young Survivors Network, Inc.; Florida

"What a blessing, as the years have rolled by, soon approaching
number twenty! I have retired from being a school nurse and am

doing volunteer work at a local hospital. One of the greatest blessings has been to watch my grandchildren grow up and wait for the newest arrival in June.

"What a blessing to walk with sister survivors, as new friendships bonded over the years."

Doris Cantrell; diagnosed in 1992 at age 52;
registered nurse; Michigan

"I am now nineteen years out, and so much more has come into my life in the past ten years. I reside in a fairly small rural community. Because of my dedication as an ACS Reach to Recovery volunteer, I was recruited to join the local affiliate board of Susan G. Komen for the Cure, acting as an education and race survivor center cochair for three years. I learned to write grants to obtain funding for yoga, postsurgery camisoles, education and support materials for patients. Most important, I am able to share my life with so many wonderful women."

Susan Sanford; diagnosed in 1992 at age 48;
retired; Nevada

"I was in the first edition of *UPLIFT*, and I'm now an eleven-year survivor. Yippee! I'm the one who bought the 450 SL as a treat to myself after I finished treatment.

"I try to be available to anyone who has been diagnosed or is going through treatment, because I know I had sooooooo many questions before I started my treatment. I'm still selling real estate and also spend my free time volunteering at Wellspring Women's Center here in Sacramento."

Patti Martinez; diagnosed in 1999 at age 54;
realtor; California

"This is my twelfth year after diagnosis. A happy survivor, I retired and joined a group of women who support the Shriners Hospitals for Children. We are all volunteers. I am responsible for leading over 450 members in our area. I can't think of a more rewarding way to spend my retirement. I am happy as a clam."

Cynthia Ferus; diagnosed in 2000 at age 57;
retired; Massachusetts

IT'S MORE THAN JUST A RACE

"I am a twenty-year breast cancer survivor. To celebrate that anniversary in April of 2010, I walked in the Susan G. Komen Race for the Cure, in the pouring rain, in Rogers, Arkansas. I felt so elated and uplifted!"

Billie Bules; diagnosed in 1990 at age 54;
homemaker; Arkansas

"Last October, I began my thirty-ninth year as a breast cancer survivor—and I'm still here! I have walked the Komen 5K every year since its inception here in San Diego. This year, I am branching out and walking in two other 5Ks around the USA. My lofty goal is to walk the Komen 5K in every state. I have done ones in Florida and Ohio, and this year am thinking of doing ones in Louisiana and West Virginia. I'll keep you updated!"

Beatrice Flannagan; diagnosed in 1972 at age 30;
realtor; California

"In the eleven-plus years since my diagnosis, my life has irrevocably changed. Twenty-seven years ago, my father was suffering with pancreatic cancer and couldn't reach out to others for help. When I was diagnosed with breast cancer, I was determined to do this. Once my treatments ended, it seemed that many friends and acquaintances were diagnosed. I felt it was vital to me to help each one as much as possible. I bought copies of *UPLIFT* to give to every new member of this unique 'sisterhood.' I'm proud and happy to say that the book not only helped my friends, but they found it so beneficial that they also paid it forward and gifted other 'sisters' as well.

"Besides advocating for breast cancer survivors, I have supported walks and products and other fund-raisers, like Stand Up To Cancer. I also finished thirty-five years teaching high school French and Spanish, traveled a bit, and finished two novels.

"Every day is a gift, every survivor is a miracle, and every ounce of prevention makes me believe that breast cancer will be wiped out someday soon."

Christine Foutris; diagnosed in 1999 at age 49;
retired educator; Illinois

"On April 3, 2011, I will celebrate eleven years as a breast cancer survivor. Everyone who is a survivor realizes how blessed she is to be able to change her life for the better. Priorities immediately change, little things take on new meaning, your family and friends become more precious. The need to help find a cure for breast cancer becomes a part of your everyday life. Whenever I go to the gym, I wear a shirt that has some breast cancer message. My hope is that some woman who has not had a mammogram will read the shirt and get one. By participating in the Race for the Cure every year, I hope to encourage my family and friends to make sure that they take care of themselves.

"My husband and I always talked about celebrating when I reached my tenth anniversary. When the time came, I decided that the way I wanted to celebrate was to ask a dear friend of mine, who is a priest, to celebrate a Mass of Thanksgiving. Sitting in church that day made me once again realize that breast cancer has made me appreciate life so much more."

Ceil Gallucci; diagnosed in 2000 at age 52;
retired occupational therapist; New Jersey

"I am an eleven-year survivor, and I have a wonderful husband, Eric, and an eight-year-old son, Carson. For almost seven years, I have worked part-time at the Susan G. Komen for the Cure Affiliate in Fort Worth, Texas. Each year, during our Race for the Cure 'season,' we register Carson as the team captain of our family's Race team. As the team captain, Carson is in charge of fundraising, meaning that we write the team web page about Carson and why he wants to erase breast cancer from the face of the earth. Carson has raised more than $10,000 over the last six years. He is really beginning to understand what it means to donate money and time to a good cause.

"I still don't mind driving east in the morning and west in the evening with the sun in my eyes both ways. For some reason, that just doesn't bother me like it did before breast cancer."

Jennifer Wersal; diagnosed in 2000 at age 30;
race and communications manager, Komen Greater Fort Worth; Texas

LIVING THE DREAM

"A few months after I finished my initial treatments, I decided to get a pink ribbon tattoo on my hip. It's just a little something I wanted for me. I knew that no one aside from my husband and me would see it unless I chose to show them. After my tenth 'cancerversary' last year, I decided I wanted another one. I am a survivor who fought for her life and I wanted everyone to know it. So I had a local tattoo artist design something for my left wrist, and what he came up with was perfect! I now have the word 'Survivor' in script, with a pink ribbon above it and pink boxing globe hanging down below. I have gotten so many positive comments on it, and every one of them fills my heart and soul with pride.

"In April 2010, I celebrated my ten-year 'cancerversary.' We had a huge party with pink everywhere you looked. All of our guests wore pink, too. What can I say—we were superexcited and needed to celebrate!"

Kimberlee Richardson; diagnosed in 2000 at age 26;
special education para-educator, student; Washington

"I am a seventeen-year survivor, and there isn't a day that goes by when I don't think of how blessed I am."

Pamela Miltner; diagnosed in 1993 at age 40;
insurance agent; Indiana

"As a ten-years-plus breast cancer survivor, I've learned that girlfriends make your life worth living. They held my hand throughout the treatment and told me that 'with a hat and an attitude, you can go anywhere.' Although the hair has grown back and I no longer need the 'hat,' the positive attitude is here to stay. Thank you, my friends."

Rosemary Liebmann; diagnosed in 2000 at age 54;
retired; Pennsylvania

"For the last nineteen years, life has been so exciting. I have met so many special people."

Mary Ann Budnick; diagnosed in 1991 at age 44;
retired school bus driver; Florida

"I had surgery in 1983, yet I've seen my children graduate from high school and college. They both are married, and I have four wonderful grandchildren. I started my own business and after twenty-five years sold it and moved to Texas to be close to our children and grandchildren. I am truly blessed."

Rita Madison; diagnosed in 1983 at age 39;
retired business owner; Texas

"Wow, it's been almost eighteen years since I was diagnosed with breast cancer, and the expression 'Time heals everything' holds true. Of course, there's always a little bird sitting on my shoulder, reminding me of yesterday. However, the bird keeps getting smaller and smaller as each year passes.

"My friends are having bouts with cancer these days, and I try to be there to guide and encourage them. I find helping others is so rewarding.

"We keep an active lifestyle between my husband's golf and my classes, canasta games, and babysitting for our four-year-old granddaughter. We recently went to Disney World with all the family and it was wonderful. We toured, had fun with the kids, and loved being together. These were very special moments. I am so very grateful for the love with which our family and friends surround us. How lucky we are!"

Alyce Feinstein; diagnosed in 1993 at age 58; retired; Florida

"In July 2011, I will be a thirteen-year survivor, and I'm feeling great. Several years ago, to mark my triumph over this horrible disease, I had a one-inch pink ribbon tattooed on my upper right wrist. I've had many people comment on it, and I proudly say it's my victory sign."

Pat Mohr; diagnosed in 1998 at age 59; retired accounting business owner; Manitoba, Canada

"Ten years ago, I thought I would never be writing this story. It is not that my diagnosis of Stage II breast cancer was ominous, but that I thought I might never feel the same way I did before breast cancer. My sister and I were sitting in my oncologist's office, and I asked her, 'Do you think we will ever laugh again?' She said, 'Yes, we will.' I didn't think so, but, in fact, we do. I go to my doctor's appointments regularly, and each time I hear the words, 'You are perfect,' I walk out of the office as if I'm walking on air.

"My daughter was married the year of my diagnosis, and I had to go to the wedding wearing a wig. That was probably one of the most difficult things I ever had to do. I remember putting on the best smile I had and hoping for the best. It was a wonderful day, and I don't think many people knew I was being 'brave.' Three years later, my husband and I divorced. I picked myself up again, and my daughter gave me two wonderful grandsons. Life has its ups and downs, but I have learned what the word 'survivor' truly means.

"It is hard to believe, but February 1, 2011, marked eleven years since my diagnosis. I have never felt healthier or happier. My family is a constant source of joy in my life. Their support gives me strength, and I am grateful for it every day."

Frances Gallello; diagnosed in 2000 at age 51;

mental health assistant; New York

"I convinced my husband to rent our home to our son and move to the ocean, which was a lifelong dream."

Deb Haney; diagnosed in 1996 at age 48;

artist; Massachusetts

"One positive thing breast cancer has done is to give each of my three sons a newfound respect for woman. It has given me strength to face test results and the patience to think situations out a little more clearly. My biggest accomplishment is to wake up each and every day and be blessed to simply do just that.

"My son, then nine, was diagnosed with leukemia two days before my initial diagnosis. He is still in remission and is now nineteen and a sophomore in college. How lucky am I?

"I was honored to be in the earlier editions of *UPLIFT*. I keep five copies on hand at all times to give to women."

Cathy Hanlon; diagnosed in 2000 at age 42;

volunteer, substitute teacher; New York

"It has been over ten years since my original diagnosis, but I still get nervous awaiting the results of my yearly mammogram. Having five granddaughters, I am very much aware that I play a major role in their medical history. I am also acutely aware that without early detection, I would not be here and able to enjoy these beautiful grandchildren."

Fran Hegarty; diagnosed in 2000 at age 47;
librarian; Massachusetts

"In October 2011, I will become a thirteen-year breast cancer survivor. I am now retired and have six grandchildren. I am enjoying ballroom dancing, volunteering with the Red Cross, exercising, and all the free time I now have. Isn't life wonderful?"

Sandy Mark; diagnosed in 1998 at age 55;
retired; Connecticut

"After retiring from teaching after thirty-three years, my life has become even more busy. I am a member of a quilt group that provides Meals on Wheels with place mats and donates quilts to our community's homeless shelter. Crocheting, knitting, reading, sewing, visiting the elderly, having lunch with friends—these are some of my other activities. However, the time spent with my grandsons is what is more precious to me. Each day is a special gift. I am so thankful to have been in good health for the last ten years. This blessing has allowed me to do what I enjoy and to place a smile on the faces of others."

Barbara Mulvey; diagnosed in 2000 at age 50;
retired teacher; New York

"My mom, May Pavese Reilly, is a warrior princess—in fact, a ten-year survivor of breast cancer. It wasn't without a fight, but then, you don't get to be a warrior princess without that battle. She hasn't run any marathons, but I've walked two of the sixty-mile walks for breast cancer, not to mention lots of shorter ones. We will be victorious!"

Judith H. Reilly; daughter of survivor May Pavese Reilly;
executive director, Compeer of the Mohawk Valley; New York

"I am very proud to have written about my friend Ruth in the original edition of *UPLIFT*. Well, Ruthie is still going strong. She has twenty great-grandchildren!"

Rae Shapiro; friend of Ruth Pollack;
retired; California

"It hardly seems possible that more than ten years have passed since my breast cancer surgery. I celebrated my sixty-fourth birthday the day after my surgery, and I'm now preparing to celebrate birthday number seventy-five. How did that happen so quickly? I am a wife, mother, and grandmother, and have a ten-month-old great-grandson! What blessings have come my way. Life has been full and wonderful."

Flo Wade; diagnosed in 1999 at age 63;
retired; Arizona

"I am a twenty-two-year survivor of breast cancer, and that is just awesome to say! The most positive thing that breast cancer has done for me is to take me from a materialistic world to a life filled with renewed faith in God. I realized what a precious gift my life is. I look to the future with hope, confident that the day will come when we can all say, 'A cure has been found!'"

Lorraine Colavito; diagnosed in 1989 at age 48;
retired, full-time caregiver; New York

"It is hard to believe that I am a ten-year breast cancer survivor. As I look back on the experience, I know that my faith in God helped me. There was nothing I could do about the diagnosis, so I took the positive approach and depended on God to see me through."

Dona Crowe; diagnosed in 2001 at age 62;
retired; Kentucky

WHAT I'VE LEARNED

"Being diagnosed with breast cancer is devastating, but I found that with a strong faith, wonderful family and friends' support, and a great medical team, I came out a stronger person. I always thought I enjoyed life, but I *really* love life now. I now have the courage to reach out and try to help others with breast cancer, something I could not have done before. There is such a strong feeling of wanting to help. I'm now seventy-four years old and feel great. Life is *good* after breast cancer."

Lois Marks; diagnosed in 2002 at age 65;
retired; Ohio

"I am a single parent of three boys. I am facing foreclosure, and have a deadbeat ex-husband, but if cancer didn't get me, these little speed bumps in life sure won't. I had to make a conscious decision to be a *warrior* and not a *wimp*—to be an example of a courageous *woman survivor*. And I think that I have. Cancer has brought so many riches to my life, but most important, a thirst for more living and an outrageous kick-butt attitude."

Margaret Keever; diagnosed in 2009 at age 45;
secretary; New York

"Breast cancer made me appreciate the little things in life. I wake up every morning happy, and focus on getting one thing accomplished each day. I am not going in circles trying to do everything at once. I can leave a dish in the sink, or I can skip dusting, or I can leave my grandchildren's toys on the floor until tomorrow. I have learned how to pace myself."

Carol Bonapace; diagnosed in 2009 at age 59;
secretary; Connecticut

"I will be celebrating my eleventh year as a survivor this year. While my life hasn't changed dramatically in the last ten plus years, I have learned a few things. If you have a remaining breast, be sure to have your mammogram each year. Reach out to family members, friends, and acquaintances who have been diagnosed with breast cancer and assure them that this diagnosis does not have to be a death sentence. Offer to take them to chemo treatments; offer to clean their house; assure them that their hair does grow back. One of the most important things I learned when I was having surgery and chemo was to set pride aside and accept help from family and friends. These offers of help are made not out of pity, but love. Mostly know that though you've lost a breast, you are still a valuable, contributing person."

Carole Humphrey; diagnosed in 2000 at age 52;
assistant, Department of the Army; Missouri

"It has been fourteen years since I had breast cancer. What have I been doing? Hmmm, I started working at the library that I love so much.

"Emotionally, in the beginning, breast cancer knocked me on my butt. But I have settled into this new life and to me I am a much better person. I listen—I mean, really listen to others now. I appreciate them more. I try to be more patient, but since I'm the mom of a teenager, that sometimes doesn't work out so well.

"I think of my breast cancer once a year, and that is when I go to see my oncologist. He gives me the all-clear sign, and then I go back to my life. Was it easy? Hell, no! But from ten years ago when I did the first *UPLIFT*, now I can say without a doubt that I am a survivor!"

Debby Whittet; diagnosed in 1996 at age 43;
library clerk; Michigan

"As a two-time breast cancer survivor, I've gained some perspective. By far, the most difficult aspect of my first diagnosis in 1995 was the fear. I couldn't let go of it. It gradually subsided, but was a three-year process. When I was diagnosed in 2008 with a new cancer on the other side, I was astounded. There is no history in my family, and my only risk factor is being a woman. However, this time I knew that this is a curable disease, and I've been able to just let go and live. I've discovered a greater ability to 'go for it' and have loved doing things like white-water rafting in Alaska, riding a camel in Jordan, and immersing myself in the Dead Sea in Israel. I think my cancer experience has helped me grow less timid. So I encourage *you* to take a deep breath and give life your best shot."

Maureen Larson; diagnosed in 1995 at age 49;

marriage coordinator; Minnesota

"I am a ten-year survivor who was diagnosed with breast cancer at the age of twenty-nine. There was no family history, so this was quite a surprise at the time. I was very lucky to have found the lump myself during what I call a miracle shower, since I was not the type that did self-exams. I thank God for my wonderful medical team and the support and love of my family. They are the reasons I am here. I feel I was given a second chance at life surviving breast cancer for the past ten years, and I need to live every moment to the fullest.

"This may sound like a cliché, but breast cancer has taught me *not* to sweat the small stuff. I can remember always worrying what my car would cost at the mechanic. Well, not anymore! I also feel that this disease has taught me to fight for myself, and that I am stronger than I thought. I am very shy, but have learned to speak up for myself more, and I have also reached out to others who are diagnosed with this disease. Every October, I raise over $4,000 in the Making Strides Walk for Breast Cancer. My shyness disappears when it comes to asking for money to fight this disease."

Christine DiGiovanni; diagnosed in 2000 at age 29;

New York

"The most positive thing about breast cancer for me: I never felt more loved, before or since."

Joyce Wiswell; diagnosed in 2003 at age 46;
writer/editor; Michigan

SPREADING THE WORD

"I am a nine-year survivor. *UPLIFT* was such a wonderful source of help to me after my diagnosis and during my treatment, and I have shared it with others."

Lois Marks; diagnosed in 2002 at age 65;
retired; Ohio

"Only two days ago, I gave *UPLIFT* to yet another person recently diagnosed with breast cancer. I found this book so helpful on my treatment journey. It inspired me so often."

Hilary Prince; diagnosed in 2009 at age 73;
retired; Prince Edward Island, Canada

"I was diagnosed in 2000. I am now eleven years out and feel blessed to celebrate the start of each new day. I found *UPLIFT* while I was undergoing radiation therapy, and it really convinced me that I could survive and thrive."

Lynn Quanrud; diagnosed in 2000 at age 54;
family medicine residency coordinator; Washington

"I was recently given *UPLIFT* as a gift and loved it! I found myself constantly saying, 'I can totally relate to this!'"

Tiffany Mannino; diagnosed in 2009 at age 36;
sixth-grade teacher; Pennsylvania

"I make sure that my women friends who have had to face breast cancer surgery and subsequent treatments each receive a copy of

UPLIFT. This is my way of letting my friends know I'm here for them and that life goes on one day at a time."

Flo Wade; diagnosed in 1999 at age 63;
retired; Arizona

"When I first read *UPLIFT*, I never would've thought that I'd be one of the sisters, too. I've learned a lot, and still do. Life is amazing."

Ester Vicent; diagnosed in 2007 at age 47;
enterprise director; Barcelona, Spain

"Wow! I am shocked that it's been ten years now that I have been recommending *UPLIFT* to my patients with breast cancer as they go through their treatment. Each and every year that I captain our Making Strides Walk for Breast Cancer walk, I first apologize to everyone by saying, 'I am embarrassed that in the year 20__ we have not found a cure for breast cancer.' I request that they help us because I swear I will not retire until we find that cure!"

Cindy L. Teeple;
oncology nurse practitioner; New York

19 • The Gene Thing

Do We Want to Know?

*U*PLIFT is not a medical book. Its focus is on the emotional side of breast cancer. We don't discuss the pros and cons of treatment protocols here, but, rather, focus on practical snippets of thought that will help us get through treatment and thrive. So I balked when my publisher suggested adding a medical update in the Tenth Anniversary Edition. I'm no doctor. I'm just one woman who has survived breast cancer.

Then I got to thinking. Medical issues are discussed, albeit indirectly, by some of the contributors to this book, and I wanted to make sure that nothing in earlier versions had become obsolete. With extraordinary generosity and care, my surgeon and her Team Uplift fellows read through *UPLIFT* and did suggest some changes. For instance, stem cell treatments are no longer used to treat breast cancer, mastectomies are not done by surprise during surgery, and silicone implants have made a comeback. I've edited earlier chapters to reflect all of this current thinking.

Though treatment options remain generally the same now as ten years ago—lumpectomy, mastectomy, chemo, radiation, medication—they have been so finely tuned that survival rates have soared. Early detection also plays a key role, as so many *UPLIFT*ers attest.

But there is one new development. When I was first diagnosed with breast cancer, few of us had ever heard of the BRCA gene. Did you know that the name originally stood for Berkeley, California (hence, B-R-C-A), where the gene was first shown to exist? A bit of trivia there, but something I've often wondered about. BRCA1 and BRCA2 have become part of the breast cancer lexicon in recent years, and the option of testing for it is offered more and more often, particularly among those with a family history of breast cancer.

It isn't an easy choice. On one hand, the results can be helpful. If we know that we have the mutated gene, for instance, and may be at greater risk of recurrence, we may skip the lumpectomy and go for a bilateral mastectomy. Likewise, our children may start screening at an earlier age.

But . . . but . . . that *sucks.* I'm sorry. There's no better way to put it. We don't *want* more invasive treatment. We don't *want* our kids fixating on getting this themselves. We're being emotional here. But this *is* an emotional issue. Which is why I've included this chapter.

Do we take the test? Will the results make us feel better or worse? Will we be stigmatized if we carry this gene? Will we feel somehow *at fault* for putting our family at risk?

I've been debating the pros and cons of having the test done since my doctor suggested it last year. Oh, I'd heard about BRCA1 and 2 well before that, but like so many of you, I worried that if I was found to have the gene mutation, health care and life insurance would be harder to get. Recent laws do protect us. Still we worry.

I also sidestepped the issue by telling myself that I have no daughters.

But I do have sons. Men can get breast cancer.

And now I have granddaughters.

For all these reasons, I was curious to know how others felt about the test. And the response has been interesting. So many of those who took the test were absolutely convinced that they had the gene, only to test negative. But in fact, studies have found that only 5 percent of all breast cancer patients carry a BRCA mutation—meaning that if you are diagnosed with breast cancer, chances are 95 percent that you do *not* carry the gene.

That said, there is nothing scientific about this chapter. I asked *UPLIFT*ers how they felt about being tested for the BRCAs. Is there a general consensus about what to do? No. But there are different reasons for considering it, and that's what I want you to read.

I haven't decided one way or another myself. Given that my mother, her mother, my sisters, and a cousin have all had breast cancer—and that I fall into a highly prone ethnic group—I pretty much assume I do carry the gene. If so, do my kids need to know yet? Do they *want* to know? Would they do anything different at this point?

For now, I'm waiting. Next year or the year after? That might be the time.

As *UPLIFT*er Renee Johannesen put it in deciding to wait, "I have made the right decision for me at this point in my life."

You all have to make the decision that's right for you. Any decision is okay. My hope is that one or another of the following thoughts will resonate and bring you comfort. That is the essence of *UPLIFT*.

YES, PLEASE

"Last October, I had the BRCA gene test. My two daughters had mixed feelings; one did not want to know the results, and the other wasn't sure. My test was negative. I am glad I did it, but it may not be right for everyone."

Sandra Haymart; diagnosed in 1990 at age 47; retired chief deputy circuit court clerk; Missouri

"I did the gene testing, as I have five sisters, two daughters, and two granddaughters. I felt it was important to know what their future might hold. I did not have the gene, but I had no family history either. None of us are exempt from this disease, although most of us (like me) think it won't happen to us. When it does, you truly know what a gift life is. I don't waste even a minute of it!"

Pamela Miltner; diagnosed in 1993 at age 40;
insurance agent; Indiana

"I was first diagnosed with breast cancer in 1975, and I am still here at the age of seventy-two! I had my only daughter in 1980, and she is expecting her first child in April. I will be undergoing genetic testing in March for her sake, as well as for the sake of my sister and her female descendants."

Dorothy Coon; diagnosed in 1975 at age 35;
retired college mathematics professor; New York

"Cancer is a disease that we cannot control, so we need to gather as much knowledge as possible in order to know how to treat it. After I had the BRCA gene test and was negative, I still opted to take off the right breast, and it was the best decision that I ever made concerning my health care. The BRCA gene test is simply another tool we can use. Information is power, and the worst feeling is being powerless. Waiting for the results of the test was frightening, but I would have regretted *not* taking the test. I wanted to have the test done for my three sons and their future families."

Cathy Hanlon; diagnosed in 2000 at age 42;
volunteer, substitute teacher; New York

"Once I was diagnosed with Stage III breast cancer, I did opt to go through genetic counseling for the sake of my daughter, my sisters, and other family members. Also to aid in research regarding breast cancer. I ended up with a negative test result. But I opted for a prophylactic hysterectomy anyway. What they found probably saved my life, as there was cancer in the fimbria of the ovaries. It turned out as a very happy ending for me, and I think that as time goes on these tests are only going to become more refined and perfected. My opinion, which I share with whoever asks me, is *do it*! Knowledge is everything in fighting this disease, so arm yourself with whatever you can!"

Ellen Christopherson; diagnosed in 2004 at age 44;
law firm office manager; Minnesota

"In April of 2000, I had a bilateral mastectomy. I have three grown children and six grandchildren. Since there was no breast cancer as far as I knew in my family, the doctor suggested I have the BRCA gene test. I met with the nurse, and after much thought decided that for the health of my children and grand-children I would have the test. Waiting for the results was stress-ful. What if I do have the gene? What will my children (especially my daughters) decide to do? But like so much else on my journey with breast cancer, I spent too much time worrying about 'what might happen.' My results were negative, but my daughters are still very aware of their chance of getting breast cancer, and we re-main our own advocates for our health."

Ceil Gallucci; diagnosed in 2000 at age 52;
retired occupational therapist; New Jersey

"I had genetic testing done, as I am a Stage IV survivor and have four daughters, aged 18–23. I needed to know for them. Doctors say I do not have BRCA1 or 2, but I have a cousin, just my age, who does. Of my generation of cousins, four of eight have had cancer. I feel there are genes out there that have not been ex-plored yet. There is so much more to discover in order to truly find a cure!"

Julie Chandler; diagnosed in 2002 at age 42;
mom, volunteer, former reading teacher; Colorado

"I was diagnosed with breast cancer at forty-two, and my surgeon and oncologist both told me about the BRCA test. We discussed the importance of the test for my future surgical decisions, as well as for my family. I have a daughter and two sisters. At first I was truly hesitant to find one more thing wrong with me, but no way was I blowing off the chance to improve my daughter's life.

"The blood work itself was pretty painless. Recounting family history was a mind task, but my counselor was patient as we went through every family member possible on both sides. I was amazed at how much I learned during that two-hour visit. For instance, myth tells you that breast cancer can't be passed on from the dad's side, but this is so not true, I learned!

"It turns out I am BRCA negative. But I wanted to do whatever I could to help others, so I chose to have my information added to the data bank. That way, any new findings and tests that become available for genetic testing will be offered to me.

"Before I was tested, my heart was telling me to do the double mastectomy. This process helped me to solidify that decision. I've been going with my gut throughout this whole process, and it proved to be a tough one. I've told many women the same thing—that you have to do what feels right for you. That's what makes living as a survivor a truly uplifting experience!"

Angela Booth; diagnosed in 2010 at age 42;
Orange Board of Education; Connecticut

"I am a survivor of twenty-nine years, but genetic testing has just recently become available as more of a 'routine test.' After discussing it with my doctor, I decided to have it done. I wanted to know what genes I carried and could possibly pass on to my daughter and my grandchildren."

Taylor Montagna; diagnosed in 1982 at age 42;
retired; Indiana

"I have been living with cancer since 1974, when I was first diagnosed. I have two daughters, and when I decided to have genetic testing done, one wanted to know and one did not. I decided it was like not having a caution sign to warn you about a bridge out on the road ahead. It just seemed that we would be better informed for future times if we knew. The test was simple, and it put our minds at ease because I did not have the BRCA gene."

Linda Almond; diagnosed in 1974 at age 27;
retired; North Carolina

"I was forty when I was diagnosed with breast cancer. After a year, my mother was diagnosed and, six months after that, my aunt was diagnosed. So it was a no-brainer for me that I should have the BRCA test done. I have an older sister who has a daughter, and I have two daughters myself. Sounds like we are a great test group. Well, to our surprise, the test was negative.

"The BRCA gene is a great finding. Just remember that it doesn't change what can or will happen. Always be preventative when it comes to your health care."

Kelly Anglim; diagnosed in 2007 at age 40;
Michigan

"After my mother, aunt, and sister all had breast cancer, the doctors had asked me to take the BRCA test, but I refused. When I was diagnosed myself, I had it done. When the results came back, all my doctors were shocked. I tested negative! To me this was a blessing, since if I had tested positive, I would have had a hysterectomy."

Carol Bonapace; diagnosed in 2009 at age 59;
secretary; Connecticut

"I decided to have genetic testing done. I thought it was important to know for my daughter and granddaughter, since my mother also had breast cancer. I found out I wasn't a carrier. It gave me a peace of mind knowing."

Judy Peterson; diagnosed in 2000 at age 58; retired RN; Colorado

"My mother, aunt, and cousin are breast cancer survivors. So when I was diagnosed in 2008, I wanted to confirm the genetics of this disease for my two daughters. I took the BRCA test in 2009 only to have it come back negative."

Maria Hammon; diagnosed in 2008 at age 53; retired government IT worker; Illinois

"My family has been affected by cancer in so many ways. Two of my daughters just had the BRCA test done, and my other daughter and I are waiting for medical insurance approvals. It isn't just curiosity that motivates us, but I have grandchildren who could be affected. Also, the outcome of the test can affect the meds if we have recurrences."

Carol Cooper; diagnosed in 2004 at age 70; senior account clerk; New York

"As an RN, I knew of the BRCA gene test, though it was not commonplace then. But my mother had breast cancer twice, so it was a responsible request. I did test positive and proceeded to have a bilateral mastectomy with reconstruction. Since I already had my children, I had my ovaries and fallopian tubes taken out a year later. This proactive stance was the best form of action I could have taken. It was right for my body, mind, and spirit."

Linda Schneider; diagnosed in 1999 at age 39; director of adult health care, author; New York

"After my sister and mother were diagnosed with breast cancer, I decided to undergo BRCA testing. I went into it assuming I would test positive. In addition to having two first-degree relatives with breast cancer, I fit the ethnic demographic. Before I began the process, I thought out in advance what steps I would take— definitely having my ovaries removed, possibly undergoing a prophylactic double mastectomy. When I found out I didn't have either of the two BRCA mutations the test identifies, the result was almost anticlimactic. A huge relief, though! The doctors reminded me that even though I don't have the BRCA mutations, I am still considered high-risk, so I am disciplined to the point of obsession about breast exams and mammograms. So far, so good!

"During her own treatment for breast cancer, my sister urged me not to have the test done. She was afraid that if I tested positive, this would be considered a 'preexisting condition' and I would have problems if I ever needed to obtain new medical insurance. I hope that with the new healthcare law now in effect, this would no longer be an issue for women considering undergoing the test."

Barbara Keiler; daughter of a survivor;
novelist, Massachusetts

"The reason I decided on the BRCA gene test is that I'm a Jew and my parents were from Eastern Europe. Even though one oncologist had done a two-hour consult with me and ascertained that I was at low risk for the gene, I simply felt that it was the responsible thing to do as the mother of two daughters.

"The most tenuous part was waiting the three weeks for the results. When the nurse called to say that the results were negative, she reiterated that because I didn't have that particular gene, it didn't mean my daughters and I were at no risk for cancer. She said our risk was the same as the rest of the population.

"I never reported my results to my daughters. I didn't want to give them the false confidence of not carrying the cancer gene and in turn neglecting to take care of their breasts."

Diana Raab; diagnosed in 2001 at age 47;
writer, nurse; California

"I was tested about three years ago for the BRCA gene, and my results were negative. I was adopted, so my doctor thought it would be a good idea, since I don't know my family history."

Jennifer Wersal; diagnosed in 2000 at age 30;
race and communications manager, Komen Greater Fort Worth; Texas

"Three years ago, my oncologist suggested I have genetic testing done to look into why I had Stage IV breast cancer at thirty-two (now I'm forty-eight). She talked about the pros and cons and told me to get back to her. I called the next day. My first thought was my seventeen-year-old daughter. Did she need to know if I carried the marker? Yes. Did I need to know for me? No. What ultimately pushed me to have it done was thinking that if I didn't and my daughter got sick and there would have been things done to prevent it, the feeling would be worse than going through chemo again.

"I decided not to tell anyone that I was having it done. I am fortunate, in that there was no marker."

B.C.; diagnosed in 1995 at age 32;
event coordinator; California

"I was diagnosed with Stage III breast cancer in December of 2009 at the age of thirty-six. Shortly after my diagnosis, I was encouraged to get the genetic testing done. Quite honestly, at that time I was in survival mode and only interested in beating the disease. It was only after a double mastectomy, chemo, radiation, reconstruction, and removal of my ovaries that I sat back and said to myself, 'Did I do everything possible to prevent this disease from rearing its ugly head again?'

"I wondered if genetic testing was even relevant at this point. I didn't have any children yet. Then my attention turned to my two younger sisters and the eggs that I had frozen before starting chemotherapy. Wouldn't knowing if I carry the BRCA gene be helpful to them? So this past fall I did have the testing done, and it turns out I don't have the mutation. I have to be honest, I was so relieved and elated. It helped alleviate my fears of recurrence, of my sisters getting breast cancer, and possibly one day my own daughter. I would encourage any woman contemplating this test to just do it. Having peace of mind goes a long way."

Tiffany Mannino; diagnosed in 2009 at age 36;

sixth-grade teacher; Pennsylvania

NO, THANKS, NOT YET

"I was the first in my family to be diagnosed with breast cancer. That was almost eighteen years ago. I have an eighteen-year-old daughter and have struggled with the decision to be tested. At this point, I have decided against it. Even if I have the gene, I do not plan to have a mastectomy, and I am already vigilant about my daughter performing self-exams and receiving mammograms. Perhaps I will feel differently in several years. If my daughter wanted me to take the BRCA gene test to give her some peace of mind, I might consider it. But I have made the right decision for me at this point in my life."

Renee Johannesen; diagnosed in 1993 at age 35;

teacher; New York

"I am a ten-year survivor who was diagnosed with breast cancer at the age of twenty-nine. There was no family history, so this was quite a surprise at the time. I have been advised to speak with a counselor regarding BRCA gene testing, but have not done so yet. I don't feel the decision will bother me either way, but I just haven't felt it was a priority right now. I have no children, so I also don't feel the rush to do this."

Christine DiGiovanni; diagnosed in 2000 at age 29;

New York

"I have decided not to have genetic testing done at this time, because I don't think it would change me or make me do anything different from what I've done."

Doris Cantrell; diagnosed in 1992 at age 52;

registered nurse; Michigan

"After being diagnosed with DCIS in April 2007, I was offered the opportunity to have genetic testing. I have always eaten healthy and exercised, am a nonsmoker, and breast-fed my children. With this background, a cancer diagnosis was a shock. My daughters exercise, eat healthy, and are nonsmokers, too, and they will start breast cancer detection at an earlier age than I did. So I did not see the need for genetic testing."

Judy Farrell; diagnosed in 2007 at age 45;

physical education teacher; Indiana

"Being the daughter of a mom who died of breast cancer makes the disease so much more real. I think that testing for the BRCA gene is a wonderful thing. However, just because you have the gene doesn't mean you will actually get breast cancer. For me, I believe I wouldn't have peace if I knew I had the gene. I also wouldn't want to do something radical, like have a mastectomy, based simply on something that may or may not happen to me in the future. I believe it's important for a woman to keep up with monthly self-check-ups and with mammograms."

Lori Smith; daughter of mother with breast cancer;

South Carolina

20 • What *UPLIFT* Does

I have written many books, but the one—*the* one—of which I am most proud is *UPLIFT*. This book helps women at a terrifying time. It boosts their spirits, convinces them that they will get through treatment and thrive. It makes them smile in the dark of the night—and this is important. There are, in fact, studies suggesting that emotions affect body chemistry, that happiness leads to an increase in illness-fighting cells in the bloodstream, that laughter can reduce pain. Does smiling actually make us live longer? I don't know about that. But it sure enhances our quality of life.

Consider these recent entries in the Survivor's Journal on my website:

"I found out that I have breast cancer four days ago. My husband bought me tons of books on the subject. They were too scary. I went to Amazon and saw *UPLIFT,* and I just got it tonight. I am laughing and crying and empathizing all at the same time. I feel like I am part of a support group already." Or this: "An old friend gave me *UPLIFT* after I had surgery for breast cancer this past summer. I would read a portion of it at a time, and reread some parts when I needed the extra reassurance." Or this: "How uplifting to read the number of years that some are postdiagnosis. You all give me the gift of hope! Thank you so very much, as I needed to hear this message today."

But there's a bigger piece to the *UPLIFT* pie that most of you haven't seen. It's the breast fellowship at Massachusetts General Hospital that *UPLIFT* helped to create and continues to fund. Under the brilliant hand of Dr. Barbara L. Smith, director of the Breast Program at MGH, the fellowship offers fully trained surgeons an additional year of training focused on innovative breast cancer treatment and research. Known within MGH circles as the Team Uplift Fellowship, the program reaches beyond one institution. Though still based at Mass General, the fellows deepen their experience by spending time at two MGH Partner institutions, Brigham and Women's Hospital (BWH) and Dana-Farber Cancer Institute (DFCI).

The first fellow began her year in July 2003. Once word of the fellowship spread, support grew within the medical community, resulting in some years when two fellows have served. Fellows have come from all over the country—actually, from all over the world. Indeed, Dr. Srila Samphao, currently a breast surgeon at Prince of Songkla University in Thailand, was a fellow in Boston during the 2008–2009 season.

As of the publication of this Tenth Anniversary Edition of *UPLIFT*, there will have been fourteen amazing participants. That's fourteen doctors spending the next several decades working to improve the treatment of breast cancer.

Each June, I get to have tea with the year's fellows and hear face-to-face about the work that they've done. Talk about uplifting! I leave that tea riding high—and, trust me, it ain't from the caffeine in the tea. These fellows are remarkable.

It occurred to me that maybe you'd like to hear from them, too. When I asked for a few words, they sent glowing reports. This is a tribute to Dr. Smith, who inspires them as she inspires

me, but it also points to the hope about the future that these fellows feel.

I'd like to share their words with you. And not only their words.
Take a look at the medical positions they're holding after their fellowship year. This will blow you away.

July 2003–June 2004
*Julie L. Jones, MD, Director, Saints Breast Care Center, Saints Medical
Center, Lowell, MA*

"The Partners Fellowship was the high point of my surgical training. Dr. Barbara Smith is an amazing mentor, and helped me to
generate an expertise for which I am grateful, and which I try to
pass on every day."

July 2003–December 2003
*Marissa M. Howard-McNatt, MD, Assistant Professor, General Surgery,
Wake Forest University Baptist Medical Center, Winston-Salem, NC*

"My experience as a breast surgery fellow was invaluable. The fellowship allowed me to gain knowledge not only about the surgical care of breast cancer patients, but also their medical
management, radiation treatments, reconstructive options, and
psychosocial concerns. I was given the tools to perform clinical
research studies in order to improve my knowledge in the field,
and learned to have a compassionate eye for the breast cancer
patient's needs and concerns."

July 2004–June 2005
*Katherina Zabicki Calvillo, MD, FACS, Associate Surgeon, Brigham
and Women's Hospital/Dana-Farber Cancer Institute, Boston, MA*

"The breast fellowship at MGH/BWH/DFCI is unlike any other
in the country. You are able to work with sixteen breast surgeons,
giving you the rare opportunity to observe different practice

styles at internationally renowned medical centers. What a breast fellowship does is teach you how to operate on breast cancer patients with the mentality of an oncologist, rather than a general surgeon, considering all aspects of a patient's care, such as medical oncology, radiation oncology, and high-risk genetics. You also have the ability to hone your imaging reading skills. These are all aspects of treating breast cancer patients that you don't really get during your general surgery training."

August 2004–June 2006
Francisco Domínguez, Cancer Surgeon, Cancer Centre Universidad Católica de Chile, Santiago, Chile

"My training at the MGH's fellowship in breast surgery was the most comprehensive and significant learning period of my medical training. The multidisciplinary approach to cancer care definitely helped me learn how to take care of my patients in the most professional and unique way. Healthcare professionals at MGH are focused on getting the best treatment with the least possible side effects for breast cancer patients. I learned how breast oncologists are always looking for better treatments, with their minds always open to clinical research, and putting into practice new diagnostic or treatment advances. They showed me different approaches to a variety of patient problems and encouraged me to make decisions based on the patient's best interest."

July 2005–June 2006
Dalliah M. Black, MD, FACS, Breast Surgical Oncologist, Sibley Memorial Hospital, Washington, DC

"The breast surgical oncology fellowship at Massachusetts General Hospital provided me with invaluable experience in the latest breast cancer techniques, contributing to the scientific arena, and most important learning how to provide each patient with personalized care and the highest level of compassion. I am honored that women entrust their cancer care to me."

July 2006–June 2007
Laurie Kirstein, MD, Breast Surgeon, Beth Israel Medical Center, New York, NY

"Deciding to do a breast surgical oncology fellowship was the best decision I have made. It was the result of a path that was influenced by personal and professional experiences. In my first rotation as a medical student, I rounded on a woman as her bandages were removed from her recent mastectomy. The scar was hideous, and there was no addressing the psychological impact this had on her. My immediate thought was, "There has to be a better way than this." Throughout my surgical residency, I had peripheral contact with breast cancer patients in the operating room or immediately postoperatively, but was never involved in their workup or follow-up. I yearned to know more about the management of the disease, but also to form a relationship with these women to make sure they were getting all of their needs addressed, not only physically but psychologically and emotionally.

"I had high expectations coming into this breast fellowship. Since there are only a handful of fellowship-trained breast surgeons in the country, I knew the education I would be receiving was special. The breast fellowship was over and away my best year of training. Because the fellowship is multidisciplinary, I was able to fill in the gaps of knowledge. Breast surgeons are the gatekeepers for care. Because of my fellowship, I know that I am referring my patients appropriately for chemotherapy and radiation, which has an impact on their overall survival. And because of the oncoplastic techniques and careful thought to incision planning taught during my fellowship, most of my patients have beautiful cosmetic results. I have often said that when my patient looks in the mirror at her chest, I don't want her first thought to be of the cancer. In my fellowship, I learned the techniques to achieve this goal."

September 2005–March 2007

Jennifer Rusby, MD, Breast Surgeon, Royal Marsden Hospital, Sutton, UK

"The research fellowship at Massachusetts General Hospital enabled me to investigate the anatomy and pathology of the nipple in detail which has helped provide a scientific basis for nipple-sparing mastectomy. Coincidentally, this week I am speaking at a conference in Washington, D.C., on the safety of nipple preservation in risk-reducing mastectomy. The invitation to speak is a direct result of the work I did at MGH."

July 2007–June 2008

Colleen D. Murphy, MD, Medical Director, Porter Comprehensive Breast Care, Denver, CO

"My breast surgery fellowship gave me the opportunity to learn from surgeons, medical oncologists, radiation oncologists, pathologists, and radiologists who are the world's leading experts in breast cancer. As I started practice, I quickly found this cutting-edge and well-rounded knowledge base gave me all the tools I needed to build a multidisciplinary breast cancer program in a community that previously lacked access to comprehensive cancer care."

July 2007–June 2008

Sara H. Javid, MD, Breast Surgeon, Seattle Cancer Care Alliance, Seattle, WA

"The breast surgery fellowship provided me a unique and wonderful opportunity to learn from many experts in their respective fields how to best care for my patients with breast cancer. I took away many skills, one of the most important being how to appropriately tailor each patient's treatment plan not only to her cancer but to fit with her own personal goals and desires."

June 2008–July 2009
Amanda Wheeler, MD, Medical Director, Legacy Meridian Park Breast Health Center, Portland, OR

"This was the most rewarding year of my academic life. The expertise I gained through my fellowship at Massachusetts General Hospital, Dana-Farber Cancer Institute, and Brigham and Women's Hospital has allowed me to offer quality care to the women in my community who are diagnosed and treated for breast cancer. Dr. Smith should be recognized; her dedication to training breast surgeons is truly heroic."

July 2009–June 2010
Elizabeth Kim, Assistant Professor of Surgery, Wayne State University, Karmanos Cancer Institute, Detroit, MI

"The fellowship was an invaluable experience for me to hone my clinical and operative skills with world-class breast surgeons. I finished my fellowship with an unforgettable life lesson about myself: There is nothing in the world that can compare with the true joy I feel when caring for breast cancer patients. I value this relationship, and it is what sustains me and inspires my creativity in the area of breast research. I am very grateful for the opportunity I had to learn from the MGH breast surgeons. My program director, Dr. Barbara L. Smith, was a role model in becoming an excellent breast surgeon and leader. This fellowship has allowed me to provide world-class breast cancer care in Michigan. I am excited for the future breast fellows who will have this opportunity at MGH."

July 2010–June 2011
Suzanne Coopey, MD, Breast Surgery Fellow, Massachusetts General Hospital, Brigham and Women's Hospital, Dana-Farber Cancer Institute, Boston, MA

"The breast fellowship at the Massachusetts General Hospital, Dana-Farber Cancer Institute, and Brigham and Women's Hospital has been an amazing learning experience. I have worked closely with breast surgeons, medical oncologists, radiation oncologists, pathologists, radiologists, and plastic surgeons who are leaders in their fields. This has given me such an appreciation for the multidisciplinary treatment of breast cancer patients and afforded me the opportunity to do collaborative clinical research projects. This has been one of the best and most important years of my life, and I look forward to the career that lies ahead of me as a breast surgeon."

Rereading these statements, I am in awe yet again. The idea that *UPLIFT* has helped bring this about is mind-boggling. I like to think that my mother, dead when I was eight but always my mentor, is smiling down on me and is proud.

Every survivor gives back in her own way. *UPLIFT* is mine. But you all have played a role as well. You are the ones who buy this book and give it to friends, and those sales are what fund this fellowship.

On behalf of the fellows, the hospital, the breast care community, and every woman who has been or will be diagnosed with breast cancer, I thank you.

Acknowledgments

Since its inception, *UPLIFT* has been a grassroots project. It is therefore fitting that my acknowledgments start and end with everyday people. I don't even know the names of some of those who spread the word (how *did* Lieutenant Governor Corinne Wood of Illinois hear about *UPLIFT*?), but I do know that the following people played a part and deserve my thanks: Carol Baggaley, Jane Bender, Dale Berthiaume, Karen Boml, Martin Bradley, Marilyn Brier, Louise Broach, Jeanne Bryner, Robin Homonoff, Autumn Hughes, Treazure Johnson, Bobbi Kolton, Cristy Peck, Lucy Pino, Sue Rabin, Martha Raddatz, Jane Salk, Linda Saulnier, Suzanne Schmidt, Jensie Shipley, Ellen Beth Simon, Lynn Smith, Phyllis Stoller, Cindy Teeple, Claire White, Cindy Wilkins, Susan Wornick, and Nancy Zlotek.

My thanks to the wonderful women and men who disseminated information about *UPLIFT* through their medical facilities and support networks: Peggie Barten at Good Samaritan Diagnostic Center North in Florida; Deb Belfato at Susan G. Komen Center in New Jersey; Corinne Cook at Inova Alexandria Hospital Cancer Center in Virginia; Wanda Diak at Cancer Hope Network in New Jersey; Kathy Dorner at the Cancer Center at Arlington Hospital in Virginia; Julie Durmis at Dana-Farber Cancer Institute in Massachusetts; James Dye at Christ Hospital Cancer Center in Ohio; Leslie Dykhouse at Fairfax Radiology Center in Virginia; Joan Frier of SHARE in New York; Francine Halberg at Marin Cancer Institute in California; Marsha Komandt at Inova Fairfax Hospital in Virginia; Helen Maurice at UConn Cancer Center in Connecticut; Catherine Owens at Carol G. Simon Cancer Center in New Jersey; and Susan Sharp at Julius Hermes Breast Cancer Center in Virginia.

Massachusetts General Hospital has been part of my life since my mother was treated there when I was a child. Though I always knew that it would remain part of my life medically, I never dreamed that there would be a professional cross-over, yet that has happened with *UPLIFT*. So, my *huge* thanks to all at Mass General who helped spread word of this project, beginning but not ending with those in the Development Office: Amy Fontanella, Beth Alterman, and Peggy Slassman. Thanks to Marie Becker, who connected with each of the Team Uplift fellows on my behalf. A very special, very personal thanks to Dr. Barbara L. Smith, who not only saved my life surgically, but saved me professionally by reading each edition of *UPLIFT* prior to publication, catching several near-bloopers and, in this Tenth Anniversary Edition, updating medical thought.

The writing community lent me a hand with an eagerness that has touched me deeply. I thank Elaine Raco Chase, Sandra Brown, and Dorothea Benton Frank. I thank Lauren Nichols, Jane Vaughan, Marcia Talley, and Blanche Marriott. I thank the *readers* of my novels, women like Nikki Provenzano, Lytrice Mains, Susan Edmondson, and Diane Williamson, who sent information on *UPLIFT* to anyone and everyone they knew who has tackled breast cancer.

And then there's the publishing world in New York. *UPLIFT* would not be the book it is today without the enthusiasm, support, and expertise of Judith Curr and Karen Mender, Michael Korda, Tracy Bernstein, Maggie Crawford, Emily Bestler, Sarah Branham, and, *UPLIFT*'s most recent shepherd, Sarah Durand. My thanks to all of these wonderful people.

I am deeply indebted to my agent, Amy Berkower. If *UPLIFT* could not have happened without my attaining the success with my fiction that I have, Amy has to take some of the credit. She is a skilled advocate, who has guided my career warmly and wisely.

Legally, I thank William Eisen. I thank Fauzia Burke and Carol Fitzgerald, both of whom have helped amazingly with online publicity. For more traditional services, I thank Barry Michaelson, Diane Charron, Scott Mason, and Wendy Page. Steve Bennett of Authorbytes.com deserves a special round of applause for designing the pages at www.barbaradelinsky.com devoted to *UPLIFT*.

Huge, *huge* thanks go to Lucy Davis. As my administrative assistant, Lucy has made life immeasurably easier for me. Without her dedication and skill, this Tenth Annversary Edition of *UPLIFT* might never have happened.

And my family? Well, folks, it's grown since the last edition of *UPLIFT*. I never had daughters but now do have *grand*daughters, which makes my goal of funding research to find a cure for breast cancer all the more urgent. That said, I couldn't have produced the *first* edition of *UPLIFT*, much less the second, third, and fourth, without the infinite patience, unremItting enthusiasm, and steady love of my husband, our sons, and their wives and kids.

Have I failed to mention others? No doubt about it, if only because *UPLIFT* was such a word-of-mouth project that friends told friends, who told other friends. I tip my hat to you all.

Lastly, mostly, I acknowledge the women and men of *UPLIFT*—survivors all—who put their hearts and souls into writing to me and whose words comprise the body of now four editions of this book. I stand in awe of their courage and generosity. If goodness counts for anything, they will live long and well!

List of Contributors

A
Jeryl Abelmann
Joyce Abercrombie
Linda Almond
Suzanne Almond
Rosamary Amiet
Eleanor Anbinder
George Anbinder
Cat Andrews
Lynne Andrus
Kelly Anglim
Gwen Angstrom
Jacki Anthony
Robert Anthony
Willie Mae Ashley
Janice Austad

B
Patricia Baker
Donna Barnett
Sallie Barron
Lori Bartz

Judy Bayha
Joanne Bellontine
Rosemary Bentley
Ruth Berler
Cindy Bird
Laurie Bishop
Gail Blackmer
Margaret Blair
Christine Bohnet
Carol Bonapace
Diane Bongiorno
Angela Booth
Dianne Bouford
Elise Bourne-Busby
Betsy Ellis Bowles
Sue Braun
Lois Brender
Polly Briggs
Cheryl Brinker
Nancy Brown
Sandra Baldwin Brown
Gerald Browne

Alice Bruneau
Mary Ann Budnick
Billie Bules
Sallie Burdine
Nancy Burgess
Linda Jones Burns

C
JoAnn Cámara
Doris Cantrell
Linda Caradec
Brenda Carr
Patricia Carr
Sharon Carr
Adelaide Carrara
Nanette Carter
Cheryl Cavallo
Glenda Chance
Florence Chandler
Julie Chandler
Elaine Raco Chase
Ellen Christopherson
Rose Marie Clark
Rebecca Clarkson
E. Mary Lou Clauss
Susan Clemente
Lorraine Colavito
Beth Compton
Nan Comstock
Joann Connor
Carol Contrino
Dorothy Coon
Carol Cooper

Miriam Cooper
Tiffany Corbell
Diane Cotting
Julie Crandall
Dona Crowe
Hope Cruickshank
Alysa Cummings

D
Virginia Danczak
Cathleen D'Antonio
Mark D'Antonio
Donna Danzis
Michele Darby
Tammy Delin
Patti Dempster
Debra DeSocio
Helene Deutsch
Marti Devich
Fran DiBiase
Christine DiGiovanni
Carol Dine
Cornelia Doherty
Gail Dorfman
Carol Downer
Carrie Drake
Jacqueline Durant
Linda Dyer

E
Maryann Eberhard
Ellinore Eckel
Marilyn Eichner

Joan Eldredge
Maybelle Timm Eley
Nancy Ellis
Carol Englund
Sharon Erbe

F

Sara Fallgren
Elinor Farber
Judy Farrell
Alyce Feinstein
Bonnie Fergerson
Janice Ferrari
Cynthia Ferus
Cindy Fiedler
Jean Firkser
Carol Fischer
Beatrice Flannagan
Michele Fleitell
Christine Foutris
Marge Fuller

G

Sandy Gabriel
Debra Gainey
Frances Gallello
Ceil Gallucci
Alan S. Gardner
Donna Garrison
Marcia Gibbons
Corda M. Gilliland
Wendy Golab
Sheri Goodman

Ann Gordon
Betsy Goree
Karen L. Graves
Susan Grayson-Johnson
Mindy Greenside
Kathleen Griffith
Richard Griffith
Jill Gross
Therese Gunty

H

Deb Haggerty
Maria Hammon
Deb Haney
Cathy Hanlon
Faye Hardiman
Betty Harris
Barbara Hartman
Carol Hattler
Wahnita Hawk
Sandra Haymart
Fran Hegarty
Dot Heimer
Helaine Hemingway
Jacqueline Hickey
Ruth Hill
Kim (Dyer) Hills
Becky Honeycutt
Judy Hooper
Annelle Houk
Caroline C. Hudnall
Pauline Hughes
Carole Humphrey

Irene Louise
Gwen Loverink
Ellen R. Luecke

M
Debbie MacLean
Rita Madison
Marcella Malamut
Katie Mandra
Suzanne Mann
Tiffany Mannino
Holly Marion
Sandy Mark
Lois Marks
Michele Marks
Sally Martel
Patti Martinez
Sharon Matsumoto
Monica May
Marianne McCaskill
Christine McNamara
Denis McNamara
Frances Meadow
Beth Meister
Carol Merrill
Joan Merritt
Holly Metcalf
Asha Mevlana
Ellie Meyers
Marshall Miller
Nina Miller
Sandra Miller
Mimi Mills

Pamela Miltner
Marian Anne Miziorko
Midge Mohler
Pat Mohr
Taylor Montagna
Angela Moore
Lynnette Moore
Barbara Moro
Jinny Morrison
Barbara Mulvey
Carleen Muniz
Sheilah Musselman

N
Lauren Nichols
Liz Nippert
Stella Norman
Louise Norville
Wanda Null

O
Nancy Oken
Judith Ormond

P
Dorothy Padilla
Wendy Page
Lorraine J. Pakkala-Lintala
Vicky Pakso
Donna Palmer
Gene Palmer
Joanne Palmer
Aileen Pandapas

Deborah Parker
Carol Pasternak
Linda Perkins
Rozanne Perlman
Judy Peterson
Arlene Petty
Barbara Phelps
Diane Phillips
Deborah Pierce
Mary Platt
Al Pobjoy
Dee Pobjoy
Suzanne Pollock
Betty Pollom
Paula Porter
Hilary Prince

Q
Lynn Quanrud
Lela Quimby
Carol Quinn

R
Diana Raab
Kathy Rabassa
Mary Raffol
Susan Ragland
Rayna Ragonetti
Judith H. Reilly
Marianne Rennie
Antonia Rhodes
Gail Rice
Kimberlee Richardson
Debbie Roberts

Sandy Rodgers
Sheila Roper
Lyn Rosenthal
Susan Rothstein
Roz Rowley
Jane Royal-Davidson
Mary Ruddell
Lynne Rutenberg

S
Susan Sanford
Judi Scally
Mitzi Scarborough
John E. Schlimm II
Sharon (Daniels) Schmitt
Bonnie Schneider
Linda Schneider
Betty Schulte
Susan Schultz
Deborah J.P. Schur
Jennifer Schuster
Dave Schwingel
Gracie Schwingel
Nancy Sena
Barb Seyl
Rae Shapiro
Ellen Beth Simon
Cindy Sloan
Earlene Smith
Lori Smith
Robin Smith
Susan Smith
Carol Snyder
Dorian Solot

Evan Solot
Leslie Solot
Rhonda Sorrell
Elizabeth Daniels Squire
Susan Stamberg
Carolyn Stein
Sheila Steinhauser
Tobi Stelzer
Mary Stewart
Dixie Stoller
Maribeth Stone
Sharon Irons Strempski
Sarah Stuart
Jeanne Sturdevant
Paul E. Sturdevant
Nancy Summersong
Barbara C. Sumner
Valerie Swett

T
Marcia Talley
Cindy L. Teeple
Laura Thomas
Angela Thompson
Nanette Thorsen-Snipes
Grace Trocco
Donna Troiani
Penny Trosterman
Joanne Tutschek

V
Jane Vaughan
Regina Vaughn
Robert David Vaughan

Kim Vermeire
Ester Vicent
Diana Vise
Judy Von Bergen

W
Pam Waddell
Florence Wade
Cheryl Wagner
Charron Walker
P.J. Wamble
Kathi Ward
Nancie Watson
Sue Watson
Kathy Weaver-Stark
Christine Webber
Cleves Daniels Weber
Barbara M. Wells
Sherry Ann Wells
Jennifer Wersal
Joy West
Pat West
Janet Whitaker
Brandon Whittet
Bryan Whittet
Debby Whittet
Bec Wiget
Helen Wilker
Marvin Wilker
Cheryl Wilkinson
Diane Wilkinson-Codon
Lee Williams
Oglatha Williams
Penny Williams

Sandy Williams
Dorothy A. Wilson
Mary Wise
Joyce Wiswell
Corinne Wood

Y
Regina R. Young

Z
Diane Zellar
Helen Zibuda
Heather Marie Zielke
Susan Zimmerman
Jane Zinda

An Invitation from *UPLIFT*

Please join us! Once you've read *UPLIFT*, you'll have thoughts of your own about what helps and what doesn't. Make note of these thoughts on the journal pages that follow. As many of the original *UPLIFT* submitters have pointed out, this can be therapeutic. Taking it a step further, if you would like to share your ideas, you can make an entry in the Survivor's Journal on the Breast Cancer Book page at www.barbaradelinsky.com, or send them to me c/o *UPLIFT*, PO Box 812894, Wellesley, MA 02482-0026.

For your convenience, I include the general guidelines that were followed by the original contributors to *UPLIFT*. Keep in mind, though, that these are only suggestions. You may have already discovered dozens of other topics that relate to having breast cancer. The following guidelines are simply to get you thinking. My only request is that you be . . . well, uplifting!

I have what!?

What was the most constructive thing you did after hearing your diagnosis?

What was the most helpful thing someone else did for you upon learning of your diagnosis?

Whom did you tell, when, and why?
Did you tell your children?
Did you tell your boss?
How did you tell the person you most feared telling? What made it easier?

Sister, friends, and bosses . . .
What single most practical thing did a friend or family member do to help?
What single most helpful thing was done for you in the workplace?
How did you juggle cancer and work? What little tricks helped?

What about the men in your life?
How did they react to your bout with breast cancer? (Can I have a quote from them, too?)
Husbands? Lovers? Sons? Brothers? Friends?

Hair today?
What most raised your spirits when your hair began to fall out?
Did you wear a hat when you had no hair? If so, what kind worked best?
Tell me about being bald. Tell me about wigs. Tell me about growing new hair.

When the going gets tough, do the tough go shopping?
What was your favorite piece of clothing during treatment, and why?
What single purchase most lifted your spirits?
How did you overcome the self-consciousness of undressing in front of others?

What was . . . what did . . . what is . . . ?
What kind of food helped curb nausea during chemo? Gave you energy? Gave you a lift?

What did you do with the tattoos on your body when radiation was done?

What made you feel the most feminine during this time? The most sexy?

What did you do to show people that you were still alive and well?

What helped pass quiet times in lieu of worrying? A hobby, perhaps? If so, what and why?

What one person, place, or thing made you feel most in control?

What was the funniest thing that happened to you during all this?

What is the single most important piece of advice you would give to a friend going through what you did?

A walk in the park . . .

What physical challenges did you face during rehabilitation? What helped most? Who helped most?

What sports did you do before breast cancer? After? How did it help?

In what ways is your post-cancer body better than your pre-cancer body?

Please do not . . .

Recount your diagnosis or treatment.

Offer medical advice.

Discuss your doctor, hospital, or health plan.

Dwell on the negative.

Again, do not be limited by the above. If you have been personally touched by breast cancer, you no doubt have many more ideas than those listed here. Think about your experience or that of the person whose experience you've shared. What practical advice would you give to a friend who is going through this now? What nuts-and-bolts kind of hints can you give? What words of encouragement of an upbeat and useful nature? Can you tell me how having had breast cancer has improved your life?